CREATING CHANGE

Also by Lisa M. Najavits

FOR PROFESSIONALS

Seeking Safety:
A Treatment Manual for PTSD and Substance Abuse

FOR GENERAL READERS

Finding Your Best Self, Revised Edition:
Recovery from Addiction, Trauma, or Both

CREATING CHANGE

A Past-Focused Treatment for Trauma and Addiction

LISA M. NAJAVITS

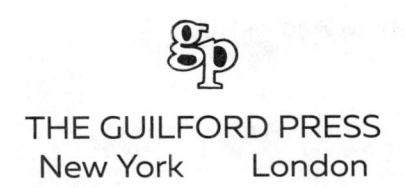

THE GUILFORD PRESS
New York   London

Copyright © 2024 Lisa M. Najavits

Published by The Guilford Press
A Division of Guilford Publications, Inc.
370 Seventh Avenue, Suite 1200, New York, NY 10001
www.guilford.com

All rights reserved

Except as indicated, no part of this book may be reproduced, translated, stored in a retrieval system, or transmitted, in any form or by any means, electronic, mechanical, photocopying, microfilming, recording, or otherwise, without written permission from the publisher.

Printed in the United States of America

This book is printed on acid-free paper.

Last digit is print number: 9 8 7 6 5 4 3 2 1

LIMITED DUPLICATION LICENSE

These materials are intended for use only by qualified mental health professionals.

The publisher grants to individual purchasers of this book nonassignable permission to reproduce the handouts. This license is limited to you, the individual purchaser, for use with your own clients or patients. It does not extend to additional clinicians or practice settings, nor does purchase by an institution constitute a site license. This license does not grant the right to reproduce these materials for resale, redistribution, electronic display, or any other purposes (including but not limited to books, pamphlets, articles, video or audio recordings, blogs, file-sharing sites, internet or intranet sites, and handouts or slides for trainings, lectures, workshops, or webinars, whether or not a fee is charged). Permission to reproduce these materials for these and any other purposes must be obtained in writing from the Permissions Department of Guilford Publications (email us at permissions@guilford.com).

The author has checked with sources believed to be reliable in her efforts to provide information that is complete and generally in accord with the standards of practice that are accepted at the time of publication. However, in view of the possibility of human error or changes in behavioral, mental health, or medical sciences, neither the author, nor the editor and publisher, nor any other party who has been involved in the preparation or publication of this work warrants that the information contained herein is in every respect accurate or complete, and they are not responsible for any errors or omissions or the results obtained from the use of such information. Readers are encouraged to confirm the information contained in this book with other sources.

Library of Congress Cataloging-in-Publication Data

Names: Najavits, Lisa M., author.
Title: Creating change : a past-focused treatment for trauma and addiction / Lisa M. Najavits.
Description: New York : The Guilford Press, [2024] | Includes bibliographical references and index.
Identifiers: LCCN 2023053996 | ISBN 9781462554621 (paperback) | ISBN 9781462554638 (cloth)
Subjects: LCSH: Addicts—Rehabilitation—Popular works. | Psychic trauma—Treatment—Popular works. | Post-traumatic stress disorder—Treatment—Popular works.
Classification: LCC RC564.29 .N33 2024 | DDC 616.86/03—dc23/eng/20240109
LC record available at *https://lccn.loc.gov/2023053996*

To my husband, Burke, forever and always, for everything—the humor, the solace, growing into adulthood together, your so-humble genius mind, for helping me change, for the honesty, the adventures, the love.

This book wouldn't be possible without you. And it perhaps wouldn't be necessary if everyone had someone like you.

About the Author

Lisa M. Najavits, PhD, is Adjunct Professor at the University of Massachusetts Chan Medical School and Director of Treatment Innovations. She was on the faculty of Harvard Medical School (McLean Hospital) for 25 years and Boston University School of Medicine (Veterans Affairs Boston) for 12 years. Dr. Najavits specializes in the development of new counseling models for trauma and addiction, clinical trials research, and community-based care. She is author of over 200 publications, including the books *Seeking Safety: A Treatment Manual for PTSD and Substance Abuse*; *Finding Your Best Self: Recovery from Addiction, Trauma, or Both*; and *A Woman's Addiction Workbook: Your Guide to In-Depth Healing*. She has served as president of the Society of Addiction Psychology of the American Psychological Association and has consulted widely on public health efforts in trauma and addiction, both nationally and internationally. She is a recipient of the Young Professional Award from the International Society for Traumatic Stress Studies, the Early Career Contribution Award from the Society for Psychotherapy Research, the Emerging Leadership Award from the Committee on Women in Psychology of the American Psychological Association, the Betty Ford Award from the Association for Multidisciplinary Education and Research in Substance Use and Addiction, and the Distinguished Alumna Award from Barnard College. Dr. Najavits is a licensed psychologist in Massachusetts and conducts a psychotherapy practice.

Preface

I came to explore the wreck.
The words are purposes.
The words are maps.
I came to see the damage that was done
and the treasures that prevail.

~ADRIENNE RICH, from the poem "Diving into the Wreck"

When clients open their hearts to revisit the past—to explore the "wreck" of trauma and addiction—treasures are possible: compassion for their younger self, release from emotional pain, and most of all, recovery. Words become purposes and maps toward those goals. It's not clear what will emerge, but putting experience into words is a process of discovery. Clients can't change what happened but can change their perspective on it.

The work moves into difficult feelings and memories. Some clients value the opportunity and want to do it; for others, it's a leap of faith. *Creating Change* provides many options for them to explore at their own pace, in their own way, while keeping sessions structured and supportive. It seeks to inspire them to delve into what matters and to take space for that.

In offering this book, I'm acutely aware that any counseling model is just one approach to the complex problems clients have suffered by the time they enter treatment. Freud said the counselor pursues a path for which there is no model (Gabbard, 2008). And despite the many models developed since his era, this remains a stark truth. Treatment manuals have much to offer but are just guides. It's the counselor who handles the unexpected, makes the difficult decisions, responds to intense needs, and faces obstacles that go beyond what any manual can fully address. There are no formulas, just material to support counselors in their work. We've had decades of treatment manuals, yet rates of addiction and trauma are as high as ever. Although manuals have improved treatment and accrued an important evidence base, it's valuable to keep a broad lens, recognizing that methods for overcoming the past have existed throughout history. There's no one right way, but many.

Creating Change has its own lengthy history. I began it in 2005, when my first manual for trauma and addiction, *Seeking Safety*, a present-focused model, had already been in use for several years. I was interested in crafting what the next stage, past-focused, might look like. The first draft of *Creating Change* was completed in 2007, but I didn't want to send it into the world without a randomized controlled trial and clinical implementation in varied settings, including by independent teams. These projects took a long time, but the delay was a blessing as the field grew a lot in the interim, offering an increasingly refined understanding of how to explore the past. Chapter 1 of this book describes the rationale for Creating Change amid the many models that have already been developed; and Chapter 2 provides historical context on the treatment of trauma and addiction.

During the years I worked on *Creating Change*, I was fortunate to visit many treatment programs, which informed the development of the model and, hopefully, reflects that real-world experience. At a deeper level, I've been "writing" this book much of my life. I first faced trauma at 19 with my mother's sudden, unexpected death. As poet Dylan Thomas wrote, "After the first death, there is no other" (1945/2000, p. 85). In other words, a first trauma can be a crucible for learning to grieve. I worked through the loss of my mother without professional help, but it taught me that I had the inner capacity to heal from painful events. I also found, to my surprise, that grief isn't the dark, bottomless pain it may look like on the outside. It includes moments of clarity, poignant appreciation, and life-altering gains. Grief always gives something back. For me, it revealed sides of myself that led to a career that has been meaningful beyond what I could have imagined. I hope this combination of professional and personal experiences can help others. As Albert Camus wrote, "We must realize that we cannot escape the common lot of pain, and that our only justification, if one there be, is to speak insofar as we can on behalf of those who cannot" (1957, p. 37).

ACKNOWLEDGMENTS

With gratitude to the teams that implemented Creating Change as part of clinical or research projects. They provided invaluable feedback to help refine the model.

- St. Luke's-Roosevelt Hospital—Crime Victims Treatment Center, led by Kay M. Johnson, LICSW
- The Washington, D.C. Vet Center, led by Cary Smith, LMSW
- St. Monica's Behavioral Health Services for Women in Lincoln, Nebraska, led by Rebecca Beardsley, PhD; Coral Frazell, PhD; and Mary Simbarcelos, MA
- The Charles George Veterans Affairs Medical Center in Ashville, North Carolina, led by Gus Diggs, PhD, and Amanda Yeck, MS
- The California Center of Excellence for Trauma Informed Care, led by Gabriella Grant
- The Centre for Alcohol and Drug Research at Aarhus University in Denmark, led by Sidsel Karsburg, PhD
- The Veterans Affairs Boston Healthcare System, led by me; Karen Krinsley, PhD; Christopher Skidmore, PhD; Joni M. Utley, PsyD; and Kay M. Johnson, LICSW
- McLean Hospital/Harvard Medical School, led by me and Martha Schmitz, PhD

With appreciation to additional colleagues who so generously gave feedback on the manuscript or parts of it along the way—especially Summer Krause, LPC, CADCIII, and Renee Schneider, PhD, for their exceptionally sensitive, close read; and also for very helpful comments from Joseph Albeck, MD; Joan M. Cook, PhD; Donna M. Dahl; William H. Gottdiener, PhD; Ricky Greenwald, PsyD; Terry C. North, PhD; Andrée Pagès; Beverly J. Patitz, PhD; Meredith Powers-Lupo, LICSW; Eva Skolnick-Acker, LCSW; Nancy S. Tamburo-Treviño, LCSW; and Fran Williams, PsyD.

Thanks also to William L. White, MA, and Francis R. Abueg, PhD, pioneers in addiction and/or trauma treatment, who responded to queries and shared from their work.

In memory of Niki Miller, MS (1957–2022), for her friendship and advocacy for those with trauma and addiction. Her work is expressed in one of her favorite quotes: "Never forget . . . who you are and where you stand in the struggle" (Bob Marley).

With abiding respect for David Seaman, for his feedback on this book, and for saying, "Feel free to use anything I've ever written, said, muttered, cried, or screamed, if it will help. I do not mind if my name is in print because I refuse to be ashamed of myself for what happened to me. I have pride in the healing I've done with substance abuse and PTSD. By passing along anything I can to others, it allows my own experiences with the very difficult and rewarding road to recovery to have reason and meaning. Too many victims live with shame and do not heal."

To the many colleagues and programs over the years that hosted me and my team, and to those who contacted me to thank me for my work, *thank you*. Words in a book are inert until you bring them alive by what you do day-to-day.

Contents

1. **Overview of Creating Change**   1
   Getting Started   2
   Seeking Safety and Creating Change   2
   The Link between Trauma and Addiction   2
   Three Types of Recovery Models (Past, Present, Future)   4
   Creating Change Content   6
   Implementation Aspects   6
   Key Principles   8
   Why a New Model?   11
   Convergence with Seeking Safety   14
   Why Is It Called Creating Change?   15
   The Development of Creating Change   16
   Evidence Base   16
   Overall   18

2. **The Larger Context**   20
   Two Major Types of Counseling   20
   Wisdom from the Past   27
   Co-occurring Trauma and Addiction: Challenges and Progress   32
   The Future   36

3. **How to Conduct Creating Change**   37
   Trying It Out   37
   Key Implementation Questions   38
   Conducting the Treatment   40
       The Session Format   40
       Starting Out   41
       During the Session   44
   Working with Emotion   48
   Implementation Decisions: Modality, Setting, and Clients   51
   Conducting Creating Change with Other Models   57
       How to Combine Creating Change with Seeking Safety   57
       Considerations for Other Models   58
   Detailed Guide to the Session Format   59
   Materials to Use across Sessions   64

4. **The Counselor**   76
   Best Practices in Treating Addiction and Trauma   76
   Positive Processes   81

TREATMENT TOPICS

Introduction	95
Create Change	109
Trust versus Doubt	120
Honor Your Survival	129
Relationship Patterns	139
Why Addiction?	149
Respect Your Defenses	161
Break the Silence	173
Darkness and Light	183
Emotions and Healing	194
Tell Your Story	206
Influences: Family, Community, Culture	216
Knowing and Not Knowing	231
Your Personal Truth	241
What You Want People to Understand	250
Listen to Your Body	264
Memory	277
Power Dynamics	288
Deepen Your Story	300
Growth	312
Extra Topic: Understanding Trauma and Addiction	321
Extra Topic: Recovery Strengths and Challenges	336
Extra Topic: Your Relationships	348
References	357
Index	371

Purchasers of this book can download and print copies of selected handouts, as well as online appendices and other supplemental resources, at www.guilford.com/najavits3-materials for use with your own clients or patients (see copyright page for details).

1

Overview of Creating Change

The farther back you can look, the farther forward you are likely to see.
~Winston Churchill, 20th-century British leader

Talking about the past can create a better future. This idea has been at the core of counseling since its formal beginnings in the 19th century. Long before this—throughout history and across cultures—exploring the past has been a way to overcome emotional pain, using methods such as storytelling, folk customs, and religious confession (Jackson, 1994; Nichols & Zax, 1977).

Creating Change was developed to address trauma and/or addiction, which are some of the most common and devastating current mental health issues. The goal is to help clients come to terms with what they experienced by exploring it in detail, sometimes called *processing*. The model can be conducted in individual or group treatment.

In the words of a client: "Not only is the work freeing, but as you do it, you start to understand why you did what you did and come to see yourself as someone who was trying but didn't have many options. What holds you back now, such as inability to speak up for yourself, was perhaps a wise choice in a violent childhood home. What was once helpful may now be holding you back. You also uncover strengths you never gave yourself credit for and learn ways to build on those strengths."

In the words of a counselor: "Creating Change is a gentle, past-focused approach that's helpful for discussing the past without getting swallowed up by it. It feels really different from other past-focused models I'm trained in—unique, with a different, empowering, softer approach. It's also intriguing to have a past-focused model that incorporates the addiction element."

This chapter has the following sections:

- Getting started
- Seeking Safety and Creating Change
- The link between trauma and addiction
- Three types of recovery models (past, present, future)
- Creating Change content
- Implementation aspects
- Key principles
- Why a new model?
- Convergence with Seeking Safety
- Why is it called Creating Change?
- The development of Creating Change
- Evidence base
- Overall

Subsequent chapters describe how to conduct the model and provide understanding of Creating Change in relation to the history of past-focused therapies. Looking back as a way to move forward is relevant to clients and also to the field broadly.

After these initial chapters, there are 23 session topics with handouts that can be shared with clients.

GETTING STARTED

Glance through the book to get a feel for it. You can read the chapters in any order and don't have to read the whole book before trying it with clients, but be sure to see Chapter 3 for guidance on how to conduct Creating Change. Definitions of terms (*trauma*, *addiction*, and others) are in Appendix A, "Key Terms," which is online at *www.guilford.com/najavits3-materials*. The website *www.creating-change.org* has additional information on the model, including training options. Note that training is available but is not required unless it's a research study.

SEEKING SAFETY AND CREATING CHANGE

Some counselors are already familiar with the author's book *Seeking Safety* (Najavits, 2002c), which is a widely used *present-focused* coping skills model for trauma and/or addiction. Creating Change and Seeking Safety are "twins": They're identical in format and style, but their focus is different (the *past* vs. the *present*). They're completely separate models; thus, a counselor implementing Creating Change doesn't need to know Seeking Safety. However, the two models can be used together, if desired, and counselors who are familiar with Seeking Safety will find that Creating Change capitalizes on their existing knowledge and skills. For more, see the section "Convergence with Seeking Safety" later in this chapter; see also Appendix C (online at *www.guilford.com/najavits3-materials*), which compares the models. Both models are evidence-based (Lenz, Henesy, & Callender, 2016; Najavits, Krinsley, Waring, Gallagher, & Skidmore, 2018; Sherman et al., 2023).

THE LINK BETWEEN TRAUMA AND ADDICTION

The wish to escape emotional pain through addictive behavior is universal (Lowinson, Ruiz, Millman, & Langrod, 1997). Trauma and substances thus represent a natural pairing: "[T]he child of an active, violent alcoholic parent receives modeling that life is dangerous, parentscan be dangerous and cannot be relied upon, and that addictive processes somehow might make life more manageable. One of my clients with this background made a conscious decision by age twelve to become alcoholic" (Potter-Efron, 2006, p. 78). As Blume notes, it's remarkable that all trauma survivors don't turn to substances for the illusion of control it offers (Sterman, 2006, p. 265).

In Creating Change, the goal is to address any addiction the person has, but substance addiction is emphasized as it's one of the most common and the most studied in relation to trauma. Nonsubstance *behavioral addictions* are also important, including problem gambling, shopping, pornography, gaming, eating, sex, exercise, and social media. The extra topic "Understanding Trauma and Addiction" offers a scale to assess these, which often go undetected in treatment programs.

Reasons for Using

It's key to also explore the meanings addiction holds for clients. It serves many functions and often opposites that speak to the extremes of their experience. The goal is to listen closely to each client's reasons:

- To forget or to remember
- To connect or to detach
- To conform or to rebel
- To slow down or to speed up
- To escape the past or to repeat it
- To nurture or to punish
- To survive or to give up
- To avoid or to approach
- To feel more or to feel less

In clients' own words: "It's how I get energy and feel alive." . . . "Meth is my way of saying f_ you to the world; I do what I want." . . . "My uncle would give me a drink before abusing me." . . . "There's no way to relate to this world without using." . . . "Different sides of me use for different reasons." . . . "I drank to stay with my abuser, so when he hit me, I wouldn't feel it."

Pathways

One of the benefits in exploring the past is helping clients understand, if they have both trauma and addiction, how each arose in their life history and how each impacted the other. There are various pathways. The most common, for two-thirds of clients, is that *trauma leads to addiction*; known as "self-medication," it's using to numb out, escape, or cope (Briere, 2019; Najavits, Weiss, & Shaw, 1997). But it's also true that *addiction leads to trauma* (unsafe people, places, and situations make clients vulnerable to trauma). It's also sadly common that *trauma and addiction can arise together*, such as when a child grows up in a home where both are present. Once the client has both trauma and addiction, moreover, each tends to worsen the other in a *downward spiral*.

Rates

Posttraumatic stress disorder (PTSD), the psychiatric disorder most associated with trauma, co-occurs at high rates with substance use disorder (SUD). For example, among people seeking SUD treatment, about 40% have current PTSD. And among people who develop PTSD during their lifetime, the majority (58%) also develop SUD at some point (Simpson et al., 2021). Some subgroups have especially high rates of co-occurring PTSD/SUD, including women, adolescents, military and veterans, sex workers, emergency room patients, the incarcerated, and the homeless (Najavits & Hien, 2013; Ouimette & Read, 2014). Repeated trauma is also common, with one study finding an average of nine traumas among clients with PTSD and cocaine use disorder (Najavits et al., 2003).

Serious Needs

In Creating Change, the goal is to address all unsafe behavior, as well as to offer referral to as much additional care as possible. Treating "the whole person" is key. Clients with PTSD and SUD, for example, have elevated rates of all sorts of problems compared to those with just one of these disorders. The list goes on and on: They have more suicide attempts; inpatient admissions; criminal behavior; HIV risk; drug overdose; interpersonal, medical, and employment problems; cognitive distortions; worse treatment outcomes; more positive views of substances; lower functioning; less compliance with aftercare; less motivation for treatment; quicker relapse; greater use of hard drugs; more substance use in relation to stress; more additional psychiatric disorder; and greater vulnerability to further trauma. For some, the disorders are chronic for many years; many experience marginalization and stigma as well. Certainly, PTSD or addiction alone creates significant issues, but the combination is sometimes called "double trouble" because of the heightened impact of both together.

Commonalities

Trauma and addiction have much in common, further underscoring how their combination can be so devastating.

- *Both represent a loss of control.* Addiction is the inability to control one's behavior, and trauma is an uncontrollable external event.
- *Both are often kept secret* out of deep shame.
- *Both have been labeled a personality defect* or "weak character."
- *Both carry across generations.* Family history is one of their biggest predictors, due to genetic and social factors.
- *Both lead to turning against the self:* self-hatred, self-harm, self-neglect.
- *Both can become a person's identity*, the focal point of their lives.
- *Both create internal splits:* lack of connection between sides of the self, resulting in ambivalence and dissociation.
- *Both are minimized or denied.* It often takes a while to become fully aware of them, to "own" them.
- *Both are triggering.* More than many other disorders, reminders can trigger intense reactions.
- *Both require exposure to an external event:* to a substance, to a trauma.

Yet their most important commonality is optimistic: *Both are highly treatable.*

THREE TYPES OF RECOVERY MODELS (PAST, PRESENT, FUTURE)

Creating Change fits into a major recovery framework: the *stage-based approach*, which originated in the trauma field but applies to addiction as well. From the earliest writing on trauma treatment in the 19th century through to the present era, stages of recovery have been repeatedly identified, especially for complex clients (Herman, 1992; van der Hart, Brown, & van der Kolk, 1989). The stage-based approach has sometimes been called a *consensus model*, as a majority of trauma experts have endorsed it (Cloitre et al., 2011; Courtois, 2004). In recent years, however, there's less focus on moving through the stages in sequence; instead, they're now understood as different types of work. Some clients do just one and don't ever need another; others do a mix or move back and forth between them.

One of the most well-known frameworks is from Herman (1992), consisting of three parts: *safety, mourning and remembrance,* and *reconnection.*[1] The terms *present, past,* and *future* are added below

---

[1] Herman (2023) recently identified a possible fourth stage, *justice*, with emphasis on repair through societal validation and related processes such as apology, rehabilitation, and restitution. In Creating Change, these are addressed in various topics; see, for example, the section in "Broad Social and Historical Context Beyond the Individual."

for clarity but are not originally from Herman. (Appendix A, online at *www.guilford.com/najavits3-materials*, has additional terms for the three types.) Seeking Safety fits the first type, *present-focused*; Creating Change fits the second, *past-focused*. Chapter 2 provides an extensive list of different models within each category as well.

1. Present-Focused (Safety)

This type of counseling is about stabilization in the present. It offers education on the basics of trauma and addiction and increases clients' ability to cope safely with current life challenges—such as how to gain control over negative feelings, improve self-care, build healthy relationships, and respond to problems in a responsible way. There's strong emphasis on learning to protect oneself from the many destructive aspects of trauma and addiction, both external (unsafe people and situations) and internal (self-harm, impulsivity). Seeking Safety is an example of this type of model.

2. Past-Focused (Remembrance)

Here, clients come to terms with their life history—what happened and why. They explore how trauma and addiction developed over time and take pride in having survived. They share what they were up against and who was or wasn't there for them, gaining insight into long-standing relationship patterns. They grieve losses, pain, and regrets. Creating Change is an example of this type of treatment.

3. Future-Focused (Connection)

This work is usually part of the prior two types (present- and past-focused), rather than a specific model. The goal is to build a better future by connecting with the world in healthy ways: finding meaning and purpose in life and relating well to others. Clients are able to maintain and even thrive in their roles at work and in their family and community, and sometimes embark on "giving back" to help others who struggle with trauma or addiction.

Past-Focused Treatment Specifically for Trauma and Addiction

Until recently, clients with addiction were consistently excluded from past-focused trauma treatment and research (Leeman et al., 2017; Watts et al., 2014). The idea was that clients already out of control in their behavior, as demonstrated by their addiction, would become even more unsafe if intense memories and emotions were stirred up—there'd be increased substance use, harm to self or others, treatment dropout, and impaired functioning (Foa, 2000; Keane, 1995; Pitman et al., 1991; Solomon, Gerrity, & Muff, 1992). These concerns were accurate as there were reports of worsening when clients with addiction were guided to tell their trauma story (Pitman et al., 1991; Solomon et al., 1992). Foa (2000), the developer of Prolonged Exposure (PE) therapy, stated that it wasn't a first-choice treatment for clients with addiction. Coffey, Dansky, and Brady (2002) identified PE as inappropriate for clients with addiction if they had repeated childhood trauma, a high level of anger or dissociation, or other vulnerabilities. Thus, most studies of past-focused trauma treatment excluded clients with addiction or at most allowed for only mild problems. In treatment settings, clients were routinely told to "get sober first" and given ultimatums ("Attend AA or I won't treat you"), before they could get help for trauma. Some clients lied and hid their addiction to get help.

It's now known, however, that some clients with trauma and addiction want past-focused treatment and can benefit from it (Back et al., 2019; Najavits et al., 2018). Yet treatment needs to be substantially modified to be safe and effective for them. As mentioned earlier, they have greater impairment and worse outcomes than those with just trauma or just addiction (Najavits et al., 1997; Ouimette & Read, 2014). The principle "first, do no harm" is key.

Creating Change was developed specifically to address the need for a past-focused treatment that would be feasible and appealing for both trauma and addiction.

CREATING CHANGE CONTENT

Treatment Topics

There are 23 treatment topics, as listed on page 7. Each offers a way to explore some important aspect of the past. If clients respond less to one topic, the next gives them another angle to try.

You can conduct as few or many topics as time allows. The term *topics* is used rather than *sessions* as each can be conducted over more than one session. They can also be conducted in any order as each is independent of the others. The goal is maximum flexibility to increase client engagement and respect counselors' clinical judgment.

Three of the topics are labeled *extra topics* as they provide options for clients who need additional support and education. They can be conducted at any point in treatment.

All topics address trauma and addiction at the same time if clients have both, helping them understand the relationship between the two. They can also be used with clients who have problems with just one or the other.

The list on the facing page offers brief descriptions. You can share it with clients to let them choose the session topic, if desired, and you can use it to track the topics you've covered.

Chapter 3 provides additional guidance on how to implement the model.

Beyond the Narrative

The narrative—the linear story of trauma and addiction—has a place in Creating Change, particularly in the topic "Tell Your Story." But rather than being the centerpiece of treatment, which is the case for many past-focused models, in Creating Change it's just one of many ways to heal the past. Offering different methods is convergent with lessons from the history of past-focused models (see Chapter 2 for more). It's also consistent with research indicating that clients with PTSD and addiction are typically less likely to benefit from narrative-based approaches than clients with PTSD alone (e.g., Foa et al., 2013). Some trauma experts, such as Peter Levine, assert that narrative approaches aren't necessary for healing at all (Levine, 2010). From clinicians' standpoint, some clients benefit from sharing their story, but for others it's not appealing or not helpful (Becker, Zayfert, & Anderson, 2004), and major research trials are increasingly showing the limitations of purely narrative approaches (Steenkamp, Litz, & Marmar, 2020). Moreover, clients may have too many painful life events to process. One client with complex PTSD and chronic addiction said, "There's no 'me' before trauma. It was the fabric of my life from the start. I can't just peek behind the curtain and be done with it."

IMPLEMENTATION ASPECTS

Creating Change was developed for a **broad range of clients**. They can be any gender, with any type of trauma or addiction, in any setting. It's been evaluated with adults but may be helpful for older adolescents as well. Clients don't have to be abstinent from substances or even committed to

List of the 23 Creating Change Topics

Introduction
Overview and practical information

Create Change
A list of over 70 skills for exploring your past

Trust versus Doubt
Trusting the process, plus a list of support helplines

Honor Your Survival
Taking stock of what you lived through

Relationship Patterns
How you relate (past and present)

Why Addiction?
Explore your addiction story (and links to trauma)

Respect Your Defenses
Self-protection methods you developed

Break the Silence
Silencing versus feeling heard

Darkness and Light
Shifting between extremes

Emotions and Healing
What you learned about dealing with feelings

Tell Your Story
Share about your past

Influences: Family, Community, Culture
The big picture—how larger forces impact trauma and addiction

Knowing and Not Knowing
Gaining awareness

Your Personal Truth
A new look at your past

What You Want People to Understand
Real-life and imaginary conversations that help you heal

Listen to Your Body
Your relationship with your body

Memory
Coping with memory issues in trauma and addiction

Power Dynamics
Feeling powerful versus powerless

Deepen Your Story
30 ways to share about your past

Growth
Look back on how far you've come

***Extra Topic*: Understanding Trauma and Addiction**
Brief information and the message that recovery is possible

***Extra Topic*: Recovery Strengths and Challenges**
Strengthen your ability to participate in Creating Change

***Extra Topic*: Your Relationships**
Improve relationships to support your recovery

From *Creating Change* by Lisa M. Najavits. Copyright © 2024 Lisa M. Najavits. Published by The Guilford Press. Permission to photocopy this material, or to download and print additional copies (*www.guilford.com/najavits3-materials*), is granted to purchasers of this book for use with your own clients or patients; see copyright page for details.

reducing their use before starting Creating Change. Sometimes motivation is the result of treatment rather than the start of it. However, they can't be intoxicated during the session, which is a general rule in addiction counseling. If there are concerns about a client's fit for Creating Change, there are several extra topics at the end of the book that offer ways to evaluate and strengthen clients in relation to participation in Creating Change. It's also highly recommended to engage clients in additional treatments and supports as needed throughout the treatment. It can be conducted at the same time as any other modalities, including present-focused therapy. In general, the more treatment options, the better for this population.

Who can facilitate Creating Change? That, too, is broad. There are **no specific degree, experience, training, or licensure requirements for counselors**. This is based on research showing that such variables don't predict success in counseling (e.g., Najavits & Weiss, 1994; van de Ven, Ritter, & Roche, 2020). The term *counselor* is used throughout the book as it fits many settings, but this doesn't imply that a particular type of degree is necessary. What matters are the counselor's genuine interest in helping people with addiction and trauma problems; commitment to carrying out the work responsibly; and willingness to learn the model. Chapter 4 offers guidance for deciding if Creating Change is a good fit for you; you can also simply try it out.

Creating Change can be conducted as a **stand-alone treatment or along with any other treatment**. There's no model that's at odds with Creating Change.

The **session length and pacing are flexible**. Creating Change was designed to fit a wide range of settings, understanding that clients with trauma and addiction enter treatment through many doors, including mental health and addiction agencies, criminal justice, hospitals, and private practice. Typically, session length is 45–50 minutes for individual sessions and 60–90 for groups, held weekly or twice weekly. But whatever length or pacing you choose, you can adjust the amount of material you cover in the session based on time available and can repeat a topic over two or more sessions, if desired.

Creating Change has a **structured session format** that encourages good use of time and offers a predictable sequence, which can feel reassuring amid clients' chaotic lives. The session format is the same whether conducted in individual or group modality. There's a *check-in*, *quotation*, *handouts*, and *check-out*, as described in Chapter 3.

KEY PRINCIPLES

Creating Change is based on six principles: (1) skill development, (2) balancing positive and negative life experiences, (3) broad social and historical context beyond the individual, (4) choice, (5) safeguards, and (6) inspiring hope.

1. Skill Development

In Creating Change, overcoming the past means clients develop skills they may never have learned growing up or may have lost along the way due to trauma and addiction. Each treatment topic is a skill relevant to both, and the topic "Create Change" also offers a list of over 70 skills they can return to at any time. The more clients work on skills, the better they'll be at responding to adversities in the future, much as physical exercise develops strong muscles. The skills framework also recognizes that clients may have experienced so many painful events that it's not realistic to process all of them—rather, it's about learning *how* to process them. By the end of treatment, they may not be done working on trauma and addiction (although they'll likely show significant symptom reduction). But they'll have the skills to continue the work safely on their own, outside of counseling. Especially for long-standing trauma and addiction, recovery is more a marathon than a sprint. The framework of skill development conveys that clients can learn new ways to heal their past, that it's within them to do this when provided with guidance and the emotional space for it.

2. Balancing Positive and Negative Life Experiences

Creating Change explores the full range of human experience—what's beautiful and moving and what's horrifying and ugly. It's challenging to hold on to both sides. There may be an impulse to gloss over the "dark side": to retreat from difficult memories or say things were better than they were. Or some clients do the opposite, staying stuck in negative memories, believing those define them ("I'm damaged," "I failed"). They lose touch with what *is* going right, who *is* there for them, the power they *do* have.

Many past-focused trauma treatments focus almost entirely on processing negative events. But that approach can reinforce distress rather than relieving it (Jemmer, 2006; Schauer, Robjant, Elbert, & Neuner, 2020; van der Kolk, 2014). In addiction treatment, research shows that focusing on positive experiences helps offset the negatives that are so discouraging for clients (Hoeppner et al., 2019; McKay, 2017). Of course, "positive" and "negative" may not always be straightforward; with recovery what seemed negative may become a positive, and vice versa (e.g., hitting bottom may ultimately save them).

Creating Change offers various ways to explore the full range of experiences. In the topic "Break the Silence," clients share about an important event; for some, positive aspects, such as what they're proud of, are more vulnerable than negatives. The topic "Darkness and Light" encourages clients to practice shifting between positive and negative. In "What You Want People to Understand," clients can create a conversation with people in their life about all sorts of experiences, including positive ones.

Throughout, they're encouraged to attend to all feelings, including those that are typically socially acceptable, such as sadness, and those that typically aren't, such as desire for revenge. Any feeling can be put into words. There's also an understanding that clients experienced harm but, in some cases, may also have caused harm. They may be both survivors and perpetrators of trauma or, as part of addiction or criminality, may have done things they now regret.

Ultimately, the goal is integration: The story becomes more cohesive rather than fragmented. Clients can relate more fully to themselves and others. They come to feel more whole.

3. Broad Social and Historical Context Beyond the Individual

Many clients feel abandoned or betrayed by society, whether by family, peers, authority figures, or societal oppression or neglect. These wider circles can cause trauma and addiction but also help heal them.

The goal is to help clients become conscious of larger forces. The topic "Influences: Family, Community, Culture" explores this theme in detail. "Break the Silence" discusses institutional silencing. "What You Want People to Understand" lets clients voice their perspective to others. "Honor Your Survival" identifies many types of adversity, including intergenerational and historical traumas, community-wide disasters, family mental illness, and genocide. Some clients are so burdened by generations of family violence and addiction that it feels like a script they can't escape.

Addressing societal issues helps clients understand their problems as not simply personal "failures" but embedded within larger spheres of influence. The puzzle pieces of culture, society, and history help clients make sense of their story and can be a source of repair. As Herman writes, recovery "must take place in community . . . [it] cannot be simply a private, individual matter" (2023, pp. 2–3).

4. Choice

Creating Change emphasizes *choice* to honor clients' (and counselors') individuality and personal path in life. It's clear that there's no one right way to heal, but many. Thus, Creating Change prioritizes respect for clients' preferences, as long as these choices are reasonably safe. The goal is autonomy: to encourage clients, with a sense that they'll open up and let go of defenses at their own pace.

Unfortunately, horror stories abound in which clients have been forced, subtly and not so subtly, into past-focused treatment or elements of it. In one program, all clients were required to tell their story, including their trauma history, at a community meeting prior to leaving the program; it was viewed as "essential to healing." In another program, a counselor instructed an incest survivor to write a letter forgiving her father for the incest or she would "never recover." More benign versions of coercion include extreme messages such as "all secrets are bad," overselling past-focused models (Morris, 2015), and assessments probing too much trauma detail (by assessors unaware that minimal trauma details are recommended on treatment entry) (Najavits, 2004). Some counselors convey inaccurate messages, implicit or explicit, that clients *must* tell their story to recover or that the only *real* treatment requires focusing on the past. (An extreme version of this is the study by Imel et al. that identifies trauma treatments that don't focus on the past as "trauma avoidant" [Imel, Laska, Jakupcak, & Simpson, 2013].)

In Creating Change, choice is offered in various ways, such as the following:

- *Many options rather than "one size fits all."* Each topic has multiple handouts that can be shared and worked on in any order, and counselors can use as few or as many as desired for a given client and setting (just as with the topics themselves). This flexibility allows you to focus on what's most relevant for the client and fluidly move between handouts during a session as it evolves. So too, the list of skills in the topic "Create Change" also offers many options; clients can choose what works for them and let go of the rest.
- *Ability to shift between past- and present-focused sessions.* This is straightforward in individual treatment but also possible in group modality. Sessions of Creating Change can be alternated with Seeking Safety, Relapse Prevention (RP; Marlatt & Gordon, 1985), or other present-focused models.
- *Implementation flexibility.* Creating Change was designed from a public health perspective to be as accessible as possible—for a wide range of staff, and without automatic exclusions for particular types of clients or settings. It's also adjustable in dosage, modality (group or individual), and other clinical parameters. In short, there's wide latitude for counselors to make implementation choices that will best serve their clients.

5. Safeguards

Various elements in Creating Change help keep the session safe, such as:

- A structured session format so clients know what to expect
- Client-centered sharing (there's no expectation of having to share the full trauma or addiction narrative)
- Session homework (called *commitments*) are a mix of present- and past-focused options so that clients can choose what they feel able to do
- Optional grounding at the end of sessions
- Extra topics for use, as needed, to strengthen clients' ability to participate in Creating Change

Overview of Creating Change

- A focus on best practices in trauma and addiction
- Strong attention to the counselor role to promote positive treatment dynamics
- A written plan for after hours and emergencies

6. Inspiring Hope

Beyond techniques, inspiration is one of the most powerful ways to create change. People "move mountains" when inspired. Throughout Creating Change, clients' greatest effort is encouraged through the use of uplifting quotations, humanistic rather than scientific language, and a pervasive optimism that life can be better. Creating Change, like Seeking Safety, is not overtly spiritual, but is strongly idealistic.

There's emphasis on possibilities. The book title and all of the treatment topics are imbued with a sense of what *can* be achieved despite the losses of the past. Clients with trauma and addiction have a great need for inspiration, given their often profound demoralization. As one client said, "It's essential to believe that we can 'make it' . . . whatever that means in our own terms" (Jennings & Ralph, 1997, p. 45).

Creating Change asks clients to explore difficult parts of their past but offers the counterbalance of a better future. For example, the topic "Trust versus Doubt" offers optimistic responses to doubts that arise about exploring the past (e.g., "I'm too far gone," "If I start to cry, I'll never stop"). In the topic "Create Change," the list of skills includes many hopeful ones such as "be the hero of your story" and "recognize growth." Ultimately, clients can transform their experience (Najavits, 2019):

- From victim to survivor
- From silence to finding their voice
- From powerlessness to a sense of control
- From isolation to connection
- From hidden to known
- From fragmented to whole

The language in Creating Change speaks to the heart: *transform, evoke, encourage, honor, heal, choose, discover, deepen, find peace*. The goal is simple human language, minimizing jargon and technical words. Terms that could be perceived as judgmental are reframed in client-centric ways: *Avoidance* becomes *self-protection*, which can be healthy or unhealthy depending on the scenario. Instead of *cognitive distortions*, it's *beliefs*.

WHY A NEW MODEL?

Various models have been developed for addiction, trauma, or both. (For a comprehensive list, see online Appendix B, "Comparison of All Models Studied for PTSD/SUD," and Appendix C, "Comparison of Models by the Author"; both at *www.guilford.com/najavits3-materials*)

With so many models available, is there need for another? Creating Change was developed to address the following gaps in the field.

Past-Focused for Both Trauma and Addiction

Creating Change is the first *fully past-focused model for both trauma and addiction*. All other models for both take solely a present-focused approach to addiction, even if some take a past-focused approach to trauma (see Chapter 2). The advantage of a fully past-focused approach is that it encourages clients to come to terms in a deep way with their addiction history too, which is often just as impactful as their trauma history.

Creating Change shines a spotlight across clients' lives to explore how trauma arose, how addiction arose, and if both occurred, how they influenced each other over time. In regular addiction treatment, there are sometimes past-focused assignments about addiction, such as having clients write an autobiography of addiction or identifying a family history of addiction. In Creating Change, there's much more extensive material (23 topics) to explore addiction history in detail and, when applicable, connect it to trauma. There are some powerful moments when clients take the long view of both.

Emphasizes Engagement Strategies

Evidence on past-focused models indicates notable engagement issues. Counselors show low adoption of many past-focused models even after receiving training in them (Cook, Dinnen, Thompson, Simiola, & Schnurr, 2014; Watts et al., 2014), and they find some models significantly more appealing than others (Najavits, Kivlahan, & Kosten, 2011). Client dropout is also a persistent problem (Hundt et al., 2020; Lewis, Roberts, Gibson, & Bisson, 2020; Najavits, 2015). Moreover, dropout "is magnified among racial/ethnic minorities and other vulnerable subgroups . . . for various reasons including stigma [and] discomfort with asking for or receiving mental health services" (Hien, Litt, Lopez-Castro, & Ruglass, 2020, p. 490). It is also higher for military and veteran samples (Varker et al., 2021).

Creating Change strives to engage clients via multiple pathways: heart, mind, body, and spirit. The quotation that opens each session draws clients in emotionally. There's emphasis on interactive, imaginative exercises (e.g., bringing in a photo or meaningful object to discuss; "opening the door" to revisit a scene from the past; creating an imaginary conversation). Topics are written to aim for fresh language and concepts to spark clients' interest, such as "Darkness and Light," "Power Dynamics," "Knowing and Not Knowing."

Other features of Creating Change described earlier are also central to the engagement strategy, such as the emphasis on *choice*, and the use of *inspiration* and *safeguards* to maintain a positive connection with the work. *Empowerment* is key as well. Both trauma and addiction represent a loss of control, so Creating Change strives to restore personal power. The focus on empowerment also serves the practical function of eliciting clients' buy-in to make attendance and successful outcomes more likely. There's a belief in the inherent power of the individual to grow when exposed to the right conditions for growth. One counselor who conducted Creating Change described it as a "kinder, gentler approach" to facing the past.

In subsequent chapters, additional engagement methods are described, including a *three-session try-out* for clients to experience Creating Change, and adapting the model based on culture. Throughout, the goal is to forge a strong bond between the client, the counselor, and the work (and among group members when conducted in groups).

Feasible in Addiction Treatment

Clients with trauma and addiction are typically routed to addiction treatment rather than mental health treatment, so from a public health standpoint it's important to offer methods that can work in either environment.

Creating Change was designed for both addiction and mental health settings. All other evidence-based past-focused models originated in the trauma field and were adapted or studied after the fact for addiction treatment (per Chapter 2). They require counselors with advanced degrees and/or extensive training and supervision, and are individual rather than group modality.[2] (In contrast, Creating Change does not have any such requirements.) Such aspects make those models challenging to implement in addiction programs, which generally have had lower funding than mental health programs, resulting in a less trained workforce with large caseloads and low salaries, high staff turnover, and greater reliance on group treatment (Najavits et al., 2020; Sherman, Lynch, Greeno, & Hoeffel, 2017). See online Appendix B for a detailed comparison of models at *www.guilford.com/najavits3-materials*.

There are three major ways that past-focused trauma models have been incorporated into addiction treatment thus far (as studied in research trials). All three of these ways can work, and study results were positive on at least some outcomes, but these approaches generally reduce feasibility in addiction settings.

- *Conduct the past-focused model as is, but in the context of high-level addiction care such as inpatient, residential, or intensive outpatient.* Eye Movement Desensitization and Reprocessing (EMDR) and Modified PE therapy are examples of this approach (Coffey et al., 2016; Perez-Dandieu & Tapia, 2014).
- *Select easier-to-treat addiction clients.* For example, a PE study excluded clients with recent opioid use (Foa et al., 2013); an EMDR study excluded clients for ongoing use of heroin or cocaine (Perez-Dandieu & Tapia, 2014); and a CPT study required clients to have a stated desire to abstain from alcohol or reduce use, and also to comply with daily assessments (Simpson et al., 2022).
- *Merge two existing models, one for trauma and one for addiction, while retaining the requirements of the trauma model.* For example, Concurrent Treatment of PTSD and Substance Use Disorders Using Prolonged Exposure (COPE; Back et al., 2015) combines PE with RP; it is solely an individual treatment model, not group, just like PE.

Creating Change takes a different approach than any of those three ways. Because it was designed from the start for both addiction and mental health/trauma programs, it was developed with the feasibility elements described earlier: group or individual modality, a broad range of counselors and clients, and no formal training requirements (unless publishable research is being conducted). It's also low-cost, requiring only the book. These characteristics make it especially relevant for addiction programs and publicly funded and nonprofit programs generally.

Increasingly, evidence-based treatment reviews are focusing more and more not just on research findings, but on relevance to practice. The review of PTSD treatments by the U.S. government Agency for Healthcare Research and Quality, for example, states, "Our findings suggest that clinicians might need to consider other factors [than research results] in selecting a treatment for PTSD: patient preference of treatment, whether the patient has care available to them, whether they can afford the treatment, whether they have tried any treatments already, or whether the patient has other co-occurring problems like substance use or depression" (Forman-Hoffman et al., 2018, p. ES-8). The Roberts et al. meta-analysis on PTSD/SUD treatments in particular draws similar conclusions, noting the early state of research in this area (Roberts, Lotzin, & Schäfer, 2022).

A Broad Approach to Client Eligibility

Offering past-focused treatment to addicted trauma survivors is quite recent. They were routinely told to "get sober" before starting trauma treatment and were consistently excluded from trauma studies, as described earlier.

---

[2] CPT can be done in group modality only if it omits the trauma narrative.

Creating Change, in contrast, takes a neutral stance toward client eligibility: Any client whom you think may benefit can be invited to begin treatment. There are no exclusions for particular types of clients or settings, but if there are concerns about a client, it's recommended to conduct some of the extra topics at the end of the book and/or the three-session try-out (see Chapter 3). This flexibility moves away from the extremes that have typically guided past-focused treatment for trauma and addiction: Either none should do it ("They're too fragile") or all should do it ("It's helpful for everyone"). In Creating Change, the decision is tailored to each client.

Other models have significant restrictions. COPE, for example, is the only other evidence-based published model for trauma and addiction with a past-focused component. Its therapist manual states that it's not recommended for clients who (1) have repeated self-injury, (2) have current domestic violence, (3) lack clear memories of their trauma, (4) don't want to stop or significantly reduce substance use, or (5) have strong urges or have made recent attempts to harm themselves or others (Back et al., 2015, pp. 10–11). The model is derived from PE and thus has restrictions based on that.

Creating Change takes a broader stance as it was designed from the start specifically for co-occurring trauma and addiction, and thus assumes that a high level of client complexity may be present.

An Evidence Base of Realistic, Complex Clients

In keeping with the point above, Creating Change was not only developed clinically for a broad range of clients, but also studied with them. The section "Evidence Base" on pages 16–18 describes the samples in detail, which is notable for *including* those who have been excluded from other studies of clients with trauma and addiction (Leeman et al., 2017; Najavits et al., 2020).

For example, studies of past-focused models in clients with trauma and addiction have excluded clients for suicidal ideation or borderline personality disorder; self-harm in the past 6 months; psychiatric hospitalization in the past month; or assault by a current intimate partner. Some even excluded for SUDs that are difficult to treat (which is quite remarkable as the goals of these programs were to treat SUD)—such as opioid use, benzodiazepine use, intravenous drug use, continuous use of heroin or cocaine, and severe substance dependence (Najavits et al., 2020).

A few studies had fewer exclusions but added elements that aren't replicable in real-world settings, such as a study that paid clients $50 per week for completing a brief assessment; held 90-minute individual sessions; and provided additional treatments and transportation for free (Back et al., 2019).

In short, a major challenge in implementing evidence-based models is that the evidence often relies on client samples that are healthier or more highly incentivized than front-line programs.

CONVERGENCE WITH SEEKING SAFETY

Creating Change is highly compatible with, yet separate from, the author's model Seeking Safety (Najavits, 2002c), which is the most evidence-based and widely implemented model for trauma and addiction. Seeking Safety is used across settings and levels of care and is translated into 16 languages. It offers 25 topics, each a safe coping skill, to help clients build greater safety in their relationships, thinking, and behavior. Examples of topics are "Asking for Help," "Compassion," "Taking Good Care of Yourself," "Coping with Triggers," and "Creating Meaning." See *www.seekingsafety.org* for a detailed description.

Commonalities

Although their focus differs—Seeking Safety addresses the present while Creating Change addresses the past—they're highly complementary. Both are optimistic, emphasizing learning new *skills* as a way to heal. Both are cognitive-behavioral therapy (CBT) approaches, but with strong awareness of psychodynamic principles (per Chapter 4). They use the same *format* (check-in, quotation, handouts, and check-out). Both are designed for a *broad range of providers and settings*, with no specific counselor license or degree required and no specific client exclusions. Both are *integrated* models, which means they address trauma and addiction at the same time for clients who have both, or can be conducted for just one or the other. Both are *flexible*: Topics and handouts can be done in any order, and the number of sessions can vary based on available time. Both *encourage adaptation* for diverse populations and emphasize client empowerment and choice. Both are *evidence based* (e.g., Lenz et al., 2016; Najavits et al., 2018; Sherman et al., 2023).

Differences

Where Seeking Safety teaches clients how to cope with their current daily lives, Creating Change helps them process events from the past. Where Seeking Safety teaches them how to gain control over negative feelings, Creating Change teaches them how to explore and move through them. Where Seeking Safety emphasizes stabilization, Creating Change emphasizes deep change. Although there's some overlap between these opposites, they're nonetheless different paths to emotional growth, consistent with differences between present-focused and past-focused models in general.

For guidance on implementing the models together, see the section "Conducting Creating Change with Other Models" in Chapter 3. Also a comparison of the models is available in Appendix C, which can be found online at *www.guilford.com/najavits3-materials*. For further understanding of present- versus past-focused models in trauma and addiction, see Chapter 2.

WHY IS IT CALLED CREATING CHANGE?

Change is the goal of all treatments,[3] but in this model *change* means, specifically, gaining a greater sense of peace with the past. Clients with trauma and addiction often have deep loss and regret about wasted years and an altered life course. They're described as "frozen in time," with impaired development after trauma and addiction began (Seidel, Gusman, & Abueg, 1994). They may feel out of step with peers, missing milestones such as an intimate partnership, children, and careers. In severe cases, change means saving their own life ("Change or die," it's said).

When successful, clients are able to experience memories and feelings without turning to substances or other unsafe behavior. The goal is captured by the phrase "mind like water" from martial arts: clear, in balanced connection to the self, neither over- nor underreacting, feeling neither too much nor too little. The nature of trauma and addiction is the opposite: chaotic, impulsive, reactive, confused, distressed.

Past-focused treatments are often described as *processing*, and physical processes are used as metaphors: to "digest," "cleanse," and "purge" (Jackson, 1994). There's a sense of unburdening and emotional relief. Some clients experience this as a deeper level of change than present-focused

---

[3] Several key mechanisms lead to change: *learning new coping, grieving, quantum change (conversion), relationship-based change, physically based change, coercion, consequences,* and *creativity* (Najavits, 2017). See also the classic framework by Prochaska, DiClemente, and Norcross (1992).

treatment, which is about improving current functioning. However, both are useful and produce positive results in research (as discussed in Chapter 2).

The word *creating* in the book title is also meaningful. Creativity and healing emotional pain are interconnected (Rogers, 1993). Both require imagination—steering into new territory, with a willingness to entertain new ways of seeing and the courage to experiment. They're also active processes; they can't be done *to* or *for* someone but must be created by the individual. Finally, Creating Change includes specific creative methods as one of many channels for growth, including art, storytelling, and metaphor.

In the end, change is mysterious and humbling. Some clients who seem the least likely to change are able to, while others who seem more likely to, don't. Often, it's a matter of timing—a spark of the right moment, treatment, and counselor combined in a way that clients respond to even if they weren't able to before. Witnessing this is profoundly gratifying.

THE DEVELOPMENT OF CREATING CHANGE

The model was developed based on clinical experience, feedback from clients and counselors, research studies, and various literatures, including a deep dive into the history of past-focused models. It draws wisdom from all of these, maintaining respect for what's come before but also offering unique features not present in other models.

Creating Change was the first past-focused model ever developed for trauma and addiction, starting in 2005 with an exploratory version and pilot study (Najavits, Schmitz, Gotthardt, & Weiss, 2005), followed by a summary of the model and larger pilot study in 2014 (Najavits, 2014; Najavits & Johnson, 2014); a randomized controlled trial (RCT) in 2018 (Najavits et al., 2018); and several clinical implementation projects. All are described in the next section, "Evidence Base." Lessons learned along the way led to various refinements, including the following:

- There was originally a three-part sequence: *before* (preparation), *during* (the main topics), and *after* (wrap-up). The "before" segment had seven topics to help prepare clients for the upcoming emotional work. But most clients didn't need preparation and for those who did, seven topics was too many. It also had the unintended effect of creating anticipatory anxiety, with some clients becoming concerned about why they had to do so much preparation, creating a "falling off the cliff" feeling. Now there are just three optional preparation topics. The "after" segment also became condensed into the topic "Growth" as that was sufficient.

- The initial exploratory version in 2005 was heavily influenced by Exposure Therapy, which was the predominant past-focused trauma model at the time. Indeed, the initial version was called Exposure Therapy Revised (Najavits et al., 2005). But with increasing clinical experience and subsequent studies, it became apparent that broader themes relevant to trauma and addiction were more compelling and allowed the model to be conducted in group treatment. Various topics, such as "Tell Your Story" and "Deepen Your Story," still offer a narrative emphasis, but the model goes beyond the narrative as well.

- The handouts were edited to be shorter, and more exercises were added to promote interaction and engagement.

EVIDENCE BASE

Summary of Evidence

Creating Change is an evidence-based model with three published studies and several clinical implementation projects. It has shown significant positive results in all of the studies, and feedback from the implementation projects was also highly enthusiastic. Creating Change was conducted in 1-hour individual sessions in the studies and group or individual modality in the implementation projects.

Study clients had current, severe, and chronic PTSD and SUD; recent active substance use; and additional psychiatric problems. To obtain clients who were typical of front-line settings, clients were outpatients, were not required to be in any additional treatment, and could participate even if they had current suicidality, self-harm, personality disorder, drug use disorder, homelessness, or severe dissociation. (In contrast, most prior past-focused studies of PTSD/SUD had multiple such exclusions and/or required clients to be in concurrent stabilizing treatments [Najavits et al., 2020]) Samples included varied populations (military veterans, crime victims, and child abuse survivors), and two of the three studies had very strong minority representation.

Results indicated improvement in multiple domains, and attendance and satisfaction were high across the studies, with no safety concerns. The 2018 RCT (Najavits et al., 2018), moreover, indicated that Creating Change achieved gains at a level equal to Seeking Safety, which is already established as an effective, evidence-based, cost-effective model (e.g., Lenz et al., 2016; Litt, Cohen, & Hien, 2019; Sherman et al., 2023; Washington State Institute for Public Policy, 2018), and gains were sustained at 3-month follow-up. Each study and its results are described in the sections that follow.

Randomized Controlled Trial (2018)

A RCT is the gold standard of scientific testing. Creating Change was compared to Seeking Safety in a sample of 52 outpatient male and female military veterans with current PTSD and current SUD (Najavits et al., 2018).

The majority of the sample was severe and chronic in both PTSD and substance dependence. A third had two or more SUD diagnoses, and there was a substantial rate of drug use disorders, with cocaine dependence the most common. The rate of lifetime traumas was very high: an average of 10 out of 23 trauma types. Despite the focus on veterans and the majority being male, sexual trauma was more common than combat trauma. Most of the veterans met criteria for additional mental health disorders (62%), and 37% met criteria for one or more personality disorders. The sample had strong (40%) minority representation, primarily Black.

Half of the veterans received Creating Change and the other half received Seeking Safety, delivered in 17 individual 1-hour sessions. They were assessed at baseline, end-of-treatment, and 3-month follow-up. Results were highly positive: Both treatments showed improvement at the end of treatment, with no difference between them, indicating that Creating Change did as well as the established evidence-based model Seeking Safety (in statistical terms, "no worse than" Seeking Safety). Significant improvements were found on PTSD, alcohol use, and drug use (the primary outcomes) as well as mental health symptoms, quality of life, beliefs related to SUD, and self-efficacy. The amount of change, known as effect size, was large for alcohol use and medium for the other measures. Improvements were sustained at 3-month follow-up after the end of treatment, and on alcohol they even continued to improve during that time. Both treatments were found to be safe; attendance, treatment satisfaction, and alliance with the counselors were also very strong.

The data also indicated that both treatments were safe. There was no increase in self-harm or suicidal ideation or actions, no pattern of worsening, and no adverse events related to either treatment. Attendance was very strong at 67% of Creating Change sessions and 68% Seeking Safety sessions. This attendance rate is especially noteworthy as clients generally reported very low attendance at other professional therapies and 12-step groups throughout the study.

Pilot Study (2014)

A pilot is a first step to see how well a treatment does in a small sample. Creating Change was conducted with seven men and women outpatients in a crime victims program. The sample was current and chronic in both PTSD and SUD and was predominantly minority (71%) and low-income (Najavits & Johnson, 2014). Creating Change was conducted as 17 individual weekly 1-hour sessions. Assessments occurred at pre- and posttreatment. Significant improvements were found in multiple domains including some PTSD and trauma-related symptoms (e.g., dissociation, anxiety, depression, and sexual problems); other mental health symptoms (e.g., paranoia, psychotic symptoms, obsessive symptoms, and interpersonal sensitivity); daily life functioning; beliefs related to PTSD; coping strategies; and suicidal ideation. The amount of change (effect sizes) was consistently large, including for both alcohol and drug problems. Attendance and satisfaction were strong, and no adverse events were reported.

Pilot Study (2005)

This first pilot study was conducted with five men (Najavits et al., 2005). The treatment model was called Exposure Therapy Revised (a precursor to Creating Change) and emphasized adaptation of classic Exposure Therapy to make it relevant for comorbid PTSD and SUD, including enhanced safeguards and attention to painful memories of both trauma and addiction. The clients (all White) had current, chronic, and highly severe PTSD and SUD, all with childhood-based PTSD. The study had fewer exclusionary criteria than any prior exposure study of PTSD/SUD. For example, suicidal ideation was not an exclusionary criterion (80% had suicidal ideation; 60% had a suicide plan). The five men were offered 30 individual sessions in 5 months and were invited to select, at each session, whether they wanted to focus on the present (Seeking Safety) or the past (Exposure Therapy Revised). Results showed 100% attendance, and significant positive outcomes in numerous domains, including trauma and SUD symptoms, as well as excellent treatment attendance and satisfaction. On average, the participants chose 21 Seeking Safety sessions and nine sessions of Exposure Therapy Revised. Notably, clients were assessed at the start of treatment on their preference for present- versus past-focused methods. They rated present-focused as more appealing than past-focused before starting treatment, but by the end, expressed strong satisfaction with both. They also reported that the exposure sessions helped equally with both their PTSD and SUD. Treatment satisfaction was high, and there were no safety concerns.

Implementation Projects

In eight different treatment programs, teams implemented Creating Change and offered feedback, questions, and some session recordings, all of which helped refine the model. The list of programs appears in the Preface to this book and represents various populations, including veterans, crime victims, clients with childhood trauma, addiction program clients, mental health program clients, all genders, and highly diverse ethnicities. Five teams were independent of the author, and three (the studies described above) were by led the author.

OVERALL

In brief, Creating Change offers the following features:

- Designed for clients with addiction and trauma or either alone.
- Highly interactive learning with extensive handouts and exercises.

- The first fully past-focused model for trauma and addiction (explores difficult addiction memories as well as trauma memories, and the impact of each over time).
- Conveys a warm, compassionate tone rather than a highly technical one.
- Public health–oriented: for a broad range of clients, counselors, and settings; all types of trauma and addiction; and group or individual modality.
- Skill building: teaches clients how to face the past in a wide variety of ways.
- Flexible: Counselors choose session length and dose as well as the order and number of topics and handouts (all are independent of the others).
- Combines easily with Seeking Safety and other models.
- Each topic is a unique theme relevant to trauma and addiction.
- Optional extra topics enhance clients' ability to benefit from past-focused counseling and can be done at any point in treatment.
- Designed to be easier to tolerate than models focused on repeated retelling of the trauma narrative. Numerous safeguards help anchor the work.
- Evidence-based for PTSD and SUD, including with severe, chronic, complex clients (e.g., active current substance use, drug disorders, suicidal thoughts, self-harm, recent hospitalization, personality disorders), and with strong minority representation.
- Addresses harm the clients may have done to others, in addition to harm done to them.
- Builds engagement via inspiring quotations; real-life examples; creative exercises; and poignant language.
- Draws wisdom from the history of past-focused therapies.
- Empowers clients to choose what, when, and how they want to share.
- Reframes *avoidance* as *self-protection* that is healthy or unhealthy depending on the situation.
- For any provider (advanced degree or license not required) but emphasizes best practices in trauma and addiction per Chapter 4.
- Low cost, requiring only the book (counselors each need a book and then can share handouts with their clients).
- Training is available but not required, except for formal research.
- A freely downloadable fidelity measure and other resources are available at *www.creating-change.org*.

One client who participated in the treatment wrote: "My ability to speak about past trauma was one way to get over the guilt I felt about being a 'drug addict.' By admitting what happened and talking about it, we gain understanding of our behavior—not just the substance abuse, but the poor relationship choices and the vast array of other issues we've dragged along behind us all our lives. Talking about sexual abuse (which filled me with shame) has been a crucial part of my recovery."

The book title *Creating Change* conveys, in two words, the optimistic perspective that clients with trauma and addiction can come to terms with their past. In doing so, they can reclaim a better present and future.

2

The Larger Context

The ancients stole our best ideas.
~Mark Twain, 19th-century American writer

Past-focused counseling has a fascinating history that informed the development of Creating Change. As the quote above humorously suggests, the same ideas get rediscovered across time.

This chapter explores some of these core ideas—time-tested truths—that offer broad context relevant to Creating Change.

TIP: If you plan to conduct Creating Change, it's helpful to read this entire chapter. But at a minimum, see these chapter sections that relate directly to Creating Change implementation:

+ Wisdom from the past (ideas underlying Creating Change)
+ Co-occurring trauma and addiction (challenges and progress)

TWO MAJOR TYPES OF COUNSELING

To set the framework for understanding past-focused models, it's helpful to start with a comparison of *present-focused models* and *past-focused models*, which were briefly described in Chapter 1. They're different ways of working and are experienced as different by both clients and counselors. Yet the distinction between present-focused and past-focused isn't always pure: There's overlap at times, and some models combine the two types.

Various terms have been used over time for present- versus past-focused approaches:

- *Coping* versus *processing*
- *Stabilizing* versus *exploratory*
- *Containing* versus *emotionally arousing*
- *Supportive* versus *uncovering*
- *Coping skills* versus *exposure*
- *Safety* versus *mourning and remembrance*
- *Non-trauma-focused* versus *trauma-focused*[1]

---

[1] Currently, the terms *trauma-focused* versus *non-trauma-focused* are common, but this unfortunate terminology is equivalent to calling women *non-men* or children *non-adults*: It negates present-focused models, rather than stating what they do provide (Najavits & Hien, 2013). It's also inaccurate as present-focused trauma models directly address trauma, but via coping rather than processing.

These terms aren't always exactly parallel as they arose across various theoretical orientations, but they speak to the idea that they represent fundamentally different types of treatment.

Addiction models are typically present-focused and trauma models are typically past-focused, but both types exist in each field and research shows that both produce positive results in people with co-occurring addiction and trauma issues. Indeed, they achieve overall equivalent results (Simpson et al., 2021).

Present-Focused Treatment

Fall down seven times, get up eight.
~Japanese Proverb

The goal of present-focused models is to help clients improve current functioning—to help them "get through the day in a healthy way." These stabilizing treatments are used either for their own sake or sometimes as a first stage prior to past-focused work. Rather than telling the detailed story of trauma or addiction, they address how to cope right now. For example, a client having flashbacks (intrusive visual or physical reminders) is guided back to the present using grounding rather than exploring the content of the flashbacks, which could further destabilize the person.

Present-focused models offer education and a wide variety of coping skills. This may include cognitive restructuring to promote adaptive thinking, social skills training, self-soothing for distress, and enhancing awareness of trauma and addiction symptoms.

Clients can share trauma and addiction memories, but this sharing is usually limited to a brief recap, not details. Present-focused models don't encourage clients to explore the past in detail for its own sake or as the primary method of healing. The treatment is not devoid of emotion, as emotion is central to all counseling models. But the idea is to address emotions in the present rather than through intensive exploration of the past, to stay within a moderate range of emotion, and to use emotion to guide current coping.

Trauma Treatment (Present-Focused)

Present-focused trauma models go by many different names, including the following adult models[2] from the trauma field:

- Stress Inoculation Training (Veronen & Kilpatrick, 1983)
- Cognitive-Behavioral Therapy (Foy, 1992)
- Imagery Rehearsal Therapy (Krakow, Kellner, Neidhardt, Pathak, & Lambert, 1993)
- Affect Management (Zlotnick et al., 1997)
- Anger Management (Chemtob, Novaco, Hamada, & Gross, 1997)
- Trauma Recovery and Empowerment Model (Harris, 1998)
- Trauma Affect Regulation: Guide for Education and Therapy for Adults (Ford, Kasimer, MacDonald, & Savill, 2000)
- Beyond Trauma (Covington, 2003)
- Cognitive Therapy (Ehlers, Clark, Hackmann, McManus, & Fennell, 2005)
- Relaxation Training (Stapleton, Taylor, & Asmundson, 2006)
- Mind Body Skills Group (Gordon, Staples, He, & Atti, 2016)
- Present-Centered Therapy (Wattenberg, Gross, Niles, Unger, & Shea, 2021)

---

[2] This chapter focuses on adult treatment (not child or family treatment, which are different specialty areas).

Addiction Treatment (Present-Focused)

Most addiction models are present-focused. Their goal is to reduce addictive behavior while increasing clients' personal strengths for ongoing recovery. Typical methods include rehearsing how to refuse substances, naming pros and cons of using, identifying addiction triggers, and increasing motivation. Examples of present-focused addiction models are:

- Relapse Prevention (RP; Marlatt & Gordon, 1985)
- Motivational Interviewing (MI; Miller & Rollnick, 1991) and, later, Motivational Enhancement Therapy
- CBT for Substance Abuse (Beck, Wright, Newman, & Liese, 1993)
- 12-Step Facilitation (Nowinski, Baker, & Carroll, 1995)
- CBT Coping Skills (Kadden et al., 1995)
- Contingency Management (Petry, 2000)
- Helping Women Recover (Covington, 2000)
- BRENDA (Volpicelli, Pettinati, McLellan, & O'Brien, 2001)
- Group Treatment for Substance Abuse (Velasquez, Maurer, Crouch, & DiClemente, 2001)
- Community Reinforcement Approach (Meyers & Miller, 2001)
- Combined Behavioral Intervention Manual (Miller, 2004)
- Matrix Model (Rawson & McCann, 2005)
- Individual Addiction Counseling (McGovern, Lambert-Harris, Alterman, Xie, & Meier, 2011)
- Alcohol Support (Sannibale et al., 2013)
- Mindfulness-Based Relapse Prevention (Somohano & Bowen, 2022)

Integrated Models for Both Trauma and Addiction (Present-Focused)

Some present-focused models address both trauma and addiction at the same time by the same provider (*integrated models*):

- Addiction and Trauma Recovery Integration Model (Miller & Guidry, 2001)
- Trauma, Addictions, Mental Health, and Recovery (Gillece & Russell, 2001)
- Seeking Safety (Najavits, 2002c)
- Triad (Clark & Fearday, 2003)
- Integrated CBT (McGovern et al., 2009)
- Mindfulness-Based Relapse Prevention—Trauma-Integrated (Somohano & Bowen, 2022)

There are also several other early present-focused approaches that are not treatment models per se, for example, Dayton (2000), Evans and Sullivan (1995), Meisler (1999), and Trotter (1992). (For a list of models that have been empirically studied, see Appendix B online, "Comparison of All Models Studied for PTSD/SUD," at *www.guilford.com/najavits3-materials*.)

Past-Focused Treatment

> *To get to the healing, you have to break your heart first.*
> ~Dorothy Allison, 20th-century American novelist

Throughout history, working through painful experiences has been described over and over, going as far back as ancient Greece (Jackson, 1994). An example from the 17th century is the following from van Helmont: "Experience informs us, that Persons over-taken with some great grief or affliction, when they cannot discharge their Sorrow by Weeping, do often fall into some Distemper or Sickness" (quoted in Jackson, 1994, pp. 474–475). In other words, expressing feelings helps overcome disturbing memories, and if this process is blocked, illness arises.

In the late 19th century, Breuer and Freud described the process as part of the newly emerging field of psychotherapy: "[Each] symptom . . . permanently disappeared when we had succeeded in bringing clearly to light the memory of the event . . . and in arousing its accompanying affect, and when the patient had described that event in the greatest possible detail and had put the affect into words" (quoted in Jackson, 1994, p. 476; see also Bemak & Young, 1998; Jackson, 1994; van der Hart et al., 1989).

Herman offers a modern version in relation to trauma recovery:

> Out of the fragmented components of frozen imagery and sensation, patient and therapist slowly reassemble an organized, detailed, verbal account, oriented in time and historical context. . . . The patient must reconstruct not only what happened but also what she felt. . . . Reconstructing the trauma story also includes a systematic review of the meaning of the event. . . . The traumatic event challenges an ordinary person to become a theologian, a philosopher, and a jurist. The survivor is called upon to articulate the values and beliefs that she once held and that the trauma destroyed. . . . The survivor must . . . reconstruct a system of belief that makes sense of her undeserved suffering. (1992, pp. 177–178)

Herman's description speaks eloquently to several components: telling one's story, connecting to emotions, and coming to terms with the meaning of the event. This work was part of psychotherapy for most of the 20th century with terms such as *catharsis, mourning, grieving,* and *working through.* Such methods were used in therapy beginning in 1850 and were applied on a large scale beginning in World War I (1914–1918) for war trauma (Jackson, 1994).

Trauma Treatment (Past-Focused)

There have been many different versions of past-focused models, all of which were specifically applied to trauma. The earliest ones were psychoanalytic, but over time the orientations broadened to psychodynamic, humanistic, behavioral, and cognitive.

- Hypnosis (e.g., Hoek, 1850)
- Catharsis (e.g., Janet, 1886)
- Psychocatharsis (e.g., Sauer, 1917)
- Psychoanalytic catharsis (e.g., Simmel, 1918)
- Abreactive therapy (e.g., Brown, 1920)
- Historical group debriefing (e.g., Marshall, 1945)
- Narcoanalysis (e.g., Grinker, 1945)
- Gestalt therapy, such as the empty-chair technique (e.g., Perls, 1951)
- Psychodrama (e.g., Moreno, 1951, 1964)
- Emotive therapies of the 1970s (see Nichols & Zax, 1977)
- Rap groups (e.g., Shatan, 1974)
- Emotional flooding therapies (e.g., Olsen, 1976)
- Grief therapies (which are applied to traumatic or unresolved grief, e.g., Re-Grief Therapy [Volkan & Showalter, 1968]; Time-Limited Dynamic Psychotherapy [Horowitz et al., 1973]; Focal Psychotherapy [Raphael, 1975]; a behavioral model [Ramsay & Happée, 1977]

a CBT model [Gauthier & Marshall, 1977]; Grief Resolution Therapy [Melges & DeMaso, 1980]; Guided Mourning [Mawson et al., 1981]; and Complicated Grief Therapy [Shear et al., 2005]).[3]

Modern-era past-focused trauma models include the following, which are primarily cognitive-behavioral and empirically studied (to varying degrees). All those listed below are either fully past-focused or include at least a strong component of past-focused techniques:

- Flooding (e.g., Keane, Fairbank, Caddell, & Zimering, 1989; Rachman, 1966)
- Implosive Therapy (e.g., Stampfl & Levis, 1967)
- Systematic Desensitization (e.g., Bowen & Lambert, 1986; Wolpe, 1958)
- Testimony Therapy (e.g., Cienfuegos & Monelli, 1983)
- Critical Incident Stress Debriefing/Psychological Debriefing (e.g., Mitchell, 1983)
- Expressive Writing (Pennebaker & Beall, 1986); and various adaptations of it (e.g., Written Emotional Disclosure: Written Disclosure [Batten et al., 2003]; Structured Writing Therapy [Schoutrop et al., 2002]; Written Exposure Therapy for PTSD [Sloan et al., 2013])
- Prolonged Exposure (PE; Foa, Rothbaum, Riggs, & Murdock, 1991)
- Cognitive-Behavioral Therapy for PTSD (Foy, 1992)
- Image Habituation Therapy (Vaughan & Tarrier, 1992)
- Cognitive Processing Therapy (CPT; Resick & Schnicke, 1993)
- Eye Movement Desensitization and Reprocessing (EMDR; Shapiro, 1995)
- Trauma-Focused Group Therapy (Foy et al., 1997)
- Cognitive-Behavioral Therapy for Acute Stress Disorder (Bryant et al., 1998)
- CBT for PTSD after Motor Vehicle Accident (Fecteau & Nicki, 1999)
- Brief Eclectic Psychotherapy for PTSD (Gersons et al., 2000).
- Skills Training in Affective and Interpersonal Regulation/Modified Prolonged Exposure (Cloitre, Koenen, Cohen, & Han, 2002)
- Cognitive Therapy for PTSD (Ehlers & Clark, 2003)
- Cognitive Trauma Therapy for Battered Women (Kubany et al., 2004)
- CBT for Motor Vehicle Accident PTSD (Blanchard & Hickling, 2004; adaptation of Fecteau & Niki, 1999)
- Group CBT for Motor Vehicle Accident PTSD (Beck & Coffey, 2005; adaptation of Blanchard & Hickling, 2004; Fecteau & Niki, 1999)
- Narrative Exposure Therapy (Schauer et al., 2005)
- Trauma Model Therapy (Ross, 2005)
- Counting Method and Progressive Counting (Greenwald, 2008; Johnson & Lubin, 2006)
- Brief CBT for Acute Stress Disorder (Sijbrandij et al., 2007; adaptation of Foa et al., 1995)
- Individual Intensive Trauma Therapy (Gantt & Tinnin, 2007)
- Trauma Informed Guilt Reduction Therapy (Norman et al., 2014)

What the various models have in common is a paradox: Clients move into painful memories as a way to overcome them. Exploring the past means revealing some or all of the following:

---

[3] These various models are compiled from literature review as well as various sources (Bemak & Young, 1998; Crocq & Crocq, 2000; Jackson, 1994; Rando, 1993; van der Hart & Brown, 1992). For an outstanding discussion of catharsis models in general, see Nichols and Zax (1977), and for a historical description of trauma treatment, see Herman (1992) and Weisaeth (2002).

- what happened ▪ how it felt (e.g., abandoned, betrayed) ▪ who hurt them ▪ impact on their mind, body, behavior, and spirit ▪ messages they took from their experiences ▪ enduring issues (e.g., symptoms, functioning)

In Creating Change (and occasionally other models, such as Narrative Exposure Therapy [Schauer et al., 2020]), there's also explicit emphasis on poignant positive memories such as people who helped along the way, and resilient moments that speak to their survival and personal strength. Awareness of positive experiences can be just as important as painful ones.

Past-focused work sometimes brings up strong emotions and even physical reactions such as nausea and heart racing. It's been described in many different metaphors such as cleansing, purging, unraveling, releasing toxins, lancing a boil, eruption of a volcano, layers of an onion, opening Pandora's box, and purification of the emotions (Chu, 1992; Jackson, 1994; Nichols & Efran, 1985; van der Hart & Brown, 1992). There's a sense of completion and resolution when it's successful.

What makes the work therapeutic is that it's planned, there's a clear objective of helping the client move carefully in and out of the past, and it achieves progress rather than just a reexperience of distress. Instead of pointless suffering, it's pain that serves a purpose, as in the Buddhist phrase, "changing poison into medicine." Like surgery or childbirth, it's intentionally entering into pain toward a larger goal.

Clients discover they can face memories, tolerate them, grieve them, and eventually these memories no longer hold such emotional power over them. It's often described informally as "The only way out is through," "You'll feel worse before you feel better," and "You need a good cry." Normally, people learn these processes on their own or as part of growing up in a healthy family. But for many people with trauma and addiction, the natural ways of learning these processes were blocked if they grew up in an environment without truth-telling or validation of feelings. One client said, "As a child, if I was upset, my parents would say, 'Go to sleep and when you wake up your problems will be gone.'"

Clients who successfully do past-focused work often describe it as liberating. They feel more alive, more aware, and more loving. They feel less stuck and confused. They're able to access a wider range of feelings, including joy, which previously may have been out of reach. They move from distress and danger to a greater sense of peace. Ultimately, "We cannot change the traumatic event, but we can change our relationship to that experience" (Carruth & Burke, 2006, p. 4).

Past-focused therapies differ from one another in some ways, too. Some go low-and-slow with gradual exploration of memories and emotion; others dive right in to the most upsetting material. Some are highly sequenced; others are open-ended. In some, clients tell their story out loud; in others, they explore it only in their mind. Some are purely verbal; others incorporate writing, artwork, or other nonverbal techniques. Some are individual; others use group. Some combine past- and present-focused interventions approximately equally—for example, Skills Training in Affective and Interpersonal Regulation followed by Exposure Therapy (Cloitre et al., 2002), Cognitive Trauma Therapy for Battered Women (Kubany et al., 2004), and Dialectical Behavior Therapy/Prolonged Exposure (DBT/PE; Harned & Linehan, 2008); many include at least some amount of present-focused work such as basic trauma education.

Models also contain unique elements. EMDR includes eye movements (back-and-forth visual tracking) to promote trauma processing. PE includes *in vivo* exercises for clients to confront current trauma reminders, such as touching clothes worn during trauma or going back to the location where it occurred, if it's safe to do so. Interoceptive exposure guides clients to tolerate body sensations related to trauma, such as holding one's breath for 30 seconds to re-create the experience of smothering or dizziness (Taylor, 2006). In virtual reality therapy, clients put on goggles to view a computer-generated trauma scene, such as "a virtual Huey helicopter flying over a virtual

Vietnam, and a clearing surrounded by jungle" (Rothbaum, Hodges, Ready, Graap, & Alarcon, 2001, p. 617).

Addiction Treatment (Past-Focused)

The addiction field doesn't have as clear a distinction between present- and past-focused models as the trauma field, but both exist.[4]

Past-focused methods, even if not formally called that, are in widespread use, usually just as one component of a model. Telling one's story is part of 12-step groups and therapeutic communities (the "drunkalog" and Alcoholics Anonymous [AA] speaker meetings). Twelve-step programs also ask participants to explore the past in other ways, such as making amends in steps 8 and 9. Writing an addiction autobiography is common in rehabilitation programs as a way to come to terms with the impact of addiction. Treatment addresses clients' life story—who they were before, during, and after the addiction—and how to build a new identity going forward.

Grieving has long been described as part of addiction recovery. Clients need to face the loss of a substance, for example, which is described as like the death of a friend or lover (Knapp, 1996). They also need to face other losses and destruction, such as how the addiction harmed their physical health, capacity for intimacy, responsibility to self and others, opportunities in life, spirituality, development, and sense of integrity and purpose.

Integrated Models for Trauma and Addiction (Past-Focused)

Several models include a past-focused component, address both trauma and addiction, and have at least one empirical study:

- Trauma-Relevant Relapse Prevention Training, later named Enhanced Relapse Prevention Training (Abueg & Fairbank, 1991; Seidel et al., 1994)[5]
- Substance Dependence PTSD Therapy (Triffleman, Carroll, & Kellogg, 1999)
- Transcend (Donovan, Padin-Rivera, & Kowaliw, 2001)
- Integrated Treatment (van Dam, Ehring, Vedel, & Emmelkamp, 2013)
- Creating Change (Najavits, 2014)
- Concurrent Treatment of PTSD and Substance Use Disorders Using Prolonged Exposure (COPE; Back et al., 2012; formerly named Concurrent Treatment of PTSD and Cocaine Dependence)
- Modified Prolonged Exposure (Coffey et al., 2016)

Among these, Creating Change is the only integrated model that is fully past-focused and developed from the start as a new model rather than combining existing models. The others include both present- and past-focused components, and combine models that were already developed by others (e.g., a past-focused trauma model such as PE and a present-focused addiction model such as RP). See the section "Why a New Model?" in Chapter 1 for more detail.

---

[4] There's also an exposure model in the SUD field called *cue exposure* but it's not past-focused in the usual sense. Rather, it's confronting current SUD triggers such as seeing drug paraphernalia (O'Brien, Childress, McLellan, & Ehrman, 1990).

[5] The inpatient version of the Abueg model included trauma exposure (Dr. Francis Abueg, personal communication, October 19, 2022).

WISDOM FROM THE PAST

Across the long sweep of past-focused methods, several ideas serve as foundations in Creating Change.

Emotion Alone ("Spilling") Is Not Enough

There's often a view by clients, and sometime counselors, that simply expressing feelings about the past is enough. "Emotional memories continue to be thought of as foreign bodies lodged in the human psyche and requiring purgation" (Nichols & Efran, 1985, p. 46). This has been termed the *ventilation school* in the history of science and is widely critiqued (Jackson, 1994). Simply expressing feelings about past events can be unproductive and even destructive (Chu, 1992; van der Hart & Brown, 1992). Thus, experts in past-focused treatment distinguish *expressing* feelings from *processing* feelings. Expressing feelings is also called *abreaction, emotional discharge,* and *grief*.[6] Processing feelings is also termed *working through, mourning,* and *accommodation* (e.g., Bemak & Young, 1998; Jackson, 1994; Rando, 1993; Shapiro, 1995). (The widely used term *catharsis* has been used for both expressing and processing feelings.)

In short, expressing feelings is not sufficient. Additional necessary elements include accessing memory, attaining insight, releasing physical distress, connecting memory and emotion, new learning, and integrating memory into one's life narrative. These elements do not all have to occur together or in every session, as long as they are included over the course of treatment.

Clinical evidence supports the idea that emotional expression is not enough. First, it can lead to short-term relief but doesn't generally endure over the long term (Jackson, 1994; van der Hart & Brown, 1992). In the 1970s, encounter groups and other human potential therapies discovered that "letting it all hang out" didn't produce lasting changes. This was actually a rediscovery as Freud, Jung, the World War I military therapist McDougal, and others had already observed this phenomenon in the early 20th century. Second, spontaneous *abreaction*—outbursts of emotion related to memory, such as flashbacks and triggers—occurs frequently in PTSD and addiction and is not productive per se. They are "closed . . . loops that offer no relief, but are only repeated over and over again" (Petersen, quoted in van der Hart & Brown, 1992, p. 129). This, too, was described by McDougal in the 1920s. Thus, it's not just emotional expression but the right context, planned and meaningful, that makes it therapeutic rather than retraumatizing. Third, and finally, emotional expression sometimes obscures important underlying feelings, such as a client who shows only rage, which serves as a defense against sadness.

Various writers have observed that "emotional arousal should be accompanied by a cognitive change to achieve maximal therapeutic effectiveness" (Bemak & Young, 1998, p. 169; see also Hembree & Foa, 2000; van der Hart & Brown, 1992). Terms for the cognitive component include *reframing, insight, recontexualization, reconceptualization, cognitive restructuring,* and *meaning-making*. Clients say, "It helped me to understand how I felt and why," and "I never realized how it affected me before" (Pennebaker, 1990, per Bemak & Young, 1998, p. 172). So, in addition to expressing feelings, clients need to achieve some new understanding about the past. Put differently, clients are ideally both participant and observer—they experience their feelings (participant) but also evaluate the meaning of them (observer) (Moreno, 1964). Yet counseling doesn't always need a formal cognitive restructuring component; for example, it occurs informally during sessions of PE (Riggs,

---

[6] The distinction between *grief* and *mourning* varies (Zisook & Shear, 2009). Sometimes *grief* refers to an internal experience and *mourning* the public expression of it (funerals and other rituals). Elsewhere, grief is the expression of pain and mourning is the processing; and sometimes the two terms are used interchangeably.

personal communication, November 16, 2007). Interestingly, research has been mixed on the value of adding a formal cognitive restructuring component to PE (e.g., Moser, Cahill, & Foa, 2010).

Memory Alone Is Not Enough

Simply recalling memories (telling the trauma and addiction story) is not therapeutic unless other elements are present. You may have seen this in clients who tell their story in a cold, numb fashion, detached, just stating the facts. As Conn wrote in 1953, "It is not the recall of the traumatic experience which is of therapeutic value, but the patient's acceptance of what he thought, felt, and did" (quoted in van der Hart & Brown, 1992, p. 135). Thus, true healing involves *integrating* memory and emotion rather than either one alone (Herman, 1992; McCullough, 2003). This may seem obvious to us, but the history of past-focused treatment has had two major schools of thought: one that emphasized accessing emotion (the *abreaction model*) and one that emphasized accessing memory (the *dissociation–integration model*) (van der Hart & Brown, 1992). The latter focused on the difficulty some trauma survivors have in remembering what happened to them (e.g., *splitting* or what used to be called *divided consciousness*). At this point, it's understood that both emotion and memory are helpful when addressed in balanced fashion.

Yet there's still uncertainty about how memory is best addressed to promote healing. Some say that trauma memories need to be integrated into the life story. Others say memories can be "put into a capsule separated from other parts of the life story" (Shamai & Levin-Megged, 2006, p. 693). Others emphasize that just the attempt to create a coherent narrative is helpful rather than needing to complete one (van Dijk, Schoutrop, & Spinhoven, 2003). The topic of memory is covered in greater detail in the Creating Change topic, "Memory." Note, too, that having the client tell the trauma or addiction story in the absence of emotion may serve a limited purpose, such as providing testimony in a legal case or compensation claim.

Processing Emotional Pain Is a Basic Human Capacity

In our era, major strides have been made to help people overcome pain from their past (including trauma and addiction). We have treatment manuals and research on how people recover. But we didn't invent the basic human capacity to face the past. Throughout history, processing painful experiences has been part of the human experience. There's evidence that it's genetically hardwired and also occurs in some animal species, such as elephants who grieve their dead.

Descriptions of mourning go back to ancient literature, such as the *Iliad* (Shay, 1994). Ancient Greeks and Romans held purification rituals called *lustration* after community-wide traumas such as plagues and massacres. Many versions arose in folk customs and religion, including confession, shamanism, exorcism, magic, healing rituals, and trance induction (Nichols & Zax, 1977). One current treatment, Pennebaker's Writing Therapy, was invented based just on observing confessions during criminals' lie detector testing: "[P]articipants often thanked the polygraph operator and some operators received Christmas cards from those they had helped to convict" (Bemak & Young, 1998, p. 171).

Thus, one way to understand past-focused treatment is that it helps unblock a natural process that was thwarted. During the Vietnam War, for example, the military didn't offer support for grief: "Mourning was dreaded, perfunctory, delayed, devalued, mocked, fragmented, minimized, deflected, disregarded, and sedated" (Shay, 1994, p. 67). Substances were widely used to manage feelings that couldn't be expressed.

In short, with counseling we're not doing something *to* the client nor creating a dramatic new procedure, but rather creating conditions for the client to access what's internal. It's teaching clients how to tap into processes that are instinctively their birthright.

It's the Individual But Also the Community

Current treatments are primarily focused on the individual: Clients are engaged and assessed as individuals and are often seen in individual therapy. From this perspective, recovery is the client's personal task to take on. But trauma and addiction are broader than the individual. They originate in a community context—family, peers, neighborhood, society—and can also be healed, in part, through that context.

Some of the most important progress in the trauma field arose from larger societal contexts. Trauma was recognized as a real and serious issue for women and children primarily due to the women's movement of the 1960s; prior to that, it was identified with men and war trauma (Herman, 1992, 2023). After the Vietnam War, veterans disenchanted by government veterans programs formed their own trauma support, called rap groups, which helped establish more empowered approaches to treatment. In the 1970s, testimony therapies arose in Chile in response to community-wide torture and genocide and later spread to other countries (Cienfuegos & Monelli, 1983). In 1995, the South African government established a truth and reconciliation commission after apartheid to hear testimony by both victims and perpetrators of violence. This model is especially interesting as a form of past-focused "counseling" applied to an entire society to promote healing and national unity. An earlier effort in post–Nazi Germany was *vergangenheitsbewältigung* or "coming to terms with the past."

Modern addiction treatment also had its most important development in a grassroots community movement: 12-step groups, founded as AA in 1935. These groups brought addiction into public awareness, gave them legitimacy as an illness rather than moral weakness, and offered a fellowship of free mutual assistance.

Helping clients make sense of the past is strengthened by awareness of how trauma and addiction arise in a larger societal context (not simply within the individual) and can be aided by community-based support and advocacy.

There's No One Right Way

A famous article on counseling outcomes is titled "Is It True That Everybody Has Won and All Must Have Prizes?" (Luborsky, Singer, & Luborsky, 1976). Over 60 years of research shows that manualized mental health counseling models typically perform equally well (Lambert, 2013). This also holds true among trauma models and among addiction models (e.g., Foa et al., 2018; Hoge & Chard, 2018; Imel, Wampold, Miller, & Fleming, 2008; Maguen et al., 2021). In short, there's no one right way, but many. Thus, counselors can select models based not just on evidence but also on their own and clients' preferences and treatment setting.

It's also interesting to explore the range of techniques that have been attempted to help clients access memory and emotion in the service of healing. These include some that are no longer used, such as *narcoanalysis* (medications such as ether, adrenaline, and sodium amytal) and harsh verbal confrontation with provocative statements, which was used both in the trauma and the addiction fields (see examples in the next paragraph). Other methods still in use are listening to a trauma narrative repeatedly; *in vivo* (real-life) exposure to reminders of trauma or addiction; stimulus methods such as watching a poignant movie; "mechanical" methods (e.g., changing body postures); creative arts such as drawing or collage; autobiographical timelines; and writing exercises (Bemak & Young, 1998; Jackson, 1994; Nichols & Zax, 1977; van der Hart & Brown, 1992). So too, various techniques help clients shift *away* from emotions and memory when needed, such as grounding, relaxation, safe place visualization, hypnosis, breathing exercises, interpretation and reframing. The wide range of methods reinforces the idea that there are many different pathways to healing.

Clients Can Improve or Worsen in Past-Focused Treatment

Past-focused counseling in both the trauma and addiction fields can produce positive results, but it's important to also recognize the potential for clients to worsen. This has been observed for over a hundred years in the form of regression, self-harm, dropout, and increased substance use, for example (Chu, 1988; Jackson, 1994; Pitman et al., 1991; Solomon et al., 1992). In the 1920s, McDougal described clients who "have been put through their paces again and again [by counselors], i.e., have been made to live through the disturbing experience repeatedly . . . and have shown increase rather than relief of symptoms" (van der Hart & Brown, 1992, p. 132).

Some historical versions of past-focused treatment appear absurd and almost humorous if they weren't so tragic. Shorvon and Sargant "were so convinced of the importance of emotional expression that they would suggest false or exaggerated trauma scenarios [to clients] just to obtain more emotion" (van der Hart & Brown, 1992, p. 134). Nichols and Zax describe an example from implosive therapy: "As Stampfl hammers his clients with melodramatic descriptions of their greatest fears and most painful fantasies, they shudder in fear, cry out in anger, and dissolve in tears. Nor does he relent when patients beseech him to stop. Instead, he generates the scenes again and again, until the emotional outburst subsides" (Nichols & Zax, 1977, p. 163). In one study of a 4-week residential program, Lebanese war veterans with chronic PTSD were given intensive exposure to military cues, including "living in tents, wearing uniforms, weapons, artillery, and hand to hand combat training" (Solomon & Johnson, 2002, p. 950). Results showed significant worsening among the treated veterans compared to an untreated control condition. So, too, addiction treatment has used numerous harsh methods such as forcing clients to wear diapers if they felt sorry for themselves (White & Kleber, 2008)—essentially negating the past, rather than addressing it.

Worsening during past-focused work is more likely to happen if counselors:

- Pressure clients into it, beyond just encouragement and support
- Leave clients in a high state of distress at the end of the session
- Don't plan for what clients should do for crises between sessions, such as suicidality
- Engage in the work when there isn't enough time to complete it (e.g., a drop-in group that clients may not return to)
- Let clients remain in states that may not be productive or safe, such as severe dissociation or rage
- Don't manage group dynamics, such as triggering or scapegoating in group modality
- Don't evaluate clients for a history of abuse or violence toward others

Past-focused counseling has great potential to help, but safeguards are needed. The goal is balanced awareness of both its positive and negative potential, being neither overly afraid nor overly oblivious to such impact and moving in stepwise fashion. By staying flexible and adjusting as needed, it can be life-changing work.

We Don't Know Why Past-Focused Models Work

There are many theories on why past-focused models work, and these vary by orientation. Theories have included, for example, *learning theory* (Stampfl & Levis, 1967); *bilateral processing* (Shapiro, 1995); *emotional processing theory* (Foa & Rothbaum, 1998); *constructivist self-development theory* (McCann & Pearlman, 1990); *discharge of pent-up emotion (the hydraulic model)* (Jackson, 1994); *insight* (Bemak & Young, 1998); *dissociation–integration* (van der Hart & Brown, 1992); *schema theory* (Gray, Maguen, & Litz, 2007); *interpersonal processes* (e.g., Klein, 1949, in van der Hart & Brown, 1992); and *habituation/extinction* (Maples-Keller & Rauch, 2020). The bottom line is that we still don't know why past-focused models work.

Clinical Experience Has Much to Teach

Yet across the many models of past-focused treatment, there are numerous clinical insights. No one model has everything so reading broadly is useful. Moreno observes that "life happens too fast or too slow, too much or too little," so when exploring the past, the client can be guided to speed up or slow down to attain a desired level of emotion (Bemak & Young, 1998, p. 176). Shapiro (1995) identifies that working on the worst trauma also helps heal other traumas even if they aren't directly discussed. Ross and Gahan (1988) indicate that after intense emotional expression, debriefing is needed to promote reassurance and meaningful understanding. Resick, Monson, and Chard (2008) suggest noticing what the client leaves out of the story as well as what's included. Back, Dansky, Carroll, Foa, and Brady (2001) find that at least three past-focused sessions are necessary to produce therapeutic effect. Frank notes that interventions during clients' peak emotional arousal are less effective than those as emotion subsides (Bemak & Young, 1998). Herman emphasizes that the counselor's stance can never be neutral regarding trauma but must convey empathy for injustice (Herman, 1992, 2023).

Lessons of the Past Tend to Be Forgotten

For past-focused treatment, lessons of each era keep getting "discovered" in the next era as if brand new. As the saying goes, "What we learn from history is that we do not learn from history." In the military, past-focused trauma therapies emerge strongly during major wars but fade away in peacetime (Jackson, 1994). There's even regression sometimes: Trauma therapies were more advanced after World War I than World War II (van der Hart & Brown, 1992). So too, the diagnosis of PTSD comes and goes. In 1952, DSM-I had *gross stress reaction*, a precursor of PTSD, based on observation of World War II soldiers and concentration camp survivors. It was absent from the DSM-II in 1968, but then returned in DSM-III in 1980 as *PTSD* in response to advocacy by Vietnam veterans (Andreasen, 2011; Crocq & Crocq, 2000).

Stage-based trauma recovery originated with Janet in the 19th century (van der Hart et al., 1989) but was mostly forgotten until the 1980s and 1990s, when very similar stage-based frameworks emerged, such as the well-known three-stage model of Herman (1992); the four-stage model of Parson (1984); and the five-stage model of van der Kolk, van der Hart, and Burbridge (1995).

Treatment manuals typically don't describe their origins in earlier works. Current past-focused trauma models have elements of Wolpe's *systematic desensitization* from the 1960s, a form of behavior therapy and, even earlier, psychodynamic catharsis therapies. *Catharsis* in particular is almost never mentioned in trauma exposure CBT models despite its strong overlap with them. Theoretical orientations often position themselves as reactions to each other and strive to separate from, rather than acknowledge, the past.

Most ironic is that each era discovers that it is rediscovering the past. Kardiner noted the problem of historical forgetting in his 1941 book on trauma (Kardiner, 1941). It was observed again by Nichols and Zax in 1977, who do not cite Kardiner, and then again by Herman in 1992, who cites Kardiner but not Nichols and Zax. Herman notes, "Repeatedly in the last century, similar lines of inquiry have been taken up and abruptly abandoned, only to be rediscovered much later. Classic documents of fifty or one hundred years ago often read like contemporary works. Though the field has in fact an abundant and rich tradition, it has been periodically forgotten and must be periodically reclaimed" (1992, p. 7). Herman observes that this historical forgetting mirrors clients' own psychological splits about remembering trauma.

In the addiction field too, some important learning is forgotten over time. Cocaine was viewed as a safe drug in the early 1980s without awareness of the tragic cocaine epidemic of the late 19th century (Das, 1993). Various addiction treatment models have also come and gone for over 150 years, largely without reference to each other (White, 1998). The Washingtonians, for example, were a major national addiction recovery self-help movement begun by six alcoholics in 1840 to promote abstinence and mutual support. It died out so completely by the late 19th century that two alcoholics, Bill W. and Dr. Bob, founded AA in 1935 with the same goals—without any knowledge of the Washingtonians.

Terms Can Be Unclear

Another challenge in the literature on past-focused treatment is that terms shift or are ill-defined. Sometimes the same term is used for different phenomena, which we might call "same word, different thing." For example, *catharsis* can mean just emotional venting (*abreaction*). At other times, it means deep processing ("purgation or purification; and rebirth or initiation into a new state"; Nichols & Zax, 1977, p. 2). Even more broadly, it refers to an entire five-stage trauma recovery model (Steele, 1989). The terms *addiction*, *alcoholism*, *chemical dependency*, and *substance misuse* are all widely used, but there is no agreed-on definition and none have ever been in the DSM.

The opposite problem is when different terms refer to the same phenomenon: "different word, same thing." PTSD has had many names over time, most in relation to war: *soldier's heart* in the American Civil War, *shell shock* in World War I; and also *combat neurosis, combat fatigue, war hysteria, masculine hysteria*, and *nostalgia* (Crocq & Crocq, 2000; Weisaeth, 2002). Females who suffered child abuse in the Victorian era had *hysteria*. New terms also arise over time based on theoretical orientation. The psychodynamic word *catharsis* became the CBT word *exposure*, and *resistance* became *avoidance*, broadly speaking.

Terminology matters because words can evoke very different responses. For example, PTSD is a medical term that validates emotional pain from trauma, whereas earlier terms often signified personal weakness, such as *masculine hysteria* (Micale, 1989).

CO-OCCURRING TRAUMA AND ADDICTION: CHALLENGES AND PROGRESS

Creating Change also incorporates current understanding of how co-occurring trauma and addiction change treatment delivery. For clients with both issues, it's not just about *more* treatment, but at times *different* treatment adapted to the realities of the combination.

Challenges

Counselors perceive clients with addiction and trauma problems as more difficult to treat than those with either alone. Areas of particular difficulty are clients' self-destructiveness, dependency, and case management needs (Najavits, 2002b). They also have high treatment utilization (Najavits, Sullivan, Schmitz, Weiss, & Lee, 2004). Many counselors, in both mental health and addiction programs, don't feel adequately trained to treat them (Washton & Zweben, 2022).

Treatment systems are often split. Addiction treatment and mental health treatment have historically been separate, and clients with co-occurring problems may be rejected for being too severe in one domain or the other. Suicidal clients have been rejected from addiction treatment, for example, while severely addicted clients have been rejected from mental health treatment. Clients with both trauma and addiction can feel that they don't fit in anywhere—"[T]he two treatment bureaucracies compete to avoid them" (Treaster & Tabor, 1993, p. 18). Even in the current era, splits remain. Some programs still lack routine validated screening for both addiction and trauma problems. Old messages are still heard such as viewing methadone or other medication-assisted treatment as "substituting one addiction for another."

Approaches that work for trauma or addiction alone may not work as well when a client has both. Clients with both issues have more intense needs and less likelihood of success in treatment; thus, traditional treatment approaches may not work as well (Bailey, Trevillion, & Gilchrist, 2019; Najavits, 2022). For example, classic trauma treatment such as PE and CPT, when studied in PTSD/SUD samples, do not outperform SUD treatment alone (Foa et al., 2013; Simpson, Goldberg, et al., 2021; Somohano & Bowen, 2022), even on PTSD symptoms. Moreover, these classic trauma treatments have intensive, expensive provider training requirements (and are typically designed for individual modality), putting them out of reach for most addiction clients. Classic addiction models such as 12-step groups, RP, and MI are important yet don't address trauma directly, which represents a lost engagement opportunity for clients who also want trauma treatment (see Najavits, 2002c, on "leveraging one disorder to treat the other"). Even providing both trauma and addiction treatment in parallel has known pitfalls: the burden on clients to attend two programs, potential confusion on who holds accountability for clients' progress, and sometimes conflicting philosophies (Carruth & Burke, 2006).

Old-school beliefs persist. Some widely held views arose within the tradition of older types of treatment but no longer appear accurate when treating addiction and trauma together. Despite major progress, some of these myths endure.

- *Belief 1: "Clients have to reduce their addiction before starting any trauma work."* This has been a core belief for a long time and is still commonly heard. "Get sober first and then we'll address trauma." Yet there was good reason for this belief. Classic trauma treatment manuals for PE, CPT, and EMDR specified that they should *not* be used with addicted clients (Foa & Rothbaum, 1998, p. 110), especially severe ones (e.g., Resick et al., 2008, p. 3), or would need a period of abstinence first (e.g., Vogelmann-Sine, Sine, Smyth, & Popky, 1998, p. 8). There were reports of significant worsening when clients with active addiction explored their trauma narrative without adequate attention to how to adapt the trauma work (Pitman et al., 1991; Solomon et al., 1992). Now, after several decades of clinical insight and research, it's been shown that clients with active addiction *can* work on trauma at the same time—they don't have to reduce addiction first—but treatment needs to be done carefully so that it's sensitive to addiction. Examples include developing novel models to address addiction and trauma in ways that don't overwhelm clients (e.g., Seeking Safety, Creating Change); combining existing addiction and trauma models at the same time (e.g., Substance Dependence PTSD Therapy, COPE); conducting trauma models only in the context of intensive addiction treatment (Coffey et al., 2016; Perez-Dandieu & Tapia, 2014); and/or selecting less severe or complex SUD clients (Foa et al., 2013; Norman et al., 2019; Perez-Dandieu & Tapia, 2014; Sannibale et al., 2013).
- *Belief 2: "Addiction treatment is the 'real work.'"* The idea is that because addiction is so important, the focus should be solely that. One father questioned his daughter's addiction treatment. She had developed PTSD from a sexual assault at age 12, then turned to drugs. "The staff still treated the two illnesses separately, feeling that substance-free was far more important than all other issues—rather than wondering, 'What was so bad that would cause a 12-year-old girl to snort Vicodin?'" The current best practice is that if a client has both trauma and addiction, each should receive direct attention just as if the client had two medical issues, such as cancer and diabetes. There's also an important phenomenon to keep in mind: Trauma symptoms sometimes *worsen* with addiction recovery. Clients can be flooded with painful trauma memories and emotions once the addictive behavior no longer masks ("medicates") them. A client may have increased trauma nightmares when no longer drinking, for example.

- *Belief 3: "Trauma processing is the 'real work.'"* Some counselors view past-focused trauma work as the ultimate goal, with other aspects less important, such as coping skills, psychoeducation, case management, and addiction treatment. These are perceived as sometimes necessary but not the "real work" that drives lasting change. Many counselors aren't aware of research showing that both present- and past-focused models work—and of the weak results thus far for classic trauma models in the context of PTSD/SUD samples (Foa et al., 2013; Simpson et al., 2022; Somohano & Bowen, 2022).[7] Moreover, when clients are told that trauma processing is the key to recovery, they may feel pressured into it to please the counselor or believe they've failed if they can't do it. One counselor pushed a client who was 6 months sober to try Exposure Therapy. When she relapsed on alcohol after a few sessions, the counselor told her she wasn't "motivated enough." Although extreme, such damaging scenarios do occur. In short, there's no one right way to work on trauma. Past-focused models can help but so can present-focused ones. Many people recover without ever telling their story or focusing on the past.

- *Belief 4: "If clients want to talk about the past, they're ready to."* Some clients are highly motivated to explore their past and may want to move forward quickly. They may think that simply telling or "purging" their story will resolve it; or they underestimate what the work will bring up. The counselor needs to serve as gatekeeper and guide, pacing the work based on clients' current clinical presentation—not just on their wish to talk about the past. The extra topic "Recovery Strengths and Challenges" addresses these issues in more detail.

- *Belief 5: "The more intensity, the better."* Sometimes there's an assumption that the greater the emotional intensity in sessions, the better the outcome. This has intuitive appeal as intensity is sometimes associated with therapeutic breakthroughs. But intensity, in and of itself, doesn't predict a positive outcome. For example, a highly depressed client may cry a lot but doesn't necessarily improve. Freud famously distinguished *mourning* versus *melancholia* (the latter was the term for depression in his era). Mourning leads to growth; it's working through emotional pain in ways that lead to new insights and feelings of relief. In contrast, depression is a "stuck" place; it too can be emotionally intense but is ruminative—repetitively cycling over the same content without progress or relief. So, too, a client who's highly triggered experiences intensity over and over, but triggering per se doesn't lead to growth. See Chapter 3 for guidance (specifically the section "Working with Emotion"; see also the section "Watch for progress and worsening").

Progress

Despite the challenges, there have been major advances in treating addiction and trauma over the past several decades.

- *The development of trauma-informed care.* There's been a revolution in consciousness on the importance of trauma and its many ripple effects on the lives of individuals and society. It's worth remembering that for most of the 20th century the concepts of trauma and PTSD largely did not exist outside of war combat; that child abuse was initially interpreted as an intrapsychic experience (fantasy) rather than a tragic reality (van der Kolk, 2000); and that until recently, trauma was not considered a topic to address in addiction treatment.

---

[7] For example, CPT was not significantly better than RP on PTSD, and performed worse on SUD (Simpson et al., 2022). COPE versus RP showed the same pattern (Ruglass et al., 2017). When CPT was added to Mindfulness-Based Relapse Prevention—Trauma-Integrated (MBRP-TI), it had worse outcomes than MBRP alone (Somohano & Bowen, 2022). PE did not outperform the SUD model BRENDA on either PTSD or SUD (Foa et al., 2013). See also van Dam et al. (2013) and Simpson et al. (2021).

◊ Attention to addiction. Where addiction was once considered untreatable and abandoned by most professional counselors, it's now much more prominent as an area of treatment and research. There's greater awareness of addiction as a public health problem; recognition of a broader range of addictions (e.g., gambling, internet, nicotine); and expanded study of the neuroscience of addiction.

◊ Treating both together. It used to be a radical idea to address trauma and addiction at the same time (*integrated treatment*). Clients were told they needed a year of addiction recovery before working on trauma, and counselors weren't trained to treat both. The past 20 years have seen a burst of new counseling approaches, resources, and research on treating them together. Addressing trauma from the start can also increase clients' motivation for addiction treatment as most want to work on both if they have both (Back et al., 2014; Najavits, 2011; Najavits et al., 2004). Counselors now perceive a strong need to address both together as well (Nass, van Rens, & Dijkstra, 2019).

◊ Greater empathy. The counselor role is now more client-centered—less authoritarian, more collaborative and empowering. Old harsh confrontation methods in addiction treatment—"break 'em down to build 'em up"—are no longer acceptable, such as yelling profanities, having the client wear a dunce cap or clean the floor with a toothbrush to learn humility (White & Kleber, 2008). Attention to trauma has also led to improvements in mental health treatment, including decreased use of isolation and restraints in mental hospitals, and more careful boundaries in terms of counselor self-disclosure.

◊ Assessment. In the past, clients weren't routinely screened for addiction and trauma. This was sometimes due to lack of training or lack of access to validated measures. But it also stemmed from the view humorously stated by Shem (1978), "If you don't take a temperature, you don't have a fever" (if you identify a problem, then you have to do something about it). Now it's become the standard of care to routinely assess all clients at intake (Substance Abuse and Mental Health Services Administration [SAMHSA], 2014).

◊ Cross-training. Formerly, trauma was seen as outside the scope of practice for addiction counselors. So too, most mental health counselors believed they weren't qualified to address addiction (Washton & Zweben, 2022). The concept of cross-training arose with the focus on co-occurring disorders that began in the 1990s.

◊ Research. Research has uncovered some surprising findings. For example:
- Trauma problems improve more quickly than addiction (Najavits et al., 2020).
- Some addiction treatment models have shown a positive impact on PTSD (not just addiction) in research studies (Simpson et al., 2021).
- Clients with trauma and addiction are just as likely to attend 12-step groups as those with addiction alone, contrary to earlier speculation (Ouimette & Read, 2014).
- Counselors perceive those with addiction and trauma as more gratifying to treat than difficult (Najavits, 2002b).
- Counselors in recovery from addiction don't produce better outcomes than those not in recovery (McLellan, Woody, Luborsky, & Goehl, 1988).

In general, there's now a substantial body of knowledge on addiction and trauma, including rates, outcomes, assessment, and neuroscientific aspects.

◊ Hope. Clients with trauma and addiction often give up on themselves, and families and even treatment programs have sometimes viewed them as unlikely to get better. With new treatment options and a stronger sense of best practices, there's now greater optimism that clients can improve. The field has moved beyond previous all-or-none messages: that clients can't tolerate working on both addiction and trauma, or that there's only one way to do it. Having options builds hope, which is crucial as client needs are often great and resources often low.

THE FUTURE

Although past-focused methods have existed for a very long time, research on them is quite recent. Many questions remain: Do some clients benefit more than others? What aspects of models produce the greatest benefit? Should present- and past-focused models be combined and if so, how? As Bemak and Young wrote, "The debate about the role of catharsis, or emotionally arousing and expressive methods . . . has been described as one of the longest-running debates in the social sciences" (1998, p. 166). Creating Change offers a new perspective on this dialogue across time.

3

How to Conduct Creating Change

This chapter describes Creating Change implementation. Next, Chapter 4 identifies skills for a counselor to be effective with it (and personal characteristics that are helpful). The rest of the book consists of the 23 treatment topics.

Creating Change is easy to learn and conduct. This doesn't mean clients' recovery is easy; it rarely is. But the model itself is straightforward. It typically takes just a few sessions for counselors to feel comfortable with the format and, if you already know Seeking Safety, many elements will be familiar.

The content will likely come naturally, too. Many counselors say it provides, in an organized way, ideas that align with what they're already doing. Each Creating Change topic is a skill that helps clients face the past and, like any skill building, some clients will learn more quickly, some more slowly. Some topics may appeal more, some less. But on the whole, the program addresses the past in a gentle, paced way that allows clients to open up as they choose to, and thus is designed to minimize their feeling overwhelmed while also bringing to light experiences and pain that need attention.

This chapter has the following sections:

- Trying it out
- Key implementation questions
- Conducting the treatment
- Working with emotion
- Implementation decisions: modality, setting, and clients
- Conducting Creating Change with other models
- Detailed guide to the session format
- Materials to use across sessions

Each treatment topic also provides specific guidance on how to conduct that particular topic

Trying It Out

You can skim this chapter and some of the treatment topics to get a feel for them, then return here for more detail on how to conduct sessions. After that, try out a session. Some suggestions:

- Start with topics that most appeal to you.
- If you conduct both individual and group treatment, begin with an individual client and then expand to group.
- You can use just the handouts for a few sessions, and then add in the format.

- Role-play a session with a colleague.
- Visit *www.creating-change.org* for training options, to ask questions, or to send feedback. (*Note:* Training is optional unless you're conducting research.)
- See Chapter 4 for more on the counselor role.

Most of all, make it your own—honor your strengths as a counselor and your personal learning style. The key is to get started, to "dip a toe in the water." It's a straightforward model to learn and you'll keep discovering more as you go.

Key Implementation Questions

Who can conduct Creating Change? Any provider can conduct this model, including professionals and peer support workers from any background, training, and theoretical orientation. Most important are an interest in the work and capacity to relate to clients with compassion. Creating Change aims to make the most of your existing expertise, whatever that is, and expand on it. In some settings, counselors haven't yet tried past-focused treatment; in others, they already do it but without a formal model. Some have experience with trauma models but not addiction models or vice versa. The term *counselor* is used throughout the book as it's a standard term in many settings, but any other term can be used if preferred (*facilitator, therapist, provider, treater, clinician, peer support worker*). See also Chapter 4, "The Counselor."

Can it be done in groups? Yes. Creating Change was designed for individual or group modality. Groups can be open (clients start at different times) or closed (all start at the same time). Groups can have one leader or co-leaders if desired. For more on group implementation, see the section "Consider the Modality: Individual and/or Group" later in this chapter.

Must clients have current addiction/trauma problems? No. Some may have current active addiction or trauma issues; others may have a history of one or both; and still others may want to explore their past in general without focusing on prior trauma or addiction. You can guide them to apply the treatment topics to whatever they want to address, whether their problems are past, present, or both. Creating Change is for a broad array of clients, even within the same group if you're conducting groups.

Do clients need to be abstinent from substances? Creating Change is for clients at any stage of recovery, including those still using substances—but this will depend on your comfort level, client preferences, and setting. Also, as with most addiction treatment, clients can't be intoxicated at the time of the session. If they show up under the influence, ensure that they have a safe way to return home or are monitored by staff. However, there may be exceptions, such as clients on prescription opioids or marijuana for legitimate physical health conditions, assuming this doesn't impact their ability to participate.

Do clients have to focus on a particular trauma? No. The goal is to help clients with any painful events from the past that remain a problem for them, including addiction-related losses and harm. At each session, they can explore any experience that relates to the session topic. Clients typically have complex histories with many adverse events; narrowing the focus to just one event for most of the treatment is less likely to be successful than allowing exploration across events, based on client and counselor judgment. Also, each topic is a skill to work on, so the overall philosophy is that they're learning *how* to emotionally heal from difficult events, which will serve them now and in the future.

How about other mental health issues? Many clients have additional mental health problems as well as family, social, legal, or financial concerns. You can use the extra topic "Recovery Strengths and Challenges" to identify and address these at any point in treatment. The main consideration is to ensure that clients receive referrals as needed and that major conditions are monitored. Clients can also apply the Creating Change skills to any other issues in their life.

How long are sessions? Individual sessions are usually 50 minutes or an hour though some counselors do 45 minutes. Group sessions are typically 1 to 1.5 hours, depending on the setting and number of clients. Try to ensure enough time to conduct the session format and address the topic with sufficient depth. Plan time for check-in (typically, 2–3 minutes per client) and check-out (1–2 minutes per client). You can also conduct a topic over multiple sessions as each topic offers a lot of material to work with.

Should topics be done in order? You can do them in any order as each is independent of the others. However, the topics "Introduction" and "Create Change" are recommended first as they provide a foundation. Some topics are potentially more intense than others so you might choose to do them later (e.g., "Deepen Your Story"). You don't have to do all of the topics; use your clinical judgment as to what will work best for your clients. Finally, "Growth" is typically last as it's a summary of how far clients have come in treatment.

How long is the treatment? The treatment can be as long or short as you want—there's no requirement for a particular number of sessions or topics to be completed. But in general, the more the better, according to research, especially for addiction and more severe clients (American Psychological Association [APA], 2017; National Institute on Drug Abuse [NIDA], 2018). Longer treatment also promotes deepening of the work although clients can benefit from even a few sessions to let them experience what it's like.

Should clients attend other treatments? Creating Change can be used as a stand-alone treatment but more commonly is one of many treatments clients receive. Some topics in the book directly address supportive resources and referrals. In general, the idea is to strongly encourage, but not require, additional treatments (but if your agency has mandatory policies, it's important to respect those, such as AA attendance).

Do clients get dismissed for substance use or other addictive behavior? Addiction is a chronic, relapsing disorder for many clients so it's not usually helpful to remove them from treatment when their illness worsens. However, this will depend on your setting. Also, any significant worsening requires careful thought and, in some cases, redirection of treatment. See the later section "Watch for Progress and Worsening" for more on this.

How do you engage clients in work like this that may be a "downer"? The topic "Introduction" addresses this in more detail, but the gist is that Creating Change also focuses on *positive* aspects of the past, such as clients' strength and resilience and noticing people who were supportive along the way—experiences that can be just as important as painful ones. Also, clients learn that they decide what to reveal and when; they're never pushed; and the treatment topics are written to be highly compassionate, each offering a poignant theme that brings to light areas that need healing. Ultimately, the reason to focus on the past is to bring forth a better future.

Can I adapt the treatment? Definitely—the treatment is designed for adaptation. Use language and examples relevant to your clients. Choose topics and handouts that appeal to you. Decide how long the sessions will be. All of these are examples of adaptations "within the model," meaning that they're consistent with the flexibility of Creating Change. However, some counselors, even before trying it out, attempt adaptation "outside the model," such as changing the format or removing materials. In general, try the model as is and see how your clients respond. You can obtain their feedback from the session check-out, as well as the End-of-Session Questionnaire and Creating Change Feedback Questionnaire.

What if clients can't read? You can still do Creating Change with them. Although there are many handouts, the concepts are straightforward. Each topic has a main theme that's summarized in the title, such as "Break the Silence," "Tell Your Story," "Honor Your Survival," and "Emotions and Healing." Clients who can't read quickly can still get the main idea and talk about it. You can also use various methods to go over the material such as a brief summary of main points or, in group counseling, having other clients read short segments aloud.

Can I use Seeking Safety with Creating Change? Yes, the models are highly convergent. Their format, style, and flexibility are the same, but one focuses on the present while the other focuses on the past. For more on Seeking Safety, see *www.seekingsafety.org*. See the section below, "Conducting Creating Change with Other Models."

Is there an attendance requirement? Clients with trauma and addiction often have unstable lives that prevent consistent attendance. Thus, it's suggested not to have an attendance requirement for Creating Change, but rather to welcome clients back even if they miss sessions. The Certificate of Achievement at the end of this chapter offers a positive way to reinforce attendance. Clients highly value the certificate and, for court-involved clients, it serves as proof of treatment accomplishment. Let them know on the front end how many sessions are needed to earn it.

What assessments are recommended? There's no one set of measures as it depends on your goals. Assessment serves various purposes such as screening, verifying diagnoses, tracking progress, and evaluating functioning. Search online for reputable assessments. One nonprofit site, for example, offers free, valid, anonymous measures that clients can take online: *https://screening.mentalhealthamerica.net/screening-tools*. There are also several assessments specific to Creating Change, which are covered later in this chapter.

When is a client ready for this treatment? Many clients can try Creating Change and within a few sessions it'll be clear whether it's a good fit (see the paragraph on the next page, "Use a three-session try-out"). There are no automatic exclusions for particular types of clients. With its gentle approach to the past, clients share and explore only what they feel ready for and thus can do the work at their own pace. But if you have concerns about a client, try any of the three optional extra topics at the end of the book. Also, see the section on page 43 about different assessment instruments that are useful for ensuring clients get the most out of Creating Change.

Note that in the outpatient RCT of Creating Change all clients were complex: They had current active substance use disorder and PTSD, typically severe and chronic, and other diagnoses as well. Yet there were no safety concerns and there was significant reduction in both substance use and PTSD as well as other variables by the end of the study (Najavits et al., 2018). Moreover, the study didn't exclude clients for additional complex issues (suicidality, self-harm, personality disorder, drug use disorder, homelessness, recent substance use, or severe dissociation). It did, however, exclude clients with current mania or psychosis, or who had seriously assaulted someone in the prior 6 months. As you implement Creating Change, use your judgment and consult with colleagues as needed. For example, if a client has a severe current crisis, that would typically be addressed first.

Conducting the Treatment
THE SESSION FORMAT

Creating Change sessions have four elements, and they are the same for both individual and group treatment. For anyone already familiar with Seeking Safety, the format is the same.

1. **Check-in** *(clients briefly share how they're doing)*
2. **Quotation** *(inspiration for emotional engagement)*
3. **Handouts** *(one of the 23 treatment topics, each offering a different way to explore the past)*
4. **Check-out** *(end the session in a positive way)*

Optional: You can do a few minutes of grounding at the end of the session if desired, either before or after check-out, but this is not a formal part of the session.

The structure promotes good use of time and a safe atmosphere so clients can explore what's most important to them. In group, it also creates balanced sharing. At a deeper level, the format reinforces planning, pacing, and consistency, which help counteract the impulsivity and instability of trauma and addiction.

Counselors typically find that it takes only a few sessions to feel comfortable with the format. If after trying it for a while you want to change the format, obtain clients' feedback before doing so, as they may have useful insights on how it feels to them.

> TIP: See the "Detailed Guide to the Session Format" later in this chapter. There's also a one-page summary at the end of the chapter to keep in front of you during the session as a reminder.

STARTING OUT

As you begin, consider the following ideas for conducting the Creating Change sessions.

Encourage Clients to Try Out Creating Change

Past-focused treatments show long-standing concerns about dropout and engagement (Becker et al., 2004; Najavits, 2015; Roberts et al., 2022). Thus, it's important to offer choices on the front end to help clients feel comfortable. They may have fears that they'll be pushed to reveal more than they want to or won't be able to tolerate the work. In Creating Change, the following strategies are useful:

Use a three-session try-out. This "try it before you buy it" approach lets them attend up to three sessions before deciding if they want to continue. They experience the model directly and you get a sense of how they respond. It also reduces their anxiety and avoidance as it's a toe-in-the-water approach rather than a full dive. You can use any Creating Change topics, including the extra topics, but for individual treatment, it's good to start with the topic "Introduction" so they get an overview of the work. For group treatment, they can either just observe or participate directly in whatever topic you have selected for that day. Interestingly, research indicates that by the third session of any counseling model, the level of alliance clients feel toward the treatment and toward you predicts how they'll feel later, so if it's not present early on, the client may be better suited to a different treatment type or counselor. To assess alliance, you can use the free, brief, validated Agnew Relationship Measure in the extra topic "Your Relationships" (there's both a counselor and client version). The End-of-Session Questionnaire later in this chapter is also helpful even though it's not an alliance scale per se. After the three-session try-out, if the model isn't a good fit, help the client view it as a positive decision based on self-care rather than dropping out or failure. *Note:* There's a flyer at the end of this chapter for the three-session try-out that you can post in your waiting room or send out electronically.

Conduct blocks of sessions for group treatment, such as 4, 8, or 12 sessions. The idea is that at the end of each block clients can decide if they want to continue to the next one. Blocks can work for open or closed groups. In open groups, you can either have clients join only at the start of a new block or, if clients join part-way through, they would just have fewer sessions. The blocks concept is a bit like the three-session try-out described above, but for clients who are already a good fit for Creating Change.

Let clients go through the treatment more than once. Some clients like to do more than one round, which allows them to pace their degree of disclosure as they feel more comfortable with the work. They also absorb different aspects each time. The same exercise takes on new meaning when done again and allows them to explore additional past events.

Use the Extra Topics as Needed

There are three extra topics to strengthen clients' capacity for the work. Any of them can be done at the start of treatment or along the way as the need arises.

- "Understanding Trauma and Addiction"
- "Recovery Strengths and Challenges"
- "Your Relationships"

These were originally conducted with all clients, but we found that many didn't need them so they're now optional. In individual treatment, you may want to invite the client's safe family members or friend to attend one or more of these sessions to build support. In group treatment, you can do them either as individual extra sessions for specific clients or have everyone do the topic(s) together.

Identify Who's Not a Good Fit

Many clients are fine to just start on Creating Change per the paragraph on page 40, "When is a client ready for this treatment?" But if you have concerns, conduct the extra topic "Recovery Strengths and Challenges," which provides a detailed assessment to identify aspects that may need to be resolved on the front end. For example, a client who has current dissociative identity disorder, is in a major abusive relationship, or is currently psychotic or manic would need attention to those problems first. But, in general, it's important not to make assumptions that clients need to fit a particular profile before beginning, such as a certain length of abstinence or a low level of trauma symptoms. How helpful Creating Change will be depends on a unique blend of client, counselor, and setting. The same client may be able to do Creating Change in a residential program but may be unsuited to it in an outpatient setting or vice versa. If clients are interested in Creating Change, it's usually best to let them try the model briefly to see if they like it (see the section on page 41, "Encourage Clients to Try Out Creating Change"). They can typically join Creating Change even if they have active substance use or other addictions (as long as they're not intoxicated during the session), and even if they have some level of self-harm, personality problems, or other mental health issues.

Communicate Your Policies

Clients have a more positive treatment experience if they know policies in advance, such as attendance requirements, whom to contact in an emergency, and whether they'll be dismissed for substance use. They also have a deep need for policies that are fair and enforced equally across clients. Unfortunately, policies are sometimes unclear or inconsistent. For example, one client is dismissed from the program for using substances, yet another is not. Or there's a treatment contract but when the client violates it, the consequences aren't enforced. For clients with trauma and addiction, who often grew up with significant neglect or unfairness, such inconsistencies may have a negative impact on their treatment. Whatever your policies, a good place to cover them is in the topic "Introduction."

Refer Clients to Additional Treatment

Clients with addiction and trauma problems often have multiple needs and benefit from multiple services. Refer clients to as many additional services as they're willing to attend. It's also helpful to provide referrals for the clients' family members, when appropriate. For additional guidance on case management, you may want to use the Seeking Safety topic "Introduction to Treatment/Case Management," which addresses 16 referral domains, with suggestions on how to engage clients in them (e.g., psychiatric medication, self-help groups, intensive outpatient, job counseling, and public assistance). Whatever method you use, begin early and monitor throughout. Creating Change can be delivered alongside any other treatments, and the more the better. In particular, it's highly recommended to encourage 12-step groups such as AA as they are effective, low-cost, and widely available (Kelly, Abry, Ferri, & Humphreys, 2020). However, keep in mind that 12-step groups do not address trauma per se, and that there are also nonspiritual alternatives such as SMART Recovery, Refuge Recovery, and Women for Sobriety.

Consider Using Creating Change Measures

You may want to use these optional measures that are specific to Creating Change:

- *Creating Change Feedback Questionnaire* (Handout 4 in the topic "Growth"), which obtains clients' views of the treatment
- *Creating Change Fidelity Scale* (Najavits, 2007), freely downloadable at *www.creating-change.org*, to identify whether key elements of the treatment are being done

See also the list of recommended measures (in the section "Materials to Use across Sessions" on pages 64–65).

Consider Inviting the Client's Safe Supports (e.g., Family or Friends) to Specific Sessions

Safe supports are defined as close contacts who are not currently harming the client emotionally or physically, and do not have a major active addiction; they may be a partner, family, friends, an AA sponsor, or advocate. It can be helpful to invite them to one or two sessions. This can boost support of the client by increasing their understanding of trauma and addiction recovery, as well as offering referrals, if needed, as some have their own struggles with these issues. Meeting with them also gives you greater insight into the client, and—strongly recommended—you can share your contact information in case they become concerned about the person. (For two-way communication between you and them, obtain a release of information from the client, but it's also good to inform them that one-way communication from them to you is legally allowed at any time without a release, such as an email or voicemail update from them.)

Creating Change topics that are especially relevant for the client's safe supports are the extra topic "Understanding Trauma and Addiction," which includes an educational handout (Tip Sheet to Support the Client), and the topic "What You Want People to Understand." Both have specific suggestions for how to involve safe supports. However, you could invite them in for any topic, as long as the client is on board with that and you discuss in advance the goals for including them. Also make clear to everyone that the sessions are not family therapy (that would be a separate referral). Inviting others usually occurs in individual treatment, but the extra topic "Understanding Trauma and Addiction" can be done as a multifamily group.

For more, see Appendix A, "How Others Can Help—Family, Friends, Partners, Sponsors, Counselors," in the book *Finding Your Best Self* (Najavits, 2019); it offers detailed guidance written directly for clients' safe supports. Also, the Seeking Safety topic "Getting Others to Support Your Recovery" has extensive information on how to involve them in counseling sessions.

Establish Emergency Procedures

Most clients, even severe ones, can do this treatment without problems, but for any treatment model, past-focused or not, it's essential for clients to know what to do in an emergency (such as suicidal or violent intent and plan, substance relapse, or major increase in psychiatric symptoms). The following topics can help:

- "Introduction." Handout 2 includes a **written emergency plan** to fill out for each client.
- "Trust versus Doubt." Handout 2 is an extensive **list of helplines, including crisis lines**, for immediate support (all national, free, and reputable).
- The extra topic "Recovery Strengths and Challenges." Handout 3 offers a **mental health advance directive** for clients to specify their preferences when in a psychiatric emergency.

In addition, offer information on local resources such as a hospital emergency room, answering service, or on-call staff member.

Beyond the practical details, the counselor's *style* in responding to an emergency is key: being kind, professional, and appropriately reactive—neither too much nor too little. One client states it beautifully: She wants someone who "understands the coping role of suicidal thoughts, as a relief, an end to the pain, as giving a sense of some control . . . who knows the difference between 'I want to die' and 'I want to kill myself' . . . who will understand and control and prevent me from hurting myself when I am in danger, but still give me options and choices, and respect me" (Jennings & Ralph, 1997, p. 19). The same applies to any emergency situation.

DURING THE SESSION

Let Clients Choose the Session Topic (If Desired)

If you're just starting out with Creating Change, it's best for you to choose the session topic so you can read through it in advance. But once you feel familiar with the model, you may decide to let clients choose as some enjoy doing that. In Chapter 1, there's a list of all the Creating Change topics with brief descriptions. You can give the list at the start of each session to choose from or, at any point, ask which topics the client wants to prioritize. In group treatment, you can do a rating (zero to five stars) and go with what gets the highest rating, or clients can take turns choosing the next topic. Often, however, clients don't have a preference and that's fine, too; you don't have to press for it. The list can also help you keep track of which topics you've covered, especially if you're not doing them in order.

Help Clients Link Trauma and Addiction If They Have Both

As stated earlier, clients don't have to have both trauma and addiction to participate in Creating Change. It can be used either alone or even as a general model for helping clients face the past. If clients do have both, however, help them link the two as they often don't make those connections. Ask questions ("Looking back, did trauma impact your addiction?"). Generate timelines ("Which came first?"). Offer support ("It's common to feel that way if you had both trauma and addiction"). But also recognize that addiction doesn't always relate to trauma—people use substances for all sorts of reasons. They may have a family history of addiction with a heavy genetic loading for it.

Culture, peers, media, personality, and other influences play a role, too. Linking trauma and addiction may be part of the story but is often not the whole story.

Guide Clients to Grieve Addiction, Not Just Trauma

It comes naturally to most people to understand the need to grieve trauma. But addiction also has much that needs to be grieved:

- Lost time and opportunities
- Harm or neglect of others as part of addiction
- The pain of giving up the behavior
- Anger at people who perpetuated the addiction
- Damage to one's body and mind
- Regrets and shame about behavior during active addiction
- Distress about consequences (e.g., homelessness, estrangement from family, incarceration)

Validate the many aspects that may still hold pain.

Consider Doing a Few Minutes of Grounding at the End of the Session

It's nice to end the session with 3 to 4 minutes of grounding if you have the time (either before or after the check-out). This also reinforces grounding as a key skill clients can use outside of sessions when upset. Try methods that clients know work for them or ones you select. In group treatment, you could have a list of grounding techniques and take turns each session to have a different client read it aloud to the others. If grounding is not familiar to you, download the free SAMHSA resource *Trauma-Informed Care in Behavioral Health Services* (2014, p. 98). The Seeking Safety topic "Detaching from Emotional Pain (Grounding)" also has extensive education on grounding, including a grounding script to read aloud.

Empower Clients

Strive to increase clients' sense of power and choice, which are so eroded in trauma and addiction. Offer options ("Which handout appeals to you?"); ask permission ("Can we talk more about that?"); seek feedback ("Was that role-play helpful?"); and encourage clients to notice what feels right for them ("Do you want to share or prefer not to?"). Empowering approaches are important in any treatment, but all the more so in the context of trauma and addiction. In trauma, clients had to endure unwanted events that they were powerless to stop. In addiction, clients are powerless over their own behavior. Empowerment doesn't mean, however, tolerating anything clients do, letting them "walk all over you," or agreeing with everything. Equally important is accountability—conveying that they're responsible for acting in safe, respectful, healthy ways.

Increase Engagement

Some clients have low engagement in treatment, which may happen if they're mandated to treatment or just have limited motivation generally. It isn't specific to Creating Change, but some aspects of the model can increase participation. First, use active exercises rather than just discussion. There are many exercises in the handouts and some are highly visual (e.g., the tree exercise in the topic "Influences," and the door exercise in the topic "Your Personal Truth"). You can enhance these by offering colored pens or other art supplies to let clients express themselves in nonverbal ways. The commitments (homework) at the end of each topic also include nonverbal options. Second, help clients notice whether their low motivation may have roots in trauma; for more on that, see Chapter 4, specifically the section "Gently Interpret Negative Dynamics in Light of Trauma (When Possible)."

Emphasize *Self-Protection* Rather Than *Avoidance*

Past-focused models typically encourage clients to explore the trauma story in detail; thus "avoiding" it is seen as perpetuating trauma symptoms (Resick et al., 2008). However, such models weren't developed for clients with co-occurring addiction (Najavits et al., 2020). Creating Change takes the approach that rather than calling it *avoidance* (which sounds negative) it's *self-protection*, which may be *healthy* or *unhealthy* depending on the context. Saying "no" to a drug, for example, is *healthy self-protection*; it's the wisdom to stay away from unsafe people and situations. Staying isolated in the house, in contrast, is *unhealthy self-protection*; it's stuck and closed. Sterman emphasizes that clients with trauma and addiction need breaks from their painful history. "It's useful to visualize recovery of addicted [trauma] survivors . . . as a perpetual staircase, rather than an uninterrupted line. . . . In other words, in treatment these [clients] frequently need 'breaks' when their material is too overwhelming" (2006, p. 268). In short, help clients view "avoidance" as an attempt at self-protection, let them move in and out of it at times, and strive to increase their awareness of these patterns.

Adapt for Subgroups (Gender, Race/Ethnicity, Culture, Age, Spirituality, etc.)

It's important to address subgroup issues that clients bring to the work. Some may be adversities that clients are directly aware of, such as ageism, sexism, homophobia, racism, or anti-Semitism. Other aspects may be below the level of awareness; it's said that "culture is unconscious." Listen closely to how clients' beliefs help or impede recovery. For example, spiritual beliefs can be a source of support but can also become distorted ("God is punishing me for being bad"). The goal is to offer culturally relevant examples from clients' lives; language that resonates for them; and sensitivity to historical issues such as marginalization and intergenerational trauma and addiction. With adolescents, for example, you can go more slowly through the material and talk about subjects such as school, parents, and partying. Also, adolescents typically don't accept the term *addiction*; try substituting *problem behavior* or *excessive behavior*. So too, in terms of language, some trauma survivors don't like the term *recovery*; ask if *healing* or *growth* fits better. See also the topic "Influences: Family, Community, Culture" for more detail on culture, trauma, and addiction.

Be the Gatekeeper

It's the counselor's role to ensure that the work stays beneficial. A common misperception is that whatever the client wants to talk about should be talked about ("I don't interrupt because I want him to feel heard"). But sometimes it's important to steer clients toward some areas and away from others. If a client moves into untherapeutic emotion, such as dissociation or a panic attack, initiate grounding or other strategies to promote stability. During check-in and check-out, gentle interruptions are sometimes necessary to ensure that there's time for the main part of the session. Such gatekeeping moments can be done kindly yet clearly. For example:

- "Are you dissociating? How about if we try grounding to help you out of that?"
- "I know there's more to the story, but we have only 10 minutes left. Let's start shifting to check-out."

How to Conduct Creating Change

However, ensure that clients don't feel invalidated when you're redirecting them. Offer an explanation or else they may think you don't value their truth. "Let's hold off on that" can be containing and caring if done well or invalidating if done poorly.

Pace the Work

There's a common belief that if clients want to talk about the past, they can dive right in. As Nichols and Zax wrote, "Some therapists believe that individuals have built-in safety valves that keep them from becoming more emotionally aroused or venting more feelings than they can easily handle. . . . Unfortunately [this] is a dangerous half-truth" (Nichols & Zax, 1977, p. 226). The reality is that some clients underestimate what the work will bring up. Thus, a good principle is "slower is faster": Clients make more progress if pacing is slow and steady rather than immersion in too much too soon. For counselors familiar with traditional past-focused models, this may seem like reinforcement of avoidance. But for clients with both trauma and addiction, it's key to adjust the intensity ongoing. Each topic in Creating Change offers options to let you steer toward greater or lesser intensity, thus moving beyond the extremes of earlier treatment eras—the view that none of these clients should do past-focused work (they're too fragile) or all should immerse fully ("just do it").

Be Careful When Encouraging Social Support

Social support has a positive impact on mental health generally. Yet encouraging trauma and addiction clients to develop social networks sometimes backfires. Some clients repeat damaging patterns from the past, finding new people who hurt or abuse them. Others are too afraid to engage in new relationships. One study of highly disadvantaged women with trauma and co-occurring disorders found limited evidence for social support moderating their symptoms: "The results point to the need for using caution in relying on women's existing social support network to help them heal" (Savage & Russell, 2005, p. 199). For a while, the only safe people may be counselors or peer mentors. If clients have good supports, encourage them to use those. But for others, don't assume it's a primary option for now.

Convey That Focusing on the Past Is Broader Than Telling One's Story

Telling the story of trauma and addiction can help heal it. But there are also other aspects to consider. Telling the story disconnected from emotion has limited therapeutic value. Telling the story when not ready can be retraumatizing. Telling the story when it's been told—over and over—in prior therapies may have little impact unless other processes also occur (reframing, learning new ways to handle emotions, etc.). In Creating Change, clients can tell their story, but focusing on the past is broader than just the details of what happened. "Telling Your Story" is a Creating Change topic, but there are many others, too, each evoking a different part of clients' experience, a different skill—not just the narrative. A wide range of session topics also helps increase engagement

Watch for Progress and Worsening

Creating Change clinical implementation and research have consistently shown no safety concerns related to the model (e.g., Najavits & Johnson, 2014; Najavits et al., 2018). However, clients with trauma and addiction can be unstable due to the nature of their problems. Thus, "progress, not perfection" is the goal. They'll typically show some negative behavior during treatment so it's important not to convey too high a bar ("You need to be abstinent for a year, hold a job, and have no self-harm"). It's a balancing act and counselor judgment is key. A client in a long-term residential setting with minor self-cutting may be fine to continue the work. A client who's decreasing substance use with occasional slips is usually fine to continue. Stay flexible and watch for the impact of treatment. Seek supervision and more training if major dilemmas arise, if it's unclear whether treatment is helping, or if you feel stuck. Assessment with validated measures for trauma and/or addiction is also useful.

Notable worsening suggests the client may need additional or higher levels of care. Any serious destructive impulse or behavior by the client warrants evaluation, including the following:

- A plan and/or intent to act on suicidal or violent impulses
- Significant increase in self-harm such as cutting
- Major increase in addictive behavior and/or new addictive behaviors
- Important new risky behaviors such as driving while intoxicated
- Severe ongoing emotional distress that results in significant dysfunction (e.g., unable to care for a child)

You can also pace Creating Change as needed, such as alternating sessions of Creating Change and a present-focused model (e.g., Seeking Safety or RP). This is straightforward in both individual and group modality per the section "Conducting Creating Change with Other Models" on pages 57–59. But if the entire group is doing fine and just one client is worsening, you can have that client take a few sessions off and then return to group. Debrief the client and group, providing a supportive stance that conveys that there's no shame or failure in taking a break. Finally, although unlikely, if you discover that Creating Change itself is causing harm or the client wants to leave, offer suggestions and referrals just as you would for any other treatment.

Working with Emotion

Emotion is sometimes more intense in past-focused than present-focused treatment, but intensity per se is not a problem unless it translates into concerning behavior or a pervasive pattern (see the prior section "Watch for Progress and Worsening"). Here are some ideas on how to be effective with emotion in Creating Change sessions.

Educate Clients about Emotion

Clients often carry damaging messages about emotions, such as "Crying is weakness" or "Anger is the only way to be heard." Thus, they typically need education about a healthy approach to emotion. Key concepts include the following:

- You can learn to shift in and out of feelings.
- It's human to have anger, sadness, and fear.
- You may feel worse before you feel better.
- If you accept difficult feelings, they decrease over time.
- Exploring trauma and addiction doesn't mean staying stuck in those emotions.
- You can develop a positive approach to emotions.
- Others can tolerate your pain (e.g., in counseling).

You can also guide clients experientially during sessions to address emotions in a productive way. As van Dijk writes, the counselor "steers when the patient seems to avoid essential details, and . . .

slows the process down when the patient is at risk of getting overwhelmed by memories" (2003, p. 365). The topic "Emotions and Healing" offers additional education about emotion.

"Start Low and Go Slow"

Start low means encouraging clients to explore less upsetting events before more upsetting ones. If a client is less distressed about a hurricane she survived than about being molested as a child, it's best to start with the hurricane. *Go slow* means exploring small segments of the past at a time. These strategies let clients build success at their own pace.

Follow the Trail of Emotion

When working on the past, memory generally needs to connect with emotion for healing to occur (see Chapter 2 for more on this). Thus, every major model of past-focused treatment emphasizes helping the client get in touch with feelings. Watch for signs of strong emotion (teary eyes, quicker breathing, facial expressions, agitation) or lack of emotion (glassy-eyed, flat voice). Directly ask clients what they're feeling if it's unclear. Also check in at times on their level of distress: "How distressed do you feel right now, from 0 to 10 (0 = no distress and 10 = extreme distress)?" The goal is to ensure that the work is not a purely intellectual, dry experience. You can also guide them to think of an image, such as "Listen for the heartbeat" or "Follow the red line of emotion." Emotions are a trail to be followed.

Know That Clients Don't Need a High Level of Emotional Intensity

Releasing intense emotions can be therapeutic and will occur at times, but it's not the central goal. Sometimes clients will be sharing at lower levels of emotion, spending time absorbing new ideas, and reading through the handouts. As long as they generally face feelings about the past, progress will occur. Also, some clients have lower expression of emotion due to culture, gender, or personality (some clients cry, others don't). In short, emotional intensity is not something to strive for in and of itself. It's not a metric of how well the treatment is going and there's no attempt to keep clients in a highly emotional state for its own sake. It's also worth noting that in past-focused treatments generally, expressing strong feelings needs to be balanced with safety and support in the present. The client experiences feelings but also reflects on them (Moreno, 1964). The Creating Change commitments (homework) also vary in their emotional intensity.

Let Clients Work on Multiple Events

Most clients with trauma and addiction have survived numerous adverse events. One study found they had an average of nine lifetime traumas (Najavits et al., 2003). As clients talk about one part of the past, other memories will naturally arise. A client describes a combat scene and this reminds him of a beloved cousin dying from an accidental gunshot as a child. In Creating Change, clients don't have to stick with a particular event for a long time. If they have a complex history, they can't work on every difficult life event as there are simply too many. Learning what it feels like to open up about some of their experiences will generalize to others. As Chu states, the work "is likely to be a series of processes rather than a single cathartic event. It is the frequent expectation of patients that traumatic events can be . . . worked through in a brief and dramatic way. However, clinical experience suggests [otherwise]" (1992, p. 358). Yet it's also important to keep clients on track if they veer into superficial or unrelated topics, which can be a defense against facing emotional pain.

The counselor can gently guide them back ("You were talking about . . .") and offer feedback ("Do you notice you keep moving away from talking about that?").

Encourage Clients to Become Aware of Their Full Range of Feelings

Clients typically have some emotions that are more familiar or comfortable than others. Fear and guilt, for example, are more socially acceptable than rage or desire for revenge. The goal is to help clients recognize all their feelings (while also learning not to act impulsively on them). Many clients with trauma and addiction had to deny or suppress feelings to survive so being able to openly express their full range of feelings is liberating. Help clients notice what they're *not* feeling as well as what they are.

For some clients, accessing *positive* feelings such as tenderness and love is even harder than negative ones. As McCullough observed, "Each opening to tender feelings brings grief, because experiencing something wonderful for the first time carries the realization of all that was missed, as well as the fear that it may be lost in the future" (2003, p. 243).

Yet some clients can't access feelings even when encouraged to. One said, "When I start to feel, it's like a wall comes down. It's not intentional, it just happens." Some can tell their story but only coldly, without emotion. Emotional blocks typically occur when they've become numb from too much pain. As Herman notes, "The survivor's initial account of the event may be repetitious, stereotyped, and emotionless. In its 'untransformed state' it is more like a 'prenarrative.' It does not develop or progress in time, and it does not reveal the storyteller's feelings or interpretation of events. . . . [It is like] a series of still snapshots or a silent movie; the role of therapy is to provide the music and words" (1992, p. 175).

Each topic in Creating Change takes a different angle to help evoke emotional responses, such as the focus on cultural forces in "Influences: Family, Community, Culture"; the physical focus in "Listen to Your Body"; and the narrative focus in "Tell Your Story." The many experiential exercises also help clients access their inner experience.

Watch, too, for preferences you may have for some emotions over others. Based on your history, you may find some emotions easier to tolerate in yourself and clients. Notice especially emotions that are prominent when you're under stress; typically, people lean toward one of the core human emotions (fear, sadness, anger).

Bring Clients "Down" by the End of the Session

Focusing on the past involves *opening up* (talking about the past) and *closing down* (shifting back to the present and wrapping up the session). Stay aware of timing so that clients aren't left at a high level of painful feelings at the end of the session. They may still have some distress, but on a scale of 0 (no distress) to 10 (extreme distress), the goal is 5 (moderate) or below. It's good to ask them for their distress rating if it's unclear. If clients are in the midst of intense feelings toward the end of the session, you can add a few minutes of grounding. You can also gently interrupt clients as long as there's a rationale so they won't feel cut off ("I'm sorry to interrupt, but I want to make sure we have enough time to wrap up the session"). Reinforce that the material will be there to come back to in future sessions.

Help Clients Shift Out of Dissociation

A high level of dissociation prevents successful exploration of the past (Coffey et al., 2002) and, in general, it's not healthy for clients to stay "spaced out" and disconnected from the present environment. If a client dissociates during the session, it's helpful to ask what triggered it, such as a specific memory or feeling, to better understand if the client needs to work on those. But the immediate response to dissociation is usually grounding, helping the client shift out of dissociation so it can be discussed. However, if a client dissociates so much during treatment that it prevents working on the past, start with a present-focused approach first. So too, a small percentage of clients may have a diagnosis of *dissociative identity disorder* (a complex, severe level of dissociation). They can still potentially benefit from Creating Change but also need specialized treatment for that. See the International Society for the Study of Trauma and Dissociation website (*www.isst-d.org*) for more information.

Address Anger

Of all the emotions that arise in counseling, anger is one of the most challenging. A high level of client anger can be frightening no matter whom it's directed toward. If the client is angry with the counselor, even at a low level (irritation, annoyance), it can evoke defensiveness and withdrawal. Yet anger is crucial to address, as clients with addiction and trauma almost universally have some degree of unprocessed anger in light of their experiences. Some clients express *only* anger rather than softer feelings such as sadness, fear, and shame. They overlearned toughness to survive ("I'm never weak"). Other clients learned to hide their anger. They show vulnerable feelings but anger simmers below the surface. A major task of counseling is integration: helping clients learn to accept all emotions and shift between them with some level of control.

There are several misconceptions about anger in counseling. First is the view that clients need to vent their anger, such as by hitting pillows or yelling. This can actually *increase* it (Nichols & Zax, 1977). The current recommendation is to teach healthy versus unhealthy anger expression: Healthy anger is put into words rather than behavior. A second misconception is that "anger is OK and nothing to be afraid of." Yet some clients truly can't control destructive impulses. Ask them what they believe will happen if they get in touch with strong anger and take that into account along with their history of impulse control. Third, there's the idea that clients *must* express anger or they won't heal. But not all clients feel angry about their past or need to.

Stay reflective also about your own reactions to anger. Many counselors have experienced trauma, and being the recipient of anger can be triggering. If the client directs anger at you, try to honestly own your errors and perhaps apologize for them, but at no point should you be victimized by clients' anger. Seek supervision if this becomes an issue. Notice, too, whether you harbor unacknowledged anger toward some clients. Ignoring anger leads to negative effects such as the client feeling more anger (as the counselor can't), and a decline in honest interaction.

Implementation Decisions: Modality, Setting, and Clients

This section addresses the nuts-and-bolts of implementation to help you decide how you may want to start on Creating Change. There are many ways to incorporate the model, driven by your goals and setting. Here are a few examples.

Paul, clinical director of a large addiction treatment program. Paul values his counselors' skills but is concerned that some are conducting past-focused work without a manual, relying solely on intuition and life experience. He believes Creating Change may provide a more planned, structured approach. He begins staff training, encouraging counselors to try Creating Change in either their groups or individual sessions and to collect the End-of-Session Questionnaire to obtain clients' feedback. He makes a plan for the team to come together periodically to discuss how it's going.

Karin, outpatient trauma therapist in private practice. Karin is experienced with classic past-focused trauma models but only recently began to treat substance addiction; previously, she just referred clients out to AA. She's intrigued by the idea of doing combined trauma/addiction treatment and decides to try Creating Change with an individual client.

Sylvia, mental health counselor in a residential program. Sylvia has used Seeking Safety for several years with clients who have multiple mental health issues. She enjoys learning new approaches and wants to try Creating Change. She starts a group with seven clients who have completed Seeking Safety. She asks another counselor to join her as co-leader so they can discuss how it's going. They plan to do six sessions and then offer another six if it goes well.

Arturo, social work intern at a men's prison. Arturo heard about Seeking Safety and Creating Change and decides to learn both. He reads the manuals while also learning about trauma-informed care. He creates a plan with his supervisor to conduct Seeking Safety in group format and Creating Change in individual format, letting clients attend both if appropriate. He discusses his ongoing casework with his internship supervisor, building his sense of confidence in working with trauma and addiction, which are the two most common issues in his client population.

Consider the Modality: Individual and/or Group

Creating Change was designed for individual and/or group treatment. Individual allows more time per client and prevents challenges that can occur in any group, such as how to share time and clients potentially triggering each other. But group has many advantages, too, including the power of peer sharing that reduces shame and isolation and lowers cost. The majority of addiction treatment has always been provided in groups. Past-focused treatment per se has been conducted successfully in groups in both addiction and mental health settings for decades, including therapeutic communities, veterans' programs, inpatient programs, and women's center groups (Bemak & Young, 1998).

Suggestions for Groups

If Creating Change will be conducted in groups, consider the following.

Group size. Group size can fit whatever is standard in your program, but it's advisable to limit the number of clients so as to have more time per person. A large group will have a different feel than a smaller one—more educational as there's less time for everyone to speak—but is still doable. The number of clients will also depend on the length of the session, which, as stated earlier, typically ranges from 1 to 1.5 hours. Note that Creating Change offers more flexibility for groups than most past-focused models. For example, group PE in a major veterans study was limited to six clients (Schnurr, Friedman, Lavori, & Hsieh, 2001), and group CPT is done in closed groups (Chard, Resick, Monson, & Kattar, 2009).

One leader versus co-leaders. Creating Change is typically conducted by one leader, but if your program has co-leaders, they may choose to divide the tasks, such as having one leader focus on the session format and monitoring the room for client reactions while the other moves through the session content. Co-leaders can also take turns on who does what session-by-session.

Open versus closed groups. Groups can be open or closed. Closed groups (everyone begins and ends together) are preferable to forge the strongest bonds, but in many settings this isn't feasible.

Open groups work in Creating Change because session topics can be done in any order, so clients don't have to attend what came before. However, if clients join an existing group, it's best to first do an individual session with them to go over the topic "Introduction." If you have several clients joining at once, you could do this in a mini-group and then they all join the larger group. If you're conducting blocks of sessions, this is another way to have clients join only at particular timepoints (see "Conduct Blocks of Sessions for Group Treatment" on page 41). For a client who is new to you, see also the extra topic "Recovery Strengths and Challenges," to help identify whether Creating Change is likely to be a good fit.

Gender-based groups. Gender-based groups are preferred as some clients may find all-gender groups triggering, for example, if they experienced sexual assault. But all-gender groups are fine if clients know about that in advance and voluntarily choose to attend.

Group composition. A broad range of clients can potentially benefit from Creating Change and, for groups, all clients don't have to have the same diagnoses or types of trauma or addiction. So too, clients may be at different levels of functioning, including different lengths of addiction recovery, and can learn a lot from that wide range of experiences. The analogy is an AA meeting: It includes people who drank that day as well as people sober for decades. However, follow your clinical judgment and program policies.

Sharing time. Group members share time in Creating Change the way they would in any group, with spontaneous interaction and the counselor balancing across member needs. The only exception is the check-in and check-out, in which each client separately takes a turn to speak (described in the section "Detailed Guide to the Session Format" on pages 59–64). Also, for some topics, you may want to set a time limit to allow each client uninterrupted time to share (e.g. "Tell Your Story" and "Break the Silence"); guidance on how to do that is in the counselor section of those topics.

Response to triggering. In general, Creating Change doesn't evoke a lot of triggering given its strong flexibility and client-centered approach. But triggering does occur at times, and the key is to respond in a way that keeps the session productive and safe for everyone. Start by inquiring, for example, "Ali, are you OK? It looks like you're having a hard time." Then any of the following may be useful depending on the situation:

- Have the client say a bit about what was triggering and see if it can be explored in a useful way related to the session topic.
- Do a few minutes of grounding. If the client is extremely triggered, this can bring it down to a moderate level so it can be talked about, rather than the client staying stuck in it. Ask the other clients in the group to follow along with the grounding silently while the triggered client does it out loud. Validate that triggering is normal and there are ways to cope with it.
- If a particular client is triggered intensely over many sessions, it may be best to refer the client to a present-focused stabilizing treatment while attending Creating Change (taking a break from Creating Change while learning coping skills).

Group bonding: positive and negative. Trust is essential for groups, especially when addressing sensitive topics such as trauma and addiction. Clients can build positive bonds, such as warmth and support, but also negative ones that derail the group. One of the most common negative dynamics is for one client (or sometimes the counselor) to become scapegoated by the group. This is a particular risk for clients with a trauma history, who may be reenacting the devaluing and aggression that are so common in trauma. When negative bonding occurs, it's usually in closed longer-term groups and not conscious. You may notice that one client receives repeated negative feedback from the group, is ignored, or put down (often subtly, such as rolled eyes or looking away). The counselor is usually the most powerful person in the room, so if you provide an extra measure of support for the scapegoated client, this may defuse the situation and gently model positive behavior for the group. In other cases, the client's behavior may be evoking negative responses (criticizing others, ignoring social cues, overdominating, or being unassertive). In this case, the client will need one-to-one feedback on how to function better in a group. In general, watch for subtle power dynamics to ensure overall balance, with no one being repeatedly disrespected. If it's the counselor who's being scapegoated (clients band together and are persistently negative toward you), seek supervision to learn strategies for countering this. See also Chapter 4 on the concept of reenactment of trauma roles: victim, perpetrator, bystander, rescuer.

Group policies. Specifying your policies in writing encourages clients to abide by them and, for groups, helps them feel that everyone is being treated equally. The Creating Change Treatment Agreement in the topic "Introduction" identifies several policies specific to groups (e.g., confidentiality) and has space for you to add policies specific to your setting.

Conducting groups in general. If you plan to conduct Creating Change in groups and have not trained in general on how to conduct groups, find resources online and/or consult with others to support your learning. Group work is more than "doing individual work with more than one person at a time." There are important group dynamics that differ from individual treatment.

Consider the Setting

Creating Change can be done in most treatment settings, but some have particular advantages.

Length of stay. It's best if clients are in a setting where they can attend at least 8–12 sessions. But clients can benefit even if their stay is shorter as each Creating Change topic is independent of the others. Typical settings for ongoing treatment are outpatient, residential care, therapeutic communities, corrections, addiction rehabilitation, day programs, and some inpatient programs. In some of these, sessions can be conducted more frequently than once a week, which allows for a higher dose. There's no "magic number" of sessions, but in general more treatment produces more positive outcomes, in both PTSD and addiction treatment (APA, 2017; NIDA, 2018).

Staff support. Help clients identify whom to reach out to in case of a clinical crisis. Help them distinguish when to use informal support (a friend or hotline) versus professional care or emergency procedures. Creating Change doesn't require ongoing support, but it helps to identify whom they can contact if needed between sessions. Settings that may not be strongly suited for Creating Change are those without any clinical support such as some drop-in programs or sober living houses.

Trauma-informed. Trauma-informed settings recognize the importance of trauma in all aspects of their work (SAMHSA, 2014). They're characterized by the following:

- A high level of client empowerment (offering options and a collaborative approach)
- Policies that are sensitive to trauma, ensuring physical and emotional safety
- Training all staff on trauma principles
- Awareness of how providers' own trauma history impacts their work
- Routine trauma assessment

In non-trauma-informed settings, trauma isn't addressed and there may be power dynamics that unintentionally perpetuate trauma symptoms. You can do Creating Change in any setting but, if needed, find ways to strengthen trauma awareness by creating a supervision group or staff training. For guidance, see the section "Best Practices in Trauma Treatment" in Chapter 4.

Addiction-informed. *Addiction-informed care* is not a current term in the field but likely should be. Just as it's important to address trauma, it's important to create a culture of addiction awareness. Clients with substance addiction are still sometimes rejected from care until abstinent or treated only if they have mild addiction. Behavioral addictions are rarely assessed. Counselors may hold older views ("You must attend AA or I won't treat you") and be unaware of alternatives such as harm reduction and controlled use for low-severity clients. Staff sometimes hold negative or fearful attitudes toward addicted clients and may not be trained on addiction. Systems of care (addiction, mental health, primary care) often remain split due to funding and policy issues. For guidance, see Chapter 4, the section "Best Practices in Addiction Treatment."

Program culture. Culture refers to the "feel" of a program. Clients and counselors are affected by it, even if not always aware of it. Cultural aspects include:

- Emotional climate (level of warmth)
- Equal treatment
- Positive staff morale
- How conflict is addressed
- Openness to feedback

If needed, you may want to get reinforcement from outside training, support, or supervision. There's also a free 10-item version of the widely used Working Environment Scale that can be helpful (it's Appendix 1 in Røssberg, Eiring, & Friis, 2004).

Consider the Client

All types of clients can participate in Creating Change, but it's useful to consider client complexity as a factor when planning treatment.

Complexity refers to how challenging the client is to treat, such as in the grid below. It's based on factors such as mental health disorders (how many, what type, how chronic, how severe); life problems (poverty, physical illness, etc.); and level of functioning now and in the past (Brown, Huba, & Melchior, 1995; Najavits et al., 2020).

Trauma processing is easier with clients who have fewer "interfering" characteristics (high level of anger, frequent dissociation, memory gaps), for example (see Coffey et al., 2002), and if clients' distressing experiences are recent rather than long-standing (Nichols & Zax, 1977).

Creating Change studies generally had highly complex samples (see the section "Evidence Base" in Chapter 1). It's also been conducted with less complex clients.

Low-complexity client	*High*-complexity client
Mild addiction and just one type of addiction	**Severe addiction** and more than one type
Simple trauma: one trauma or a few separate traumas, typically in adulthood; remembers trauma details; if PTSD, fits DSM criteria	**Complex trauma:** many traumas, often in childhood or over a long time; symptoms are broader than DSM criteria and may include problems related to sexuality, identity, dissociation, self-injury, etc.
Less chronic: addiction and trauma problems are brief or recent	**More chronic:** addiction and trauma problems have gone on for a long time

Low-complexity client	*High*-complexity client
Minimal or no current life problems such as poverty, homelessness, serious health or legal issues	**Various current life problems** such as poverty, homelessness, serious health or legal problems
Strong prior functioning before addiction and trauma, such as stable work, relationships, housing, self-care	**Weak prior functioning** with major deficits in work, relationships, housing, self-care
Mild or no other mental health disorders: if present, generally acute, and no major mental illness	**Significant other mental health disorders:** multiple disorders, some severe and chronic, and likely personality disorder or major mental illness
No history of physical harm to self or others; may have thoughts of these, but able to contain impulses	**History of physical harm to self or others, possibly current**, e.g., self-injury such as cutting; suicidality; or assault
Reasonable self-care; generally able to manage daily activities and health	**Problems with self-care**, which may result in medical problems and an unstable living situation

With low-complexity clients, you may need fewer topics or may move through them more quickly. It's typically easier to sustain a positive attitude and to feel gratified by the work. High-complexity clients need more repetition of concepts and have more ups and downs along the way, such as unstable attendance and difficulty managing impulses. You may have more mixed feelings—liking the client, but sometimes confused, angry, guilty, or pessimistic. Yet high-complexity clients can achieve remarkable recovery, and it's deeply moving to be part of that.

Most clients fall between the two extremes with a mix of characteristics from each side of the table above. Other client factors also impact treatment, such as level of motivation and resources (financial, social, etc.).

Here are some examples:

Mike, military veteran, example of a low-complexity client. Mike is a 25-year-old military veteran who served in Afghanistan, honorably discharged. He's well-liked and has a good sense of humor but keeps his feelings to himself. During the war, several close buddies died. He developed a lot of guilt and became increasingly depressed during his second tour of duty. He was haunted by nightmares and had most of the DSM PTSD symptoms. He always liked to party with friends but, once back home, was binge-drinking alone most days and unmotivated to cut down. He was arrested twice for driving drunk. Although he did OK at his sales job, he seemed to be just marking time, uninterested in anything. His family brought him to a local veterans center for treatment. At first, he wouldn't talk about his PTSD and alcohol addiction, but was willing to try Creating Change on an outpatient basis, weekly, while also attending AA and receiving antidepressants. He attends sessions regularly and, although the work is difficult at times, he finds an increasing sense of relief. "It's like a burden is lifted that I was carrying too long. I see now that I couldn't save my friends. I was drowning my feelings with booze. I didn't know how to deal with what was going on inside and the more I ignored it, the worse it got." In 12 sessions, he showed improvements in PTSD and alcohol use but still needs help to continue his gains. He chose controlled drinking ("I can't imagine going the rest of my life without a beer") and for 8 weeks has been able to keep to the drinking limits set in his counseling.

Carla, child abuse survivor, example of a high-complexity client. Carla is 40 years old. Her mother died when she was 3 and she was abused physically, sexually, and emotionally in childhood by her alcoholic father until age 12, when he died. She was placed in foster care but, after trying to kill herself at 14, was sent to a residential program for girls. She began drinking in grade school and started drugs in middle school (marijuana and eventually polysubstances). She says she felt depressed her entire life and trusted no one. She can be charming but has a history of unstable relationships, with repeated anger outbursts and a tendency to get involved with men who end up physically and emotionally hurting her. She's intelligent, but never graduated from high school and held jobs just briefly. She has various medical problems, including asthma and diabetes, is overweight, and has a poor diet. She started residential addiction treatment 3 months ago (her sixth residential program) and received Seeking Safety twice weekly in group format and Creating Change weekly in individual format, plus other treatments. She says she never before had the opportunity to explore trauma and addiction together. She missed some sessions and had several addiction slips with her ex-boyfriend while out on pass, which required her to leave the residential program briefly and then return. She eventually moved to a sober house in the community and continued aftercare AA and weekly counseling. She still struggles with physical and emotional problems but is more committed to self-care than before. She put together 6 months' substance abstinence and reports lower trauma symptoms.

Conducting Creating Change with Other Models

This section offers options for using various models in conjunction with Creating Change.

HOW TO COMBINE CREATING CHANGE WITH SEEKING SAFETY

Many counselors are already familiar with Seeking Safety (*www.seekingsafety.org*); this section offers options for using it in conjunction with Creating Change. The two models go together extremely well—they are "twins," with the same format, flexibility, style, and integrated approach to trauma and addiction. The key difference is that Seeking Safety focuses on the present, while Creating Change focuses on the past. Each model can be used alone, but if you choose to combine them, any of the following methods work well. However, don't try to cover a Seeking Safety topic and a Creating Change topic *in the same session*. There's not enough time to do justice to the content of each, as they have different goals.

* *One, then the other (sequential).* Clients first complete Seeking Safety (building coping skills), then enter Creating Change (focusing on the past). This is consistent with the stage-based approach to recovery that emphasizes stabilization before moving into past-focused exploration (Herman, 1992). This has intuitive appeal and can be helpful, but a sequential approach is not always needed (De Jongh et al., 2016). It's one way but not the only way. If you use this method, you may choose to have clients complete a specific dose of Seeking Safety (typically anywhere from 12 to 25 sessions) or you can base it on their ability to use the coping skills rather than simply attendance.

* *Back-and-forth (alternating).* Today is Seeking Safety, the next session is Creating Change and so on. Or you can do a block of four topics from one model, then four from the other repeatedly. Alternating the models helps build different types of skills, mutually reinforcing each other

Seeking Safety sessions strengthen clients' ability to do the emotional work in Creating Change and vice versa. It also allows clients to experience both models and, if they develop a preference for one over the other, you could, especially in individual modality, then focus more heavily on that.

- *Based on check-in (choice).* You decide whether to focus on the present or the past based on how the client is doing at check-in. This was the method in the initial Creating Change pilot study (Najavits et al., 2005). It allows pacing that's sensitive to the client's progress week-to-week and is most feasible in individual treatment. After the client completes the check-in, the counselor and client decide together whether to do a Seeking Safety or Creating Change session. For example, if the client had an addiction relapse or other major setback that week, Seeking Safety might be the best choice. For this method to work, the counselor needs to feel comfortable switching in real time (having available both a Seeking Safety and Creating Change set of handouts on hand and being prepared to do either model). This method is not likely to be feasible in group, however, as clients will differ in their level of progress.

- *Concurrent treatment (parallel).* Clients attend Seeking Safety and Creating Change at the same time. This is typically done as group Seeking Safety and individual Creating Change. But it can vary (either model can be individual or group modality; so too, each may be conducted by the same counselor or different ones).

- *One model is primary (partial combination).* In this method, you decide on one model as the main one and just add in a few topics from the other rather than conducting both fully. For example, if Creating Change is primary, you might choose a few key topics from Seeking Safety to use with it. Some that may be especially helpful are:
  - "Safety"
  - "Detaching from Emotional Pain (Grounding)"
  - "Asking for Help"
  - "Healing from Anger"
  - "Coping with Triggers"
  - The Case Management section from the topic "Introduction to Treatment/Case Management"

CONSIDERATIONS FOR OTHER MODELS

All of the methods listed above can work with other counseling models, too. In addition, keep in mind the following.

Suggested models. Most models are likely to converge well with Creating Change. But the three described below may be an especially good fit as they: (1) have been developed specifically for co-occurring trauma and addiction and/or studied in that population, (2) can be implemented by almost any provider (not requiring training or certification), and (3) are published and thus widely available.

See also Appendix C online, "Comparison of Models by the Author" (*www.guilford.com/najavits3-materials*), regarding the four models developed by Lisa M. Najavits (*Finding Your Best Self, Seeking Safety, Creating Change,* and *A Woman's Path to Recovery*).

- *Finding Your Best Self (www.best-self.org).* This model (Najavits, 2019) was developed for trauma and addiction and has unique content that doesn't overlap with either Creating Change or Seeking Safety. It can be conducted by anyone—professionals, peer specialists, sponsors, friends, or family members—and also used as self-help. It lends itself easily for use with Creating Change because clients can do it between sessions on their own or with caring people in their life, or you can make it part of their treatment program in either individual or group modality.

- *Relapse Prevention.* This is a classic evidence-based model in the addiction field (Marlatt & Gordon, 1985). It's a present-focused, cognitive-behavioral approach that offers practical strategies to prevent addiction relapse, such as identifying high-risk situations and "thinking traps" that maintain addiction. It's been evaluated in several studies of co-occurring PTSD/SUD and typically shows positive results in both domains even though it was only designed for the latter (Simpson et al., 2021). It can be conducted in individual or group modality.

- *BRENDA* (2001) is an individual present-focused model that was originally designed for use with SUD medication therapies (Volpicelli et al., 2001). Its name signifies its elements: biopsychosocial evaluation; report results to the patient; empathic approach; needs that are collaboratively identified; direct advice on how to meet the needs; assess reaction and adjust advice. It focuses on SUD only yet showed impact on both PTSD and SUD in a major study comparing it to PE (Foa et al., 2013).

Checking for overlap. Try to ensure that clients don't receive the same content from different models. For example, the Creating Change extra topic "Understanding Trauma and Addiction" may not be needed if clients are learning about trauma and addiction symptoms as part of another model.

Client feedback. Ask clients, either informally or via a satisfaction scale, how much they like each model and how you're combining them. Their feedback can help you make adjustments as needed.

Detailed Guide to the Session Format

What's most essential to know about the session format is that *it's easy to do* and *clients generally really like it.*

The description below is detailed so that you have a resource to turn to, but the best way to learn the format is simply to try it with your clients. Use the two-page summary at the end of this chapter (pages 66–67) and, as you go through each element of the format, keep in mind the points that follow.

1. Conduct the Check-In

The session begins with a check-in, which is like a "temperature check" to briefly find out how each client is doing, and to identify major issues to return to during the session.

Check-In (2–4 minutes per client)

Since the last session . . .

1. How are you feeling?
2. What good coping have you done?
3. Any substance use or other unsafe behavior?
4. Did you complete your commitment?
5. Community resource update?

Suggestions for the check-in are as follows.

Let clients go through the questions on their own. Each client completes all five questions before the next client starts. This provides a sense of empowerment and also saves time. Don't read the questions out loud but prompt for an answer if a client misses a question. At the end of this chapter is a list of the check-in and check-out questions to photocopy and either (1) post on the wall for clients to see or (2) let them pass it around in turn as each does the check-in. *Note:* For telehealth, share the question on-screen.

Keep to time limits. The check-in is brief, 2–4 minutes per client. This allows clients to highlight what's most important and also reinforces boundaries. Don't ask questions unless absolutely essential, and don't do any reflective listening (repeating back what you heard) or analyzing. No meaningful interventions can be done during the brief time of the check-in.

Just listen and offer short validating responses, such as "That's great!" or "I'm concerned about that; let's come back to that later in the session."

Question 1 ("How are you feeling?") is a general update. Clients don't have to report an emotion word such as "sad" or "scared." It's for any updates the client wants to report (e.g., "I had a tough week, arguing with my partner about the kids").

Question 2 ("What good coping have you done?") reinforces strengths. Encourage clients to come up with their own answers rather than offering your ideas. (A helpful tool is the Seeking Safety list of safe coping skills in the topic "Safety." You can ask them to identify anything on the list that they did this week; they always find something.) Note that if a client names something that is personally unsafe ("Drinking helped me relax" or "I spent all day in bed"), remind the client that only *safe* coping counts. Finally, don't try to link check-in question 1 and question 2; they are entirely separate questions.

Question 3 ("Any substance use or other unsafe behavior?") may need follow-up questions. If a client reports substance use or other unsafe behavior, also ask the *amount*, *frequency*, and *type*. For example, "How much alcohol did you drink?," "How many times?," and "What type (e.g., wine, beer, or hard liquor)?" The goal is to monitor change over time. If a client has multiple unsafe behaviors, you would generally just ask the follow-up questions about the most important one(s). Keep in mind that "unsafe behaviors" can refer to any behavior that's unsafe for a particular client, such as isolation, spending time with unsafe people, rage attacks, binge eating, excessive spending, driving under the influence, or any other. Note that if you work in a correctional setting where reporting substance use would add time or charges to a client's sentence, you can ask about "substance cravings" rather than "substance use."

Question 4 ("Did you complete your commitment?") is brief. A commitment is homework clients do between sessions. Often, just a "yes" or "no" to question 4 is sufficient rather than adding detail on how it went, but use your judgment. Individual modality lends itself to more exploration, whereas group is best to keep limited unless the client had a major problem with the commitment. If the commitment was written, the client could hand it to you to read between sessions, if desired.

Question 5 ("Community resource update?") is an update on referrals. "Community resources" are referrals from the previous session that you gave to the client for support outside of Creating Change (e.g., AA, a doctor or dentist, parenting skills class, domestic violence hotline). For question 5, clients provide a simple update on whether they followed through on the referrals and, if there were none that week, they just state that.

For group treatment, there are several additional aspects:

- Teach clients not to cross-talk during the check-in; protect each client's "space." It's helpful to provide a trauma-informed explanation for this, such as "We do this to be respectful of each other, empowering everyone to be heard."
- A client who shows up late can check in, but don't provide a catch-up summary of others' check-ins. This helps keep the session on track and doesn't reinforce lateness.

How to Conduct Creating Change

- For large groups in which check-in would take up too much session time, use the *large-group check-in method:* You read aloud the first check-in question and have just one or two clients answer it; then you read the second check-in question and have another one or two clients answer that; and keep doing that for all five check-in questions with different clients for each question. This highlights the check-in questions without focusing on every client (everyone tracks their own responses internally), thus preserving time for the rest of the session.

2. Share the Session Handouts

Next, the counselor shares the handouts from one of the 23 treatment topics. All of the topics are set up so that the first few pages are the *counselor guide* (these do not go to clients), and the rest of the chapter are the *client handouts* (from the quotation page through the end of that chapter, which is always the Commitment page). Even if you can't cover everything in the handouts during the session, still give clients the full set. This is simplest for you and clinically best as it allows them to glance through everything to see what interests them most; they can also continue to read the full set of handouts between sessions if desired.

3. Go Over the Quotation

The quotation helps emotionally engage clients in the session with a brief point of inspiration.

Quotation (1–3 minutes)

~ The client reads the quote out loud.
~ The counselor asks, "What's the main point of the quotation?"
~ The counselor links the quotation to the session topic.

Note: For group treatment, one client reads the quote, and another states the main point.

Keep it brief. The quote is a brief point of inspiration, not an intervention. In both individual and group treatment, keep the entire process to 1–3 minutes. To achieve this, use the wording above, which focuses on what *the author is saying*. If you were to ask, "What does the quote *mean to you?*," it will open up clients' very personal meanings, which reduces time for the actual session topic. In group modality, ask for a volunteer to read the quote and another to state what it means. If desired, you could have one or two additional clients also state what it means, but definitely don't go around to ask each client to respond.

Link the quote to the session. Each topic offers suggested wording to link the quote to the topic (e.g., "The reason that's the quote for today is because we're going to be talking about . . ."). It's in the "Session Format" section of each of the 23 treatment topics.

Consider adding quotations. The quotes are carefully selected to connect with the session topic and are drawn from a wide range of cultures and authors. But you and your clients may have favorite quotes you'd like to add (which is especially helpful if you're conducting a second session on the same treatment topic; this way you don't have to repeat the same quote a second time). It also allows for culture-specific quotes relevant to the population you serve.

4. Engage Clients in the Handouts

Each topic brings forth a different way to help clients overcome the past. Most of the session is spent working with the handouts, relating them to clients' lives.

Handouts (most of the session)

Clients look through the handouts and the counselor helps them explore the topic.

See the specific ideas within each topic. The counselor section of each topic provides various ways to help clients work on it, including exercises and discussion questions.

Give clients a few minutes to look through the handouts (or use an alternative method). For most clients, it works best to give them a little time to glance through the handouts to get a feel for them; they don't have to read every word. However, you may prefer a different method that fits your clientele better, especially if they have difficulty reading or are highly distractible. Alternatives include:

- Focusing on just one or two handouts (you guide them to one you believe is most relevant)
- Having them read small sections aloud
- Summarizing key points

The topic names and concepts are quite straightforward (e.g., "Listen to Your Body") so even clients who can't read can still participate as they'll understand the gist of what's being covered.

Start with open-ended questions to identify what's most important to them. To begin discussion, ask questions such as "Any reactions?," "Is there anything new or surprising in the handouts?," "How does this topic relate to your life?," or "How would it feel to explore this more?"

Cover the handouts in any order you choose. All topics have several handouts. You can do them in any order and over more than one session. That's why each chapter is called a *topic* rather than a *session*; it provides a lot of material for as many sessions as you choose to do it. The pace should feel calm, not rushed. Listen closely to clients and cover the material in a deep, meaningful way.

Weave back and forth between the handouts and clients' issues. Use them therapeutically—draw out key points and try the exercises. Help clients connect the material to their experiences. Too much focus on the handouts can seem like school. Too little focus on them derails the session. Keep moving back and forth between the handouts and clients' exploration.

Focus on important issues. If the session feels bland or superficial, it's typically because clients aren't emotionally engaged. Select problems they care about and, in general, problems of at least moderate difficulty. If unclear, occasionally ask them how important a problem is to them.

For clients with both addiction and trauma, explore how they impact each other. If one gets better, does the other get better, too? Did one lead to the other? Guide them to focus on both if they have both.

Address immediate needs as well. Sometimes clients raise current issues at check-in that need attention during the session, such as recent substance use or self-harm. Even though Creating Change focuses on the past, it's also important to address current needs. Suggestions are as follows:

- Still ask clients to look through the handouts as usual (unless the immediate need is so urgent that case management is needed—getting them hospitalized, medically evaluated, etc.).
- Start by addressing the current issue in relation to the handouts, if possible. For example, if

today's topic is "Emotions and Healing" and the client used a substance this week, encourage the client to notice how substance use has become a way to cope with emotions. *Note:* Some topics will be more relevant to the client's current issue than others. Switch topics if needed.
- Identify practical steps in the present, such as increasing AA attendance. Here too, help the client link to the past (e.g., "In the past you were alone with distressing feelings, but now you can connect with others rather than turning to alcohol").

Use questions more than lecture. With so much material in the handouts, it may be tempting to provide long explanations. But it's more powerful for clients to speak rather than listen, as long as they focus on the session topic. Aim for an 80:20 ratio—the client speaks about 80% of the session, with the counselor offering brief comments and questions about 20% of the time.

5. Conduct the Check-Out

The session ends with a brief check-out to wrap up in a positive way. Just as with the check-in, clients don't cross-talk and the counselor doesn't attempt interventions or processing. The counselor offers brief statements of support and reminds clients, if needed, to answer all the questions.

Check-Out (1–2 minutes per client)

1. Name one thing you got out of today's session.
2. Any problems with the session?
3. What is your new commitment?
4. What community resource will you call? (as needed)

Question 1 ("Name one thing you got out of today's session"). This question reinforces clients' learning and helps the counselor know what had the most impact. There are no right or wrong answers—it's important to accept whatever clients say, without trying to correct it. Indeed if they state that they got nothing from the session, this too would be validated (e.g., "I'm sorry to hear that but I hope next time will feel more helpful").

Question 2 ("Any problems with the session?"). This question helps prevent dropout by encouraging clients to openly air concerns. If they name any, it's usually good to praise their honesty but not delve into a discussion during the check-out. If it requires further discussion, come back to it at the next session or in a separate meeting.

Question 3 ("What is your new commitment?"). The commitment is basically homework, but "commitment" is a more inspiring term. It's a promise to do something productive toward recovery before the next session. Commitments are voluntary but strongly encouraged. The last page of each topic has a list of commitments that vary in intensity and methods (some are verbal, some nonverbal). Clients choose from the list or can select anything else—it doesn't even have to relate to the session topic. A commitment just needs to be specific and safe for that person. For example, *journal at least once this week* is specific; *be more confident* is not. Clients write down their commitment, making a copy for both you and them using the Commitment to Recovery form at the end of this chapter.

Question 4 ("What community resource will you call?"). The goal is to refer clients to additional treatments and supports as needed, also known as *case management*. You might encourage a client to go to a self-help group, join a job training program, call a dentist, or have a medication evaluation. Then you'd find out whether the client actually followed up with the referral as part of the check-in at the next session. However, not all clients will have community resources to pursue. For additional guidance on case management, see the Seeking Safety topic, "Introduction to Treatment/Case Management."

Materials to Use across Sessions

The materials listed below are relevant throughout Creating Change.

Creating Change content (located in Chapter 1)

- List of the 23 Creating Change Topics (page 7). A list of all topics and a brief description of each. You can hand the list to a client to help them choose a topic, if desired, and/or log the topics you've covered.

For each session (located at the end of this chapter)

- **Summary of the Session Format** *(for counselors).* You can keep this in front of you during the session as a reminder of the session structure.
- **Check-In and Check-Out** *(for clients).* Make this visible to clients so they see the questions to answer. You can post it on the wall (or onscreen during telehealth) or hand a paper copy from client to client.
- **Commitment to Recovery** *(for clients).* At the end of the session, clients write their Creating Change commitment (homework) on this form so both they and you have a copy of it.
- **End-of-Session Questionnaire** *(for clients; optional).* After the session, clients can provide feedback on this brief (2- to 3-minute) optional questionnaire. It can be done anonymously in group treatment.

Weekly (located at the end of this chapter)

- **Safe Behavior Scale** *(for clients; optional).* This weekly scale is recommended but optional for tracking clients' progress.

General (located at the end of this chapter)

- **Flyer for the Creating Change three-session try-out.** This flyer encourages clients to try Creating Change. You can post it in a waiting room or share it electronically. For an editable version, go to *www.creating-change.org*.
- **Certificate of Achievement.** Clients appreciate recognition. You can award this for attending a specific number of sessions, typically seven or more.

Scales (located in specific topics)

- **Agnew Relationship Measure** *(Handout 2 in the extra topic "Your Relationships").* This free, brief validated scale assesses the quality of the counseling relationship, also known as the *therapeutic alliance* (Cahill et al., 2012). There is both a counselor and client version.
- **Excessive Behavior Scale** *(Handout 4 in the extra topic "Understanding Trauma and*

Addiction"). This screening tool for behavioral addictions is recommended for all clients as these often go undetected in treatment (e.g., problem gambling, eating, shopping, work).

- **Creating Change Feedback Questionnaire** *(Handout 4 in the topic "Growth")*. A brief questionnaire to share feedback about different aspects of Creating Change.

- **Strengths and Challenges Questionnaire** *(Handout 1 in the extra topic "Recovery Strengths and Challenges")*. You can use this optional questionnaire to explore whether a client is a good fit for Creating Change if you have doubts, such as for a client who is new to you. But, in general, the three-session try-out method is preferred (see the paragraph "Use a three-session try-out" on page 41).

Summary of the Session Format (*for Counselors*)

The format is the same for individual and group treatment.

Check-in (2–4 minutes per client)

Purpose: Clients share how they're doing by briefly answering five questions.

"Since the last session . . .

1. How are you feeling?
2. What good coping have you done?
3. Any substance use or other unsafe behavior?
4. Did you complete your commitment?
5. Community resource update?

In group treatment, each client answers all questions before going to the next client.

Quotation (1–3 minutes total)

Purpose: Emotionally engage clients in the session topic.

✦ The counselor distributes the handouts from a Creating Change topic (the quotation page through the end of the chapter).

✦ A client reads the quotation out loud.

✦ The counselor asks, "What's the main point of the quotation?"

✦ The counselor links the quotation to the session (suggested language is in the counselor section of the topic).

In group treatment, one client reads the quote, and another states the main point.

Handouts (most of the session)

Purpose: Relate the topic to clients' lives.

✦ Clients look through the handouts.

✦ The counselor helps them explore the topic and guides exercises.

(cont.)

From *Creating Change* by Lisa M. Najavits. Copyright © 2024 Lisa M. Najavits. Published by The Guilford Press. Permission to photocopy this material, or to download and print additional copies (*www.guilford.com/najavits3-materials*), is granted to purchasers of this book for use with your own clients or patients; see copyright page for details.

Summary of the Session Format (*for Counselors*) *(p. 2 of 2)*

Check-out (2–3 minutes per client)

Purpose: Wrap up the session in a positive way; clients address four questions.

1. Name one thing you got out of today's session.
2. Any problems with the session?
3. What's your new commitment?
4. What community resource will you call? (as needed)

In group treatment, each client answers all questions before going to the next client.

Optional: **Grounding** (3–5 minutes)

Purpose: Encourage a sense of emotional calm.

✤ If desired and time allows, conduct a few minutes of grounding.

Optional: **End-of-Session Questionnaire** (2–3 minutes)

Purpose: Clients share written feedback about the session.

✤ Ask clients to fill out the questionnaire (anonymously if in group treatment).

Check-In and Check-Out

CHECK-IN

Since your last session ...

1. How are you **feeling**?

2. What **good coping** have you done?

3. Any **substance use** or other **unsafe behavior**?

4. Did you complete your **commitment**?

5. **Community resource** update?

CHECK-OUT

1. **Name one thing** you got out of today's session (and any problems with the session).

2. What is your new **commitment**?

3. What **community resource** will you call?

From *Seeking Safety* by Lisa M. Najavits. Copyright © 2002 The Guilford Press. Reprinted in *Creating Change* (The Guilford Press, 2024). Permission to photocopy this material, or to download and print additional copies (*www.guilford.com/najavits3-materials*), is granted to purchasers of this book for use with your own clients or patients; see copyright page for details.

Commitment to Recovery

*A commitment is a promise—to yourself, to your recovery, and to your counselor.
If you cannot complete your commitment, or need to change it,
be sure to leave your counselor a message before your next session.*

Name: _____ Date: _____

Commitment for next session	
I will do:	**By when:**

Community Resource to call before next session	
I will call:	**By when:**

REMINDERS

- Your next session is scheduled for: _____ Date _____ Time
- Where will you put this sheet to remember it? Wallet ____ Refrigerator door ____ Notebook _____
  Other location: _____

(tear here) - *(tear here)*

COUNSELOR COPY

Patient Initials: _____ Today's Date: _____

Commitment for next session	
I will do:	**By when:**

Community Resource to call before next session	
I will call:	**By when:**

From *Seeking Safety* by Lisa M. Najavits. Copyright © 2002 The Guilford Press. Reprinted in *Creating Change* (The Guilford Press., 2024). Permission to photocopy this material, or to download and print additional copies (*www.guilford.com/najavits3-materials*), is granted to purchasers of this book for use with your own clients or patients; see copyright page for details.

End-of-Session Questionnaire

To be completed anonymously; do not fill in your name.

Session Topic: _____ Date: _____

Please be honest about your view of today's session so that the treatment can be made as helpful as possible. Answer questions 1–6 using the following scale:

0	1	2	3
Not at all	A little	Moderately	A great deal

1. How helpful was today's session for you, overall? _____

2. In today's session, how helpful were:

    a. The topic of the session? _____
    b. The handouts? _____
    c. The quotation? _____
    d. The counselor? _____

3. How much did today's session help you with your:

    a. Trauma? _____
    b. Addiction? _____

4. How much do you think you'll use what you learned in today's session in your life? _____

5. Do you have any other comments or suggestions about today's session? Please be honest about both positive and negative reactions.

    Positive reactions: _____
    _____
    _____

    Negative reactions: _____
    _____
    _____

6. How could this treatment be more helpful to you?
    _____
    _____
    _____

From *Seeking Safety* by Lisa M. Najavits. Copyright © 2002 The Guilford Press. Reprinted in *Creating Change* (The Guilford Press, 2024). Permission to photocopy this material, or to download and print additional copies (*www.guilford.com/najavits3-materials*), is granted to purchasers of this book for use with your own clients or patients; see copyright page for details.

The Safe Behavior Scale

Today's date: _____ Your name or initials: _____

This brief scale helps you build awareness of your safe and unsafe behaviors. If you have trauma or addiction problems, you may feel good but your behavior is unsafe—or the opposite, you may feel bad but your behavior is safe. Behavior "wins" over feelings in providing accurate feedback about your recovery.

Thinking about the past week, in each row circle either "not at all," "some," or "a lot" (don't focus on the numbers for now). Truly *listen* to your behavior—sometimes it may be obvious and other times it may be subtle, perhaps just short of denial.

Your behavior	Examples	Not at all	Some	A lot	Describe briefly (optional)
1. **Safe coping skills**	Positive use of skills such as asking for help, reading recovery materials, anger management, reducing stress, etc.	0	1	2	
2. **Treatment/ self-help groups/ medication**	Actively pursuing structured help (e.g., for mental health, addiction, medical, self-help groups), attending all as scheduled, and taking all medications as prescribed. ❑ Check here if you have no current need for any of these, and then circle 2 for this item.	0	1	2	
3. **Healthy living**	Good diet, sleep, exercise, balance of work and leisure, etc.	0	1	2	
4. **Major responsibilities**	Fulfilling major duties at work, at school, in your family, etc.	0	1	2	
5. **Daily tasks**	Keeping up with daily to-do's (house cleaning, car upkeep, food shopping, bill paying, staying organized).	0	1	2	
6. **Social support**	Spending time with safe people* (family, friends, colleagues, sponsor, self-help groups); positive and genuine interactions.	0	1	2	

*Unsafe people encourage addictive behavior, put you down, undermine or betray you, physically hurt you, are violent, etc.

(cont.)

From *Finding Your Best Self, Revised Edition: Recovery from Addiction, Trauma, or Both* by Lisa M. Najavits. Copyright © 2019 Lisa M. Najavits. Reprinted in *Creating Change* (The Guilford Press, 2024). The scale cannot be adapted without advance written permission from info@treatment-innovations.org. Permission to photocopy this material, or to download and print additional copies (*www.guilford.com/najavits-materials*), is granted to purchasers of this book for use with your own clients or patients; see copyright page for details.

The Safe Behavior Scale *(p. 2 of 2)*

Your behavior	Examples	Not at all	Some	A lot	Describe briefly (optional)
7. **Responding to your feelings**	Staying aware of feelings and responding to them in healthy ways. Includes all types of feelings (e.g., emotions, cravings, body sensations).	0	1	2	
8. **Managing addictive behavior**	Keeping within necessary or agreed-on limits.** For substances, the goal may be abstinence; for spending, it may be a budget, etc.	0	1	2	List the addictive behavior(s) you are rating; and if you circled 0 or 1, describe *how much* and *how often* the behavior(s) occurred***:
9. **Harm to self or others**	Actions such as cutting, burning, suicidal behavior, hitting, punching, yelling, verbal abuse, violence.	2	1	0	If 1 or 0: What type of harm? How much and how often?
10. **Avoiding triggers**	Staying away from trauma and addiction triggers (people, places, and things that are unsafe for you) as much as possible.	0	1	2	
11. **Level of effort**	How much you are actively, strongly, and consistently working to improve your life.	0	1	2	
12. **Other unsafe behavior**	Any other actions that are unsafe for you (e.g., reckless driving, unsafe sex, illegal activity, hanging with unsafe people*).	2	1	0	If 1 or 0: What unsafe behavior(s)? And how much and how often?***

*Unsafe people encourage addictive behavior, put you down, undermine or betray you, physically hurt you, are violent, etc.

**Safe limits on addictive behavior vary by type of addiction and your needs. If you're unclear what's a safe limit for you, get feedback from reputable people or resources.

***List how much the addictive behavior occurred. For example, if you drank, how much did you drink: a bottle of wine? five beers? If you gambled, how much money did you lose? If you watched porn, how many hours did you watch?

How to score it: Add up the numbers you circled (don't be concerned about which column they're listed in). The higher your score, the safer and healthier you are. Track your progress each week to see if you're getting better or worse. Strive to keep increasing your score.

Try Three Sessions of Creating Change to See If You Like It!

A super opportunity—try up to three sessions of Creating Change and then decide if you want to continue.

Creating Change is counseling that helps you explore your past.

Examples of topics:

- "Honor Your Survival"
- "What You Want People to Understand"
- "Listen to Your Body"
- "Relationship Patterns"
- "Your Personal Truth"
- "Influences: Family, Community, Culture"

It's a compassionate approach that addresses challenges you've faced. You share only what you choose to and go at your own pace.

Creating Change was developed at Harvard Medical School and Boston University School of Medicine by Lisa M. Najavits, PhD. It's an evidence-based model for trauma and/or addiction, which means that it shows positive results in scientific studies.

Just as a "picture is worth a thousand words," experiencing it is the best way to see if it can help you.

If you want to continue after three sessions, you can keep going. If not, that's OK, too. There's no one right way—there's only the way that's right for you, right now.

Interested? Speak to the staff.

You can also learn more at **www.creating-change.org.**

From *Creating Change* by Lisa M. Najavits. Copyright © 2024 Lisa M. Najavits. Published by The Guilford Press. Permission to photocopy this material, or to download and print additional copies (*www.guilford.com/najavits3-materials*), is granted to purchasers of this book for use with your own clients or patients; see copyright page for details.

Certificate of Achievement

CERTIFICATE OF ACHIEVEMENT

Awarded to

_____

For attending ____ of ____ available sessions of the *Creating Change* treatment

Presented by

_____

on the date:

_____

Further Information about Creating Change

Please visit the website **www.creating-change.org**. It provides implementation resources (including the *Creating Change Fidelity Scale*), training information, research updates, and downloadable articles.

From *Creating Change* by Lisa M. Najavits. Copyright © 2024 Lisa M. Najavits. Published by The Guilford Press. Permission to photocopy this material, or to download and print additional copies (*www.guilford.com/najavits3-materials*), is granted to purchasers of this book for use with your own clients or patients; see copyright page for details.

4

The Counselor

What your giving can do is to help your [clients] be braver, be better than they are, be open to the world again. . . . Maybe you can give her something from deep within to find or do or fight for that will break the trance for her. You'll have to find this first within you, though. And then you'll have it to give away. This woman may get to wake up. And then she will have something to give, a song to sing. Maybe it won't be a song exactly, but maybe just a little tune, a calliope tune, the tune of survival.

~Anne Lamott, 20th-century American author, *Bird by Bird*

This quotation, relevant across genders, speaks to the profound influence of a helping relationship. The counselor is one of the most important elements in a treatment such as this. The materials are inert until brought to life in sessions. Indeed, research suggests that, in general, counselor factors are more important than client factors or treatment models (Castonguay & Hill, 2017; Najavits & Strupp, 1994; Najavits & Weiss, 1994).

Counselors bring different backgrounds to the work. Some are already doing past-focused treatment but without a formal model. Creating Change offers resources to enhance that. Others are trained in past-focused trauma models, such as exposure or EMDR, but not in addiction. Some are addiction specialists who have strong knowledge of trauma but haven't yet tried past-focused counseling. Creating Change aims to make the most of your expertise, whatever that is.

No specific degree, experience, training, or licensure is required to conduct Creating Change, for reasons described in Chapter 1. But it's helpful to explore counselor aspects that are relevant throughout the treatment.

This chapter has two parts:

- Best practices in treating addiction and trauma
- Positive processes

See also Chapter 1, the section "Key Principles."

BEST PRACTICES IN TREATING ADDICTION AND TRAUMA

It's said that "[e]ven if you think you're not treating clients with addiction or trauma, you are." That is, many clients are not formally assessed for addiction or trauma problems but are suffering from them, unknown.

Trauma used to be treated only in mental health settings and addiction only in addiction settings. But recent decades have seen the emergence of a no-wrong-door approach—the willingness to treat both regardless of clients' point of entry, whether medical settings, criminal justice, schools, specialty clinics, veterans programs, faith-based communities, homelessness programs or outreach. Any entryway can be an opportunity to help, a "golden moment."

As part of this shift, it's now expected that counselors will address both trauma and addiction. Yet many training programs don't address both, and systems that are stretched thin often don't provide adequate support in working with these complex, multiply challenged clients.

The best practices here briefly summarize the current state-of-the-art, no matter which specific treatment model you're conducting. Most counselors have strengths on some, but others may be new or surprising.

Also, if desired, see Appendix B online, "Comparison of all Models Studied for PTSD/SUD" (*www.guilford.com/najavits3-materials*), for implementation information on key treatment models.

Best Practices in Addiction Treatment

★ *Star those you're already doing; circle any you want to improve.*

- ***Ask about addictive behavior at each session:*** amount, frequency, and type. This is part of the check-in for Creating Change. If a client says, "I drank," the follow-up questions would be "How much and how often?"

- ***Learn addiction concepts*** such as *denial, enabling, withdrawal, tolerance, dry versus sober, set versus relapse, harm reduction, moderation management, controlled use, the 12 steps, sponsor, hitting bottom, the pink cloud, chasing losses, co-occurring disorders.* Be able to specify the major classes of recreational drugs and to list various behavioral addictions. Know what amount of alcohol counts as a *standard drink.*

- ***Understand what addiction is and isn't.*** A brief definition is a person *can't stop, even if it's causing serious problems* (physical, social, legal, emotional, or occupational). Sometimes it's assumed people must be addicted if they use certain types of substances, such as hard drugs; or use alone or every day; or as a way to change a mood such as to relax or feel better. People with these behaviors *may* have an addiction but need formal assessment as these don't signify addiction per se. So too a person may be physically dependent on a substance, such as an opioid for pain, yet not meet criteria for substance use disorder. See formal definitions online, for example, *substance use disorder, gambling disorder, binge eating disorder.*

- ***Avoid ultimatums*** ("I will not treat you if . . . ") until most other methods have been tried. Ultimatums in addiction treatment are generally best as a last resort rather than a starting point. Rather than an awakening after "hitting bottom," the bottom may just keep dropping, especially when co-occurring mental health problems are present.

- ***Don't insist that clients have to be motivated to work on addiction.*** Motivation is often the *result* of good treatment rather than the start of it. Many clients enter addiction treatment due to coercion of some kind (the threat of losing an important relationship or job; child custody issues; or being mandated by a court). Research shows that treatment doesn't have to be voluntary to be successful (NIDA, 2018). Keep in mind that early in treatment many clients don't perceive an addiction problem even if it's obvious to others.

- ***Recognize that addiction isn't just a reflection of "deeper issues."*** If a client has addiction, treat it directly. For most of the 20th century, addiction was ignored based on the idea that treating deep-rooted psychodynamics would resolve the addiction (Najavits & Weiss, 1994). Even now, some counselors believe that if trauma is treated, addiction will heal, but research doesn't support this (Najavits et al., 2020; Simpson et al., 2021). In short, whatever problems the person has—addiction, PTSD, or other conditions—treat each in its own right.

* ***Have a written contract with agreed-on limits.*** Depending on your setting and client, the contract could specify *abstinence* (no use); *harm reduction* (gradual decrease in use); or *controlled use*, also known as *moderation management* (setting limits to return to a safe level of use). The plan will depend on the type of addiction (e.g., one can be abstinent from drugs but not from food), and the philosophy of your program or practice. The Seeking Safety topic "When Substances Control You" provides an example contract.

* ***Don't take it personally when clients relapse.*** Addiction, when severe, is considered a chronic relapsing disorder just like medical conditions such as diabetes (McLellan, Lewis, O'Brien, & Kleber, 2000). Expressing frustration or disappointment moves the focus away from the client. Notice your reactions but find ways to manage them and get support so you can be fully present as a helper. And praise clients for being honest about their use.

* ***Convey that there are many ways to recover.*** Remember the phrase "many roads, one journey" (Kasl, 1992). Whenever possible, let clients choose among options rather than forcing one path. (But always respect program policies, which may include mandatory AA or other treatment.) Also adapt treatment as needed for subgroups such as adolescents, veterans, and minorities.

* ***Educate clients that the more addiction treatment they attend, the more likely they are to recover.*** Refer them to as much as they're willing to do. Note too that outpatient treatment is generally just as effective as inpatient (Finney, Hahn, & Moos, 1996). To help find referrals, see Handout 2 in the topic "Trust versus Doubt," which has national toll-free numbers and websites. (In Seeking Safety, topics that help with referrals are "Introduction to Treatment/Case Management" and "Community Resources.")

* ***If clients have moderate or severe addiction, refer them for a medication evaluation,*** preferably by a psychiatrist or nurse practitioner who specializes in addiction. Clients may benefit from addiction-related medications such as Antabuse, naltrexone, methadone, and acamprosate, as well as antidepressants and other medication for mental illness. Medication was often viewed as another form of addiction in the past but is now understood as a positive part of treatment if given by a reputable professional and taken as prescribed.

* ***Create*** **addiction-informed care** ***in your setting.*** This term isn't common but, like *trauma-informed care*, the goal is to bring awareness of positive treatment principles to all levels of an organization. It means all clients are screened for substance and behavioral addictions, and all staff learn about addiction and how to interact with addiction clients in positive ways (especially as addiction is so stigmatized).

* ***Respond to addictive behavior with concern and problem solving,*** rather than harshness or judgment. People with addiction typically hate themselves for not being able to stop and have already heard negative messages from others, so additional negativity is unlikely to change their behavior. Engage addiction clients with motivational principles such as *roll with resistance, avoid argumentation,* and *express empathy.*

* ***Know that clients will lie to you at times*** no matter how skilled you are and how strong your connection. It's the nature of the illness. Clients also lie to themselves (denial, rationalizing).

* ***Be prepared for worsening.*** Ups and downs, and occasional slips (single unplanned addictive behaviors), are common. But significant worsening suggests a higher level of care. Criteria from the NIDA study project manual (Crits-Christoph et al., 1997) are as follows:

1. An increase in drinking or drug use above the participant's baseline level
2. The addition of new substances not used at intake
3. Engaging in new risky behaviors such as driving while intoxicated
4. Serious threat of harm to self or others, with a plan and intent

See also the section "Watch for Progress and Worsening" in Chapter 3.

- ***Understand* symptom substitution.** It means replacing one addiction with another ("I started gambling when I stopped drinking").
- ***Become familiar with self-help resources*** and attend at least one meeting to get a sense of how powerful they can be (anyone can do this). Twelve-step programs include AA and Narcotics Anonymous and other variations. Alternatives to 12-step groups include Smart Recovery, Refuge Recovery, and Women for Sobriety. In general, *encourage* but don't require self-help groups unless your agency requires it (see "Avoid ultimatums" on page 77). For family and friends, Al-Anon, Alateen (for adolescents), and Adult Children of Alcoholics are excellent. Also stay sensitive to how the 12 steps can be applied to trauma survivors (Marich, 2012).
- ***Obtain medical clearance or detoxification for severe or chronic substance addiction.*** It may not be safe for clients to suddenly stop using on their own. A severe alcoholic could be at risk for seizures, for example. Consult with medical personnel as needed.
- ***Conduct urine testing for severe substance addiction, if possible.*** It's an excellent tool if you can access it. Some agencies conduct tests or insurance companies may cover them. Some counselors are concerned that it may erode trust in the counseling relationship, but it signifies that you care enough to want to know what's really going on and allows you to do your best, most informed work.
- ***Understand the biological basis of addiction.*** Addiction is no longer seen simply as a failure of will, replacement for relationships, or learned habit, although these can all play a role. Some people are genetically more vulnerable than others. There are also brain changes that occur with chronic use, and substances vary in their addictive potential (e.g., cocaine is more addictive than marijuana).
- ***If a client doesn't accept the term* addiction, *use others.*** *Addiction* can seem extreme and raise clients' defenses. There's also no single definition of addiction, although DSM-5-TR has a few specific ones (substance use disorder, gambling disorder, binge eating disorder). Use those when relevant; for other types you can refer to *excessive behavior* or a *behavior that gets you into trouble*. But remember some excessive behaviors are not addictions, such as sleeping too much (which may be a sign of depression). See the Excessive Behavior Scale (Handout 4 of the extra topic "Understanding Trauma and Addiction"); it screens for all types of addictions but omits the word *addiction*.
- ***Explore how addiction interacts with trauma*** and other mental health issues. Monitor, and help clients notice, how improvement or worsening in one domain impacts the other and how they developed over time.
- ***Be prepared for your own complex feelings***, including strong attachment and identification; sadness and disappointment when relapse occurs; helplessness at not being able to do more; frustration and judgment at times; and loss related to client overdose or suicide. If you're in recovery from addiction, recognize too how that may have an impact, both positive and negative.
- ***Screen all clients for addiction.*** Use valid measures and, for anyone who screens positive, follow up with a full diagnostic assessment. An example of a free, brief scale for clinical use is the Brief Addiction Monitor, which assesses substance use and related problems. It's available from *https://arc.psych.wisc.edu/self-report*, which also lists other self-report scales for addiction and mental health.
- ***Offer education about addiction to clients and their families.*** Examples of reputable websites include www.rethinkingdrinking.niaaa.nih.gov and www.samhsa.gov. It's also useful to invite safe family members to at least one session to help inform your work, to offer resources, and to help them get to know you so they can reach out if the client worsens.
- ***Cross-train in addiction.*** Learn more via websites and courses. Even if addiction is not

your specialty area, you can gain basic education and referral options. An excellent starting place is SAMHSA's evidence-based practice resource center (*www.samhsa.gov/resource-search/ebp*).

✎ ***Consider joining a professional organization focused on addiction***. Most professions have subgroups on it, including for trainees and students, and there are also national and international organizations.

Best Practices in Trauma Treatment

★ Star those you're already doing; circle any you want to improve.

✎ ***Learn trauma concepts*** such as *dissociation, reenactment, moral injury, retraumatization, Stockholm syndrome, simple versus complex PTSD, secondary traumatization, foreshortened future, PTSD symptom clusters, splitting,* and *betrayal trauma*.

✎ ***Monitor trauma symptoms*** during treatment and help clients learn to identify them, such as dissociation, triggering, numbness, and reenactments.

✎ ***Refer clients for a medication evaluation.*** Some medications help trauma symptoms. Even if clients are unsure about taking a medication, encourage them to explore options so they can make an informed choice.

✎ ***Notice how trauma shows up in behavior.*** Self-destructive and "difficult" behavior (power struggles, rage, low motivation, poor self-care) can be a repetition of the trauma experience or attempts at self-protection.

✎ ***Don't require addiction to be reduced before addressing trauma.*** However, do choose a model that's safe to do, especially for severe clients (Bailey et al., 2019). Consider *integrated* treatments that help clients understand linkages between trauma and addiction.

✎ ***Highlight trauma themes in counseling.*** Themes include trust, power, control, safety, and betrayal, for example. Clients may not directly connect these to trauma, especially if they're in an addiction program that doesn't address trauma. Guide them to see how trauma has played a role in their life and relationships.

✎ ***Use an empowerment approach*** to help counteract the powerlessness of trauma. Offer choices and convey optimism. Yet hold clients accountable for their actions—trauma isn't an *excuse* but may be an *explanation* for problematic behaviors.

✎ ***Be sensitive to trauma but don't overprotect clients or lower standards.*** They need to adapt to realities that will help them grow, such as getting a job, taking responsibility for self-care, and working with staff of all genders. These can be therapeutic if done with support and guidance. Yet it's also important to adapt treatment to be trauma-sensitive, such as allowing a client to leave lights on at night to feel safer while sleeping in a residential program (Chu, 1992; SAMHSA, 2014).

✎ ***Respect clients' choice on confronting and/or forgiving the perpetrator.*** Some clients benefit from taking these steps, but they can also backfire emotionally. Help clients understand that they can recover without confronting and/or forgiving. (Forgiving *themselves*, however, is important for healing.) The topic "What You Want People to Understand" addresses these issues in detail.

✎ ***Maintain boundaries.*** Complex trauma clients may attempt boundary violations, such as wanting a special relationship with the counselor or probing for a lot of personal information. Respond with boundaried compassion.

✎ ***Understand mind–body connections in trauma.*** The brain and other body systems change in response to trauma, including heightened reactivity and difficulty regulating emotion (van der Kolk, 2014). And genetics studies show that children of parents with PTSD are more likely to develop PTSD if exposed to trauma. Help clients learn to recognize body sensations that relate to trauma and how to calm their mind and body.

The Counselor

* ***Be flexible with approaches.*** There are many paths to healing and many models. (See Chapter 2.) Ensure that you don't convey a message that there's just one right model or best way. Watch for clients' response to treatment and adjust as needed.

* ***Recognize that addictive behavior does "solve" trauma problems in the short term,*** such as getting to sleep or feeling more energy, but in the long term it's not a solution, of course. Become curious about clients' reasons for using. As Mate (2022) says, "It's not what's wrong with the addiction but what's right about it."

* ***If you have a trauma history, recognize its impact on your work,*** for better and worse. You may be more sympathetic to clients, for example, but also more triggered by them.

* ***Be prepared for intense dynamics.*** Clients may engage in push–pull control struggles; splitting; and unconscious reenactment of key trauma roles (*victim, perpetrator, bystander, rescuer*). These can occur both in the client's life and in the counseling relationship, especially with complex, long-term cases. Yet even amid such challenges, stay aware of positive dynamics, too, such as clients' ability to create attachments and their desire for growth.

* ***Screen all clients for trauma, PTSD, and related disorders,*** such as *acute stress disorder* and *dissociative identity disorder*. Use valid measures and, for anyone who screens positive, follow up with a full diagnostic assessment. Also, don't delay trauma-related assessment. In earlier times, programs would wait until a criterion was met (abstinence from substances, a strong therapeutic alliance, etc.). The current standard of care is to conduct universal, immediate assessment to help guide treatment planning.

* ***Create trauma-informed care in your setting.*** In addition to screening (per the paragraph above), educate all staff about trauma so they can be aware of it when interacting with clients. Download a free, detailed guide on trauma-informed care by SAMHSA, *Treatment Improvement Protocol #57, Trauma-Informed Care in Behavioral Health Services* (2014), which is easily found online.

* ***Refer families to trauma resources.*** For example, see the SAMHSA National Child Traumatic Stress Initiative (*www.samhsa.gov/child-trauma*); the National Child Traumatic Stress Network (*www.nctsn.org*); and for veterans, *www.ptsd.va.gov*.

* ***Cross-train in trauma.*** Learn more via websites and courses. An excellent starting place is SAMHSA's Evidence-Based Resource Center (*www.samhsa.gov/resource-search/ebp*).

* ***Consider joining a professional association that focuses on trauma.*** Some professions have subgroups on trauma, including for students, and there are also national and international trauma-specific organizations (e.g., *www.colleaga.org/article/list-ptsd-organizations-and-resources*).

POSITIVE PROCESSES

Working with clients who have trauma or addiction can be much more effective if you sharpen not only the techniques you use, but also the way you use them, your posture or style. In addition to *what* you do, the *how* is equally important.

Express Empathy Directly

It's essential to *actively* convey warm support for the client. It's not enough to offer a silent supportive presence or stay neutral. The nature of trauma and addiction is that clients were too often alone—abandoned and rejected by others, or isolated due to mental illness. Thus, part of healing is not to feel this same loneliness when they talk about the past. One client said: "When a person is feeling despair, what helps is validation of their pain, knowing they're not alone . . . and understanding that grief is part of the healing process" (Jennings & Ralph, 1997, p. 29).

Every session, offer kindness and reassurance:

- "It takes real courage to do this."
- "I feel honored to hear your story."
- "I can hear the sadness in your voice."
- "I believe you can heal."
- "It feels hard, but it really will get better."
- "I'm so sorry that happened to you."
- "I know this isn't easy."

At times, empathy means accepting that the client's view is different from yours. A client may feel happy when his abusive father dies, or positive about divorce, abortion, losing a job, or other events. Strive to understand clients' perspective, rather than imposing your own point of view. One can empathize without agreeing ("I hear you feel happy that your father died").

Honor Your Past, Too

As you help clients face their past, also honor your own history. You may have experienced trauma or addiction and everyone has, by living, experienced loss, pain, and disappointment. Counselors who honor their history recognize the strengths it can bring to the work, such as empathy and the ability to handle crises calmly. But it can also have negative impact if not sufficiently processed (taking on clients' hopelessness or feeling triggered). Indeed, the concept of the *wounded healer* goes back to ancient times and in the modern era has been a core theme in the helping professions (White, 1998). The wounded healer is double-edged: having both great strengths and potential weaknesses. Some professional contexts also heighten the connection between self, suffering, and work: when counselors endure a community-wide trauma along with their clients (such as the COVID-19 pandemic) or are traumatized at work (physical assault by a client). Whatever the context, respect your personal history and recognize how it impacts your professional life. As Horowitz wrote,

> Rare are the practitioners who are themselves untouched by the pain of loss. We must remember and perhaps relive the meaning of those moments in our lives to share deeply the anguish of our patients, who never find themselves far from reminders of the losses they have suffered. The more we keep alive memories of our own moments of vulnerability, the more vital and authentic is the support we render grief-stricken men and women embattled with mental illness. The quest for meaning is, in the last judgment, a shared journey. (2002, p. 243)

Encourage Rather Than Push

The counselor has a lot of power in the counseling situation. It's important not to misuse that power by conveying, directly or indirectly, that clients should reveal more than they're ready to reveal, focus on the past when they prefer to stay in the present, or forgive someone who hurt them. The dilemma is that clients may benefit from facing topics they've been avoiding. A balanced approach is to encourage and educate, but not push beyond what feels right to them. This approach also has the advantage of not activating defensiveness (they may feel slow or stupid for not being able to move faster). With the rise of trauma-informed care, there's greater recognition that clients need to be allowed to keep details private if they want to, even in programs that rely on principles of openness such as addiction therapeutic communities. Similarly, in the mental health field, counselors trained in classic trauma models are taught not to let clients "avoid" trauma material. Although clinically sound (avoiding painful material prevents processing of it), counselors need to adjust to the complexities of comorbid clients. In Creating Change, there's a distinction between *self-protection* that's healthy versus unhealthy. Healthy self-protection respects clients' need to pace themselves in sharing about the past. It empowers them to choose what to share and helps them gain trust so they'll want to share. *Unhealthy self-protection* is staying stuck too long, unable to move forward in addressing what needs to be addressed, even a little, with anyone. This is described further in Chapter 3 and the topic "Respect Your Defenses." In sum, rather than pushing, strive to encourage, evoke, and inspire clients to change.

Stay Real

There's a fine line between support and excessive support. Clients benefit from genuine responses, not from sentimentality or "sugar coating" what happened. As Nichols and Zax observe: "It is not therapeutic simply to have patients speak freely and have everything they say accepted and seemingly validated by the therapist. . . . [T]herapy involves urging the patient to reexperience emotionally distressing events; the therapist then accepts the feelings and encourages further exploration. . . . [I]t is important to discuss this material rationally, and for the therapist to suggest alternate ways of perceiving and acting" (1977, pp. 212–213).

As adults, clients may have made choices that led to trauma even though that wasn't their intent, such as driving drunk or walking alone in a dangerous area if they didn't have to. Addiction too can involve poor judgment ("I'll just have one"). This doesn't mean clients *ever* deserve or should be blamed for what happened, but this may be an opportunity for them to learn to protect themselves more. Convey that you're on their side in helping to understand the past, but not at the expense of the truth. Some counselors become so consumed with "It's not your fault" that they miss opportunities to explore adult self-protection that's essential for empowerment and survival. Also, it's essential to distinguish adults from children: Children were too young to protect themselves or to have the cognitive capacity to assess danger. Similarly, some adult traumas could never have been prevented. Thus, always bring sensitivity to the context.

Sustain Hope

Hope is a lifeline that makes the work possible. A wonderful image is "hope as horizon"—like the horizon in the distance, hope beckons clients to do the work they need to do in treatment (Miller 1999). Especially for clients who feel persistent and deep despair, it's essential to offer hope, both in words and in your loyalty to the treatment. Clients have said, "People who have believed in me have been the ones who have been helpful," and the best counselors "are always hopeful for me even when they are seriously concerned" (Jennings & Ralph, 1997, p. 38). Clients who are hopeful may be able to access more of themselves and persist when it's most difficult. Yet for counselors to inspire hope, they need to feel it themselves. There's a parallel process in which counselors' ability to sustain hope becomes mirrored in their clients. As one counselor put it, "Hope in treatment is like the Olympic Torch—it must remain lit regardless of weather conditions."

Respond to Moral Injury

When a client has been betrayed by others, the counselor can't stay neutral about the right or wrong of what happened (Chu, 1992; Herman, 1992). A child who was raped, a refugee displaced by war, a woman battered by her partner, or a citizen tortured by his government need to hear that these represent serious breaches of ethics and normal life. This has been called *moral injury, betrayal of what's right,* and *betrayal trauma* (Litz et al., 2009; Shay, 1994). The counselor needs to ally with the client's sense of injustice:

- "No child deserved that."
- "The torture was a breakdown of justice."
- "Nothing you did meant that he had the right to attack you."
- "You should never have had to live through that."

Some traumas are more likely to require this moral stance than others. A natural disaster rarely needs moral affirmation, while interpersonal trauma usually does.

There are also clients who have betrayed or harmed others, sometimes as part of their addiction, who may need to feel remorse and make amends. Twelve-step programs can be very healing as some of the steps help clients address harm they did to others (e.g., steps 4, 5, 8, and 9). When clients have betrayed others, don't criticize their actions. Instead, allow clients to explore the feelings and meanings the event holds for them so they can ultimately reach their own conclusions about what they did. So too, it's important not to simply "excuse" or discount clients' behavior. Litz et al. (2009) write, "Psychotherapists are often too eager to relieve guilt, and, thereby, undermine the patient's need to feel remorseful. This may invalidate [the patient's] thoughts and beliefs about the event or be distracting or annoying. The goal is to help patients consider more useful and contextual appraisals. [They] may first need the experience of telling another person about the event, without it being excused, and still be viewed as a person of value" (2009, p. 703).

Encourage "One Foot in the Present, One in the Past"

Creating Change emphasizes a healthy balance between present and past. Although rare, some clients become immersed in the past to the point that they neglect responsibilities or become over-attached to suffering or the "victim" role. Such phenomena have been observed repeatedly in the literature on past-focused treatment (Chu, 1992; Nichols & Zax, 1977). To maintain a healthy balance between present and past, there are various options in Creating Change, including grounding at the end of sessions; letting clients share only what they choose to, which helps regulate intensity; and offering options for both present- and past-focused commitments (homework). It's also recommended that clients have structure in their day and attend present-focused treatments if needed, such as Seeking Safety or RP.

Be Open to Feedback

This work requires ongoing learning for both client and counselor. Part of the counselor's job is thus to be able to hear and respond to feedback. Positive feedback is easy. Negative feedback—complaints, concerns, criticism—can be hard, yet is essential for adapting the treatment productively. Unfortunately, counselors who take criticism personally or feel insulted by it lose this opportunity for improvement. They also convey a message to clients, all too familiar to some, that they should just keep quiet and go along. Instead, gracefully accept the critique ("Thanks for sharing your feedback") and strive to understand it. Sometimes, it may reflect the client's issues and it's part of the work to see that clearly. At other times, you may have erred and should honestly own up to that. Often, it relates to both of you. Some counselors use supervision or a journal to process feedback. You can also read more about how to make productive use of feedback (Stone & Heen, 2015).

Maintain Boundaries

The addiction and mental health fields have historically had very different approaches to boundaries. The addiction field arose mostly as a grassroots phenomenon of AA and therapeutic communities, with generally looser boundaries. Addiction counselors routinely self-disclose about their own recovery and sometimes spend recreational time with clients as part of the program. There's a more informal style and greater use of paraprofessionals. The mental health field, and trauma programs in particular, generally have stricter boundaries. Counselors don't routinely disclose their history, informal contact is discouraged, and there's less use of paraprofessionals.

In working with trauma and addiction, some boundaries are always clear, such as no sexual contact or violations of confidentiality. Other boundaries are a judgment call. It's generally advised to maintain firm boundaries with trauma survivors, who may misinterpret a benign pat on the shoulder as "Is my counselor coming onto me?" So too, stay aware of "pulls" by the client. Chu observes that some clients with early, complex trauma histories may "seem oblivious to the need for boundaries and may even invite inappropriate roles that feel 'normal' to them. . . . Many competent, experienced therapists . . . fail to set adequate limits . . . [and] may tolerate a slow pattern of escalating demands and only become aware of the consequences when they find themselves overwhelmed by them" (1992, p. 363).

Maintain boundaries and seek supervision if concerning issues arise. Counselors can become ensnared in clients' intense dynamics and find themselves doing or saying things they normally wouldn't. Such processes are often subtle and easy to miss as they're happening.

Be Careful with Self-Disclosure

Related to the point above, consider carefully whether to self-disclose about your own experiences. A helpful guideline is not to disclose unless the client asks for information, and even then be cautious about what you reveal. Clients with addiction or trauma often played the role of *parentified child*—having to parent their own caretakers by taking care of them emotionally, physically, or otherwise. Although you may intend a disclosure to be helpful, it can be misinterpreted as "My therapist needs me to listen to him," "Here I am again taking care of everyone around me." If a client asks a personal question ("Are you married?," "Do you have kids?," "Have you had trauma?"), you can convey that you have a general policy with all clients: "I appreciate that you want to know more about me, but I'm here to help you. I don't share about my life with any client because I think the focus needs to remain on your issues." Even if it's a question you feel comfortable answering, such as your own trauma or addiction recovery, still try to find out what it means to the client. Some counselors believe that disclosing will gain them credibility. But if clients view their addiction or trauma as a weakness, they may then view you as weak or flawed too.

Watch for Reenactments

Some clients re-create the past in the counseling relationship. The more severe clients' history, the more likely this is. If they were treated with contempt, they may express contempt toward you. They may "mind read" based on their past ("You think I'm weak and pathetic"). They may emotionally repeat the trauma roles of *victim*, *perpetrator*, *bystander*, or *rescuer*, especially in group treatment (adapted from Karpman, 1968). Rather than taking such repetitions personally, feeling offended or defensive, use these moments therapeutically. Help clients reality-test and recognize hidden assumptions derived from their past. Provide an opportunity for them to experience healthy resolution of conflicts.

Take Care of Yourself

Being a counselor calls for being emotionally present. This is a career where you can't separate the work from who you are as a person. It also means each new client can influence you one way or another. As Jung wrote: "For two personalities to meet is like mixing two different chemical substances; if there is any combination at all, both are transformed. In any effective psychological treatment the doctor is bound to influence the patient, but this influence can only take place if the patient has a reciprocal influence on the doctor" (1966, p. 71).

Much of this influence may be positive and growth-enhancing. But letting clients into your emotional world can also overwhelm you with their pain. Some counselors develop symptoms resembling trauma, known as *secondary* or *vicarious trauma*, with work-related nightmares and depression. "The pain, isolation, and despair of abuse survivors can be contagious" (Chu, 1992, p. 368). You likely also have professional stressors, such as insurance and financial constraints, working with colleagues who don't understand trauma or addiction, and trying to help clients with repeated relapses and low motivation. You may develop burnout or compassion fatigue, feeling you have no more to give. Rather than a sign of weakness, it's usually the most caring and dedicated counselors who develop such issues. To give all to others and lose oneself is common in the helping professions.

Stay aware of how the work affects you. You can only be effective if you're emotionally present, but doing so can leave you vulnerable to reduced emotional capacity. The task then is to take good care of yourself and to follow all the good advice you've heard: seek rest and help when needed, listen to your body, and find ways to leave the work when you go home (Briere & Scott, 2014). Most counselors value this work—the opportunity to make a difference, the learning, the sense of connection with others, and the inside view of the human experience. To stay on these positive sides of the equation, *take care of yourself*. Creating Change reinforces self-care for both counselors and clients by its strong emphasis on pacing and flexibility, which provides modulation of intensity that's especially important when working with complex clients, and addiction and trauma together (Sterman, 2006).

The following resources may also be helpful:

1. The Professional Quality of Life Health Measure, which assesses compassion satisfaction, perceived support, burnout, secondary traumatic stress, and moral distress (Center for Victims of Torture, 2021). It's free, brief, and validated and can be completed online or downloaded (*https://proqol.org/proqol-health-measure*).
2. Workaholics Anonymous, as lack of self-care may reflect work addiction for some counselors (*www.workaholics-anonymous.org*).

Know You'll Make Mistakes

Comedian Stephen Wright said, "Experience is something you don't get until just after you need it." Counselors at all levels make mistakes that are only clear afterward, such as saying something harsh in a stressful moment, reacting too much or too little, or not listening closely enough. Moreover, with treatment manuals, there's sometimes a sense that if you follow them with fidelity, the treatment will succeed, with little discussion of negative impact or ways it may fall short. But no matter how skilled and caring you are, and how good a treatment manual you use, there will be mistakes. The key is to acknowledge them as soon as possible, apologize to the client if needed, and put in place corrective action, such as referring clients to additional care.

Respect Clients' Choices in the Work

Throughout Creating Change, there's no one right way but many. Clients can share small or larger aspects of their past, easier or harder parts, chronologically or out of order, focused on one event or several. So too, clients don't have to be at a high level of emotion. Some need to experience what it's like to share at all as vulnerability may be new for them, or they may not yet be ready to acknowledge the full reality of their story. A positive treatment experience in which they share, at their own pace and in their own way, builds their long-term capacity to express more. As one trauma survivor describes it:

> Ultimately, we heal ourselves, find our own paths. So, when we're lost in the middle of our ugly, scary forests, it's not helpful for a therapist to just stand outside of it, at a safe distance, and (metaphorically speaking) yell, 'This way!' because that may not be the direction we need to take. I think good therapists are willing to stand with us in that forest and witness our experience. They provide a second pair of eyes on the situation, teach navigation skills, and accept that progress will most likely be made using a hybrid of our perceptions/skills and theirs. (Trauma Survivors Share Tips for Therapists Dealing with Trauma, *www.giftfromwithin.org*)

Build an Alliance—But More Than That, Too

A therapeutic alliance (positive working relationship between the client and counselor) is essential for effective counseling of any kind. (And there's a brief validated scale to measure it in the extra topic "Your Relationships.") However, it's sometimes said that because the alliance is so important, it's all that's needed or that it's the main ingredient in treatment, but this is not accurate (Cuijpers, Reijnders, & Huibers, 2019). Alliance per se isn't enough to resolve trauma or addiction, especially if they're chronic or severe. Research shows that supportive therapy alone isn't effective for PTSD, for example (Lewis, Roberts, Andrew, Starling, & Bison, 2020). Well-developed treatment manuals, psychoeducation, and specific techniques are also needed. Indeed, these components help build the alliance because clients perceive them as beneficial and they convey that the counselor has expertise to offer.

Bring Compassion to Complex Dynamics

The more complex the clients, the more likely that challenging dynamics will arise. As Davis describes it: "Substance abusing trauma survivors often engage in styles of relating that strain the therapeutic relationship [such as] blaming others, being the victim, being disconnected from oneself, one's emotions and others, being noncompliant or oppositional. . . . These clients often inappropriately blame themselves for their trauma, and yet can't take responsibility for their current behaviors and feelings" (2006, pp. 64–65). Such patterns, Davis notes, are usually an attempt to cope with painful feelings.

A list of key challenging dynamics is provided below, but it's important to understand them with compassion. They may or may not arise with your clients, but if they do, effective responses include education, skill building, limit setting, exploration, and referral to more treatment.

- *Regression.* The client becomes dependent and childlike rather than more mature; it may reflect the client's age when a disturbing event occurred, such as trauma.
- *Continual crisis.* The client seems "addicted to drama"—leaving treatment abruptly, fired from jobs, explosive relationship breakups.
- *Paranoia.* The client may perceive you as the abuser, for example. Paranoia is also a side effect of some substances.
- *Destructive behavior.* This may be directed toward self or others (self-injury, assault, emotional abuse), or general recklessness such as driving drunk.
- *Walking into danger.* The client lacks an instinct for self-protection and repeatedly gets involved with harmful people and situations.

- *Externalizing/internalizing.* The client takes too little or too much responsibility—distancing from actions as if not responsible, or harsh self-blame over small flaws.
- *Poor self-care.* The client doesn't keep up with basics such as hygiene and reasonable diet.
- *Provoking others.* The client speaks in ways that appear designed to shock or get attention rather than to process real issues, or the client alienates others in group through negativity or confrontation.
- *Lashing out.* The client pushes others away, blows up in anger, rejects help.
- *Entitlement.* Nothing feels like enough; the counselor and others give and give, but it's a "bottomless pit" with little appreciation.
- *Overidentification with the victim role.* The client talks a lot about the past but doesn't seem to actually be working on it. Rather than movement, there's stagnation and overattachment to the past to avoid growth.
- *Failure of empathy.* The client can't take others' perspective; may ignore others' needs; may justify criminal behavior.

These patterns usually reflect early, repeated trauma; chronic and severe addiction; and co-occurring disorders. They may also be based in current stress, personality, how the client was raised, and other factors—a big "soup" of many influences.

In Creating Change, clients can present with such issues yet still do fine. Indeed, getting a chance to talk about the past can reduce some of these patterns. Next, you'll find more guidance for handling challenging dynamics.

Gently Interpret Negative Dynamics in Light of Trauma (When Possible)

When clients engage in negative processes, such as those described above, it helps to gently bring their attention to it in a face-saving way—through the lens of trauma. For example, if a client rarely participates in the session, you could say, "I notice you're often quiet in here. When people have been through a lot of trauma, they may become numb, feel shut down, and have no energy. Does that happen to you?" Or if a client keeps rejecting every suggestion, you might say, "I know you've had a really tough life. It may feel like nothing ever helps, so why bother trying. Does it feel that way for you?" These are framed as questions rather than statements to encourage clients to become curious about themselves. Of course, not every negative process relates to trauma but when it does, it helps clients "own" it rather than feeling judged (by you or themselves). Regardless of trauma, however, you never have to tolerate abusive or demeaning interactions; trauma isn't an excuse or a free pass.

Observe Your Reactions

Stay aware of what you're feeling (in mind, body, and heart) as you do the work. Sometimes you may feel emotions that clients can't yet let themselves feel: You become a temporary "container" for them (van Dijk et al., 2003, p. x). These can inform the counseling: noticing what you feel can help you guide clients to get in touch with their own feelings. At other times, your reactions may indicate parts of your own past that need healing. In communicating with clients, the goal is to be empathic yet professional. "We need to find the right balance between empathic responses to our clients' pain and professional distance that allows us to respond in a manner that is therapeutic for clients" (Foa & Rothbaum, 1998, p. 174). If the counselor expresses extremes of emotion during the session (shock, crying) or a lack of emotion (numbing, distancing), this will not serve clients. They may feel invalidated or think it's a cue to focus on you. As one client said, "Don't take on my feelings, for example, being scared when I'm scared. When that happens with a professional, I feel

I have to take care of them" (Jennings & Ralph, 1997, p. 38). Observe your reactions and transform them into responses that help clients, that relate to their needs.

Acknowledge Countertransference

At the deepest level of work, counselors acknowledge *countertransference*—their own emotional responses that reflect important truths about the treatment, clients, and themselves. It's typically evoked when treating severe or long-term clients. The term *countertransference* originated in traditional counseling models early in the 20th century. In CBT therapies, there's less focus on counselors' emotional reactions, but it's been described in terms of counselor *schemas*. It's a key aspect of counseling regardless of theoretical orientation.

What makes countertransference complicated is that it's a blend of counselor and client issues, and it can be confusing to tease apart how much comes from either source. The counselor and client each bring their own histories into the room and these at times collide or collude. The willingness to honestly explore such patterns is a sign of the highest level of counselor. As Horowitz eloquently observed: "Countertransference becomes a window or wall, either widening the therapist's experience of self, in turn deepening the connections to the client's reality, or erecting a barrier that prevents access to the internal experience of both patient and therapist" (2002, p. 240).

Some counseling perspectives suggest that with complex clients, such patterns *must* arise for clients to work through their deepest problems. They have to "bring into the room" the issues that cause problems on the outside, and these will naturally evoke emotional reactions in the counselor. If successfully acknowledged and resolved in the treatment, clients can see their patterns more clearly and act them out less in their lives. In contrast, with brief treatment, group modality, or less complex clients, counseling is often productive without such deeper resolution.

Countertransference is typically difficult to perceive. You may find yourself not knowing why you react as you do or trying to suppress uncomfortable reactions. You may not be aware of countertransference until it has taken a toll in the treatment. Once you see it, it may be painful or embarrassing, which is why it's hard to acknowledge.

Addiction and trauma tend to evoke opposite countertransference patterns (Najavits, 2002c). At the extremes, addiction evokes harshness and blame (typically, from frustration with clients who persist in addictive behavior), whereas trauma evokes overprotection and lack of accountability (typically, from empathy that's gone too far).

Remember, too, that counseling also evokes *positive* counselor responses—kindness, nurturance, protection, guidance, wisdom, and compassion. All of these can coexist with negative reactions and buffer the harder moments. Indeed, a study of counselors treating clients with trauma and addiction found they reported more gratification than difficulty in the work (Najavits, 2002b).

This section describes some common countertransference patterns in trauma and addiction counseling (Chu, 1992; Imhof, Hirsch, & Terenzi, 1983; Najavits et al., 1995; Pearlman & Saakvitne, 1995). The focus here is your own issues, but it's important to reiterate that in almost any countertransference pattern, the client's issues play a role, too. You will usually have more than one pattern, although they tend to be quite consistent as they represent automatic responses, typically based on how you were raised or your own life struggles. They are also heightened by outside stress such as a heavy workload, toxic work environment, or pressure to treat a client quickly.

All counselors have elements of these patterns at times; they're part of being human and doing this work. They become damaging when they remain unacknowledged or not used productively. The degree of difficulty will depend on how pervasive the pattern is—occasional (which is common and usually easy to repair) versus persistent (which can thoroughly derail the treatment). It will also depend on how soon the counselor sees the pattern and corrects it, either through self-reflection or in honest discussion with the client.

Superficial. Such counselors may be good-natured and build rapport but don't go deeper. They may focus just on support or surface issues, with too little exploration of challenging topics or accountability. Sessions may feel like a nice friendship rather than a growth-oriented emotional experience. Clients may like the counselor yet feel unsatisfied, sensing they should avoid difficult feelings and complaints. There may be an unstated pact in the room to keep things pleasant, at the cost of facing painful truths.

Overidentified. The counselor is empathic but becomes overattached or enmeshed and may have a sense that no one else truly understands the client. There's a loss of perspective, sometimes protecting the client from necessary growth (such as believing that the client can't hold a job or, for women, believing they can't work with male staff, when this may be possible with support and guidance).

Underidentified. The counselor becomes too detached, distant, gives up, or sees the client as "other." There's a lack of empathy and connection. It's been termed *failure to feel*. There may be negligence, such as not setting up a safety plan for a suicidal client or minimizing the client's experience ("It wasn't all that bad").

Constricted. Counselors with this pattern have a narrow emotional bandwidth and may find it hard to tolerate intense emotions in clients and in themselves. Directly or indirectly, they may convey that clients shouldn't cry or express strong feelings, especially negative ones.

Sentimental. This means not acknowledging the harsh, dark sides of life. Such counselors have difficulty with "ugly" emotions such as rage or revenge and too often feel a need to turn negatives into positives. They may express the opposite of what they're really feeling, such as becoming too nice when they're frustrated with a client. They may have trouble setting limits and being direct about sensitive topics.

Anxious. Anxious counselors have a need to know exactly how to do things, leading to excessive fear of mistakes and difficulty exploring possibilities. They may rely too much on others for guidance and lack access to their own intuitions. This may reflect emotional immaturity or being at an early stage in training. There's potential to grow out of it, although this doesn't always occur. Clients may feel they have to protect or emotionally care for anxious counselors.

Unfocused. Unfocused counselors aren't good at details or keeping track of things ("What was your homework?"). They veer off task, with sessions sometimes becoming chitchat. At times they miss big things such as follow-up on an important referral or a letter the client needs. The counselor operates from a childlike place, not accepting the full professional responsibilities that go with taking care of others. Clients may feel forgotten; there are too many loose ends.

Controlling. Some counselors have difficulty letting go. They push or coerce clients, unable to hear feedback or back off. They may pressure clients to forgive or confront a perpetrator, or to feel a particular way ("You have to get angry at him"). They can be inflexible with a do-it-my-way stance ("This worked for me, so you need to do it too"). In general, they react to the inherent uncertainty and confusion in clinical work by squashing those feelings in themselves and clients. This style disempowers clients and can create excessive dependency.

Narcissistic. This means focusing on one's own needs at the expense of the client. It includes pursuing details that aren't central to the task at hand (e.g., too many sexual questions or curiosity about a celebrity client). Narcissistic needs may be of any kind—intellectual, social, financial, sexual.

Sadistic. Every counselor has occasional moments of harsh feeling toward a client. It becomes a problem when it's persistent and destructive—put-downs, threats, or verbal abuse. These are more likely in settings prone to violence, such as corrections or institutions that serve a warehousing function with little treatment. The counselor may be burned out and view the client as less than human.

Evaluate Whether Creating Change Appeals to You

Exploration of the past is one of the most intimate types of therapy. Counselors who value it say it's some of the most meaningful work one can do—coming to know clients' darkest secrets, pain, and despair, as well as their strength and resilience in surviving. But counselors naturally have preferences for some types of work over others, for all sorts of reasons.

Give Creating Change a try, then honor your choice. Glance through the chapters. Try a variety of session topics with clients and/or role-play with colleagues to see how it feels. Some counselors find Creating Change appealing right from the start. Others are unsure but find it easier than expected once they try it. And some decide it's not for them.

Example 1. Niki is drawn to this work. Early in her career, she found she likes past-focused counseling. She knows people can overcome hardship because she's done that herself. She has compassion for clients' suffering while also being able to guide them into difficult topics. She's flexible and attentive to their multiple needs. She sets limits in a kind way. However, she isn't a "saint"—she sometimes becomes overinvolved and struggles with her own self-care. Her clients say they can tell her anything.

Example 2. Deirdre tried conducting past-focused counseling while in training. She appreciated learning it but quickly knew it wasn't for her. She's a fun-loving person who prefers to stay on the lighter side of life. When she conducts past-focused counseling, she feels uncomfortable asking clients to talk about upsetting topics. She prefers technical, structured clinical work, such as assessment. She's excellent at what she does and clients like her. But when she reads past-focused treatment manuals, she thinks, "I don't want to be doing that."

Notice Your Strengths

There are as many ways to do this work well as there are counselors. Everyone has a unique perspective that can bring it alive. There are also general strengths that are known to be helpful. No one has all of them all the time (it's important not to be perfectionistic), but the more they're present, the more the counseling will flourish. ★ *Check off any below you see in yourself.*

- Sustains hope, in clients and in themselves.
- Has experience processing painful experiences in one's own life.
- While growing up had at least one loving, nurturing caretaker.
- Is psychologically minded (interested in the inner lives of others).
- Holds to high standards, especially ethics, boundaries, and continued learning.
- Is sensitive to complex dynamics (e.g., unexpressed anger in oneself or clients).
- Can guide clients in and out of emotion.
- Wants to do this type of work.
- Feels drawn to clients with trauma and addiction.
- Can sit with a wide range of feelings.
- Sets limits compassionately.
- Is a good listener.
- Can give clients space, not overdominating the session.
- Is highly professional (remembers promises made to the client; stays on task).
- Asks good questions.
- Has some background in trauma, addiction, and co-occurring issues.
- Is empathic.

- Can retain clients (has a low dropout rate).
- Works well with personality issues such as negativity and power struggles.
- Is sensitive to nonverbal signs (behavior, body language, dissociation).
- Understands that symptoms are often an attempt to cope (e.g., substance use as self-medication).
- Is curious about the dark side of life (brutality, sadism, scapegoating).
- Gives positive and negative feedback clearly.
- Believes clients can get better.
- Strives for balance (not over- or underreacting).
- Willing to admit mistakes and explore how one's own flaws impact the work.
- Can openly discuss conflicts.
- Is flexible.
- Tolerates uncertainty and confusion.
- Is good at validation and support.
- Explores clients' meanings without imposing one's own meaning.
- Can process the relationship with the client
- Recognizes that counseling dilemmas often have no right answer (How much to encourage clients to tell their story? How much truth can someone bear?).
- Is comfortable with clients' dependency.
- Takes reasonably good care of self.
- Views clients' resistance as a natural part of the work, based in pain from the past.
- Moves onto painful topics when it's therapeutic to do so.
- Is sensitive to power dynamics and willing to share power with clients.
- Is warm.
- Can say what's hard to say.
- Develops written contracts to keep clients safe (emergency plans, substance use limits).
- Teaches coping skills as needed (e.g., RP, Seeking Safety).
- Monitors clients' progress with validated measures.
- Refers clients to additional help.

It's also important to identify what isn't central. Research shows that easy-to-measure counselor characteristics generally don't predict skill, such as age, gender, ethnicity, years' experience, degree type, setting, session fee, personal history of trauma or addiction, level of extraversion/introversion (e.g., Lambert, 2013; McLellan et al., 1988; Najavits & Weiss, 1994). Some providers are outstanding at this work without a formal degree and some with PhDs and MDs are not. So too, a personal history of trauma or addiction can be a strength or a weakness depending on how it's brought forth in the work.

The larger system also plays a role: access to supervision and support, training opportunities, caseloads, and length of stay. Many counselors practice within less-than-ideal contexts.

What Your Giving Can Do

This quotation from a client beautifully summarizes what helping means (Leslie, 2011, p. 57): "The main message was that they cared about me and that, no matter what, they would help me . . . they seemed to like me even though I didn't like myself. They kind of loved me back to life again."

TREATMENT TOPICS

Introduction

SUMMARY

This initial topic aims to engage clients in the treatment in a positive, uplifting way. It offers the opportunity to get to know each other and explore what's ahead. The handouts also address practical details of the treatment.

ORIENTATION

Clients who have lived with trauma or addiction typically feel disheartened and afraid. Today's topic is designed to inspire a sense of hope while also providing a detailed description of Creating Change. The goal is *engagement*—helping clients feel warmly welcomed into the treatment and allaying any concerns they may have. Clients may hold mistaken beliefs about the work, such as fearing that they'll be asked to reveal more than they want to. They may be concerned about issues of confidentiality or treatment policies such as what happens if they relapse. If this is your first-ever session with a new client or group, getting to know each other will also be a major focus.

Emphasizing engagement from the beginning of treatment can offset the high dropout rates of many past-focused models (Hundt et al., 2020; Lewis et al., 2020; Najavits, 2015). For clients with both trauma and addiction, preventing dropout is all the more important given their instability and fragile treatment alliances (Najavits et al., 1997). A collaborative approach—working closely in a spirit of joint exploration—also offsets the "one-down" power dynamic that can be such a reminder of powerlessness for them.

There are three handouts: (1) About Creating Change; (2) Practical Information about Your Treatment; and (3) Creating Change Treatment Agreement.

If it's unclear whether clients have addiction or trauma issues, you can conduct the extra topic "Understanding Trauma and Addiction" before or after today's introduction. This is also useful for deepening their knowledge and reinforcing self-compassion, and it has a brief screen for behavioral addictions, which are crucial to address if present—such as excessive gambling, spending, eating, sex, or work. In most treatment settings, behavioral addictions are rarely identified or treated. See Chapter 3 for additional suggestions on how to use the various extra topics, as well as the "three-session try-out" engagement approach.

In sum, today's introduction lays the groundwork for a positive treatment experience. It can be conducted in individual modality or group, or as an individual pregroup session to get to know a client before the group begins.

Your Emotional Reactions

As you help clients face the past, awareness of how you have or haven't done that in your own life may surface more. This can be a strength, letting you draw on your direct experience to increase empathy and awareness. But it can also be a weakness if you impose your own recovery methods rather than allowing clients to discover what works for them. Also, if you have major "unfinished business" from the past, such as unresolved losses, trauma, or addiction, you may be in a parallel process with your clients, continuing to do your own work as they do theirs. If this is the case, you can still do Creating Change, but place extra effort on self-care and reaching out for supervision as needed.

Acknowledgments

The session quote is from Mary Oliver's poem "Wild Geese" (1986, p. 14). In Handout 1, the concept of stages of recovery is from Herman (1992; see also van der Hart et al., 1989, for earlier versions); the second quotation in the section "Benefits" is from Aviv (2021), and the third is from Najavits (2002a).

PREPARING FOR THE SESSION

- Add a description of your professional background to the end of Handout 1 if desired.
- Identify if there are any treatment policies you want to add to Handout 3.

SESSION FORMAT

Note: Chapter 3 describes the session format in detail.

1. ***Check-in*** is not conducted today as this is the first session but will occur in all future sessions.
2. ***Quotation.*** Link the quotation to the session topic—for example, *"I'm so glad you came in. I look forward to working with you. Each session we'll start with a brief inspiring quote; today it's from a poem. It conveys that life can get better, no matter what you've been through."*
3. ***Handouts*** (relate the topic to clients' lives):
    Handout 1: **About Creating Change**
    Handout 2: **Practical Information about Your Treatment**
    Handout 3: **Creating Change Treatment Agreement**
4. ***Check-out*** (per Chapter 3).

SESSION CONTENT

Goals

- ☐ Describe the treatment so clients know what to expect.
- ☐ Discuss how stages of recovery are relevant to trauma and addiction.
- ☐ Identify which Creating Change topics clients are most interested in.
- ☐ Fill out the Practical Information handout with the client's input.
- ☐ Complete the Treatment Agreement handout.

Introduction

Ways to Relate the Material to Clients' Lives

★ *Encourage clients to share what "change" means to them (Handout 1).* Point out the name of the treatment (Creating Change). What changes do they want to see in 6 months and 1 year? For group treatment, you can go around the group asking clients to name a change they want to achieve.

★ *Focus on engagement (Handout 1).* Clients understandably may be hesitant about a treatment that focuses on sensitive areas such as trauma, addiction, and exploring the past. Help reassure them via key points such as these:

- *Pacing and choice.* Clients will decide what to reveal and when; they won't be pushed.
- *Compassionate topics.* Each session offers a poignant theme that brings to light areas that need healing.
- A *focus on the past to make the future better.* The goal is to free clients from aspects of the past that are holding them back.
- *Both positive and negative experiences.* Their strengths and courage will be emphasized just as much as their problems.
- *Direct benefits.* You may want to go over the three client quotes in the "Benefits" section of the handout. Also emphasize that all scientific studies of Creating Change have shown positive results across a wide range of clients. If you want to share more about the studies, they're described in Chapter 1 and also available at *www.creating-change.org*.
- *A three-session try-out.* Clients can try up to three sessions before they decide to join, which is highly recommended as described in Chapter 3. They can also leave the treatment at any time.

★ *Ensure clients understand emergency and nonemergency plans (Handout 2).* The handout is straightforward, but clients may need help completing it, especially if they don't have many supports. Consider adding crisis lines and helplines (there's an extensive list in Handout 2 of the topic "Trust versus Doubt"). Also ask clients to take a photo of the completed handout so they can access it easily on their phone.

★ *Discuss your treatment policies (Handout 3).* Clients need and appreciate clarity on treatment policies (missed sessions, whether clients can contact each other outside of sessions, etc.). If desired, add your treatment policies as noted toward the end of the handout.

★ *Emphasize the concept of* agreement *in the Treatment Agreement (Handout 3).* It's called an *agreement* rather than *rules* to convey a spirit of cooperation. (*Note:* Some counselors like to reread treatment rules at the start of sessions, but it's strongly suggested *not* to do that in Creating Change. It takes time away from the session goals and creates a tone of compliance, rather than a trauma-informed tone of empowerment. If a client has problems adhering to the treatment agreement, take steps to address this with gentle reminders or, if needed, a one-to-one discussion with the client.)

★ *Consider asking clients which Creating Change topics most interest them.* See the list of topics in Chapter 1 (page 7). If time allows, you could go over it today. But this is optional; you can return to it in the future or just select topics for them as you go forward.

★ *Discussion*
- "What changes do you want to see in your life?"
- "What does the term *creating change* mean to you?"
- "What appeals to you most and least about this treatment?"
- "Do you think it would help to talk about your past?"
- "Have you told your story before? How did it go?"
- "Do any feelings come up as you look through the handouts?"
- "Are you more motivated to work on trauma or addiction, if you have both?"

- "Do you believe you can honor the Treatment Agreement? What might get in the way?"
- "Why is a Treatment Agreement important?"

Suggestions

✦ *Refer clients to additional services.* This is especially important if a client is new to you or not yet sufficiently connected with services. Consider options such as counseling, medication, job training, and parenting classes. See the Seeking Safety topic "Introduction to Treatment/Case Management" for a detailed guide to case management for trauma and addiction.

✦ *Explain* integrated treatment. This means that if they have both addiction and trauma, they can work on them at the same time. The old approach was addiction first, then trauma ("Don't talk about it until you have a year sober"). But each impacts the other and can also heal together, as long as the treatment is designed for that. You can say, "If you had two physical problems, diabetes and cancer, you'd be treated for both together too."

✦ *Talk openly about concerns.* Some clients may have had prior unsuccessful past-focused treatment or may be pessimistic ("I'm too far gone"); lack motivation ("This is too hard"); feel afraid ("If I start to cry, I'll never stop"); have unrealistic expectations ("I need this to work ASAP"); or have safety concerns ("I think I may become suicidal"). Help them understand how Creating Change may be different than other treatments they've had; provide realistic reassurance; and if helpful, conduct any of the extra topics (the last three in the book). Also, the topic "Trust versus Doubt" addresses client concerns in detail.

✦ *Discuss the goal of staying safe in the present.* Emphasize that although Creating Change focuses on the past, there's still strong attention to safety in the present. Depending on the client, this may mean a limit on substance use or other addictive behavior; actively using coping skills; and continuing daily functioning such as holding a job and attending treatment. Also reassure clients that Creating Change has been found to be a very safe treatment, even among people with major active addiction and other problems (per Chapters 1 and 3). But if there's a need to interweave present-focused sessions or take breaks from working on the past, that's fine, too, and the client can request that at any point.

✦ *"Expect the unexpected."* When first meeting clients, it's natural to make judgments of how they'll do in treatment based on the severity and duration of their problems and their current context (housing, relationships, finances, etc.). But one of the most humbling parts of this work is how unpredictable progress is. Some clients who seem least likely to change will do well, while others who seem to have everything on their side won't. Keep a spirit of complete openness. Each session reveals a new layer of who clients really are rather than how they initially appear, sometimes with poignant surprises and unexpected gains.

Tough Cases

* "The past is over. I just need to move on."
* "I tell lots of people about my past, even strangers I meet on the bus."
* "I don't think change is possible. No one ever changes."
* "I told my story before and relapsed."
* "I'm afraid to talk about what happened; it's too upsetting."

Introduction

Quotation

*"Whoever you are, no matter how lonely,
The world offers itself to your imagination . . . "*

~ MARY OLIVER, 20th-century American poet

HANDOUT 1

About Creating Change

WHAT IS CREATING CHANGE?

Creating Change is a counseling model to help you recover from trauma and/or addiction by coming to terms with your past. Talking about the past has been a method of healing throughout history and across cultures.

There are 23 session topics, but you don't have to do all of them. They can be done in any order and as few or many as time allows. You can also try a few sessions to see how you like them. Your counselor may decide to share the list of session topics with you or may just choose them based on your needs.

WHY IS IT CALLED CREATING CHANGE?

It's called Creating Change because making changes in your life is a creative process. *Creativity* means generating something new and valuable. It involves discovery, trying alternatives, and clarifying what you really feel and think. It's about inspiration and intuition. When talking about the past, these concepts are especially important because you can't go back and change what happened—but you can change your relationship to it. You can gain new perspectives.

This helps you overcome long-standing patterns and frees you from emotional pain so that the future can be better than the past.

TRAUMA AND ADDICTION

Creating Change focuses primarily on trauma and addiction.

Trauma is a major negative event such as physical, sexual, or emotional abuse; bullying; natural disasters; fires; accidents; and war trauma. Many people experience trauma. It can lead to problems such as nightmares, flashbacks, rage, grief, and medical issues.

Addiction is common, too. It refers to a behavior you can't stop doing even though it's causing major problems, such as substance addiction or others (food, spending, gambling, pornography, sex, gaming, exercise, work).

(cont.)

From *Creating Change* by Lisa M. Najavits. Copyright © 2024 Lisa M. Najavits. Published by The Guilford Press. Permission to photocopy this material is granted to purchasers of this book for use with your own clients or patients; see copyright page for details.

HANDOUT 1 *(p. 2 of 5)* — Introduction

"STAGES" OF RECOVERY

There are three major ways to recover from trauma and addiction. These used to be called *stages of recovery*, but we now know they don't have to occur in a particular order and you don't have to do all three. Some people do multiple types at once; others do a sequence or just one.

Creating Change addresses the second type below: *past-focused*.

Although the three types are different, they overlap to some extent, and you may find yourself moving back and forth between them. That's fine—there are many ways to heal. You can find what works for you. You're the author of your recovery.

1. **Present-focused (safety).** You learn coping skills to become safe and stable in the present. You get better at here-and-now tasks such as managing triggers; taking care of your body; reducing addiction; honesty; setting boundaries; asking for help; and grounding (bringing down negative feelings). An example of this type of treatment is Seeking Safety.

> 2. **Past-focused (remembering).** This means exploring the past as a way to heal and move forward. It's what we'll be doing in Creating Change. You can:
> - Share your story.
> - Honor your ability to survive.
> - Identify messages you absorbed.
> - Understand relationship patterns.
> - Observe how you've changed.

3. **Future-focused (connection).** There's no specific treatment model for this; it typically occurs as part of the first two types. The goal is to build a life worth living: to develop healthy relationships; maintain self-care; and find a positive life purpose, such as nurturing others or supporting important causes. You acknowledge the past but aren't overwhelmed by it.

THE BENEFITS

People who have done past-focused counseling describe it as liberating—becoming unstuck, feeling more alive. They gain access to more positive feelings and learn to manage negative ones better. Their perspective broadens.

In the words of people who have done it . . .

"Sobriety means that you turn to a life that gives you dignity and self-respect. I can accomplish the things I used to just sit there and think about. I realize that colors are bright, and not gray and black—I thought things were gray and black when I was first in recovery."

"I figured out that I am living a life with a billion different possibilities. . . . My inner voice became stronger, my intuition that I don't have to live my life the way he [the perpetrator] taught me, that I can keep going."

"My ability to speak about past trauma was one way to get over the guilt I felt about being a drug addict. By admitting what happened and talking about it, we gain understanding of our behavior—not just the substance abuse, but the poor relationship choices and the vast array of other issues we've dragged along behind us all our lives. Talking about sexual abuse (which filled me with shame) has been a crucial part of my recovery."

(cont.)

HANDOUT 1 *(p. 3 of 5)*   Introduction

RESEARCH RESULTS

There have been several scientific studies of Creating Change, with positive results in all of them. Participants showed significant reductions in trauma symptoms, substance use, and other domains as well as strong satisfaction, low dropout, and no evidence of safety concerns.

The studies included military veterans, crime victims, and adults who suffered child abuse. Clients in the studies had severe, chronic, and current PTSD and substance use disorder. Many also had additional issues such as active suicidal ideation.

See *www.creating-change.org* to freely download the studies and discover new research and other information on Creating Change.

WHAT CHANGES DO YOU WANT IN YOUR LIFE?

✧ Answer as many questions below as you choose to.

1. Do you have any behavior you struggle to control (substance use, eating, gambling, etc.)?	Yes	No	Unsure
2. Are you still bothered by a difficult event you lived through, such as child abuse, major accident, natural disaster, or war?	Yes	No	Unsure
3. Have you often felt misunderstood or not believed?	Yes	No	Unsure
4. Do you tend to feel too much (overwhelmed) or too little (numb)?	Yes	No	Unsure
5. Do you have difficulty remembering parts of your life?	Yes	No	Unsure
6. Are there important secrets you haven't told anyone?	Yes	No	Unsure
7. Do you wonder why difficult things happened to you?	Yes	No	Unsure
8. Do you have emotional issues such as ongoing depression, anxiety, shame, guilt, or anger?	Yes	No	Unsure
9. Do you have repeated relationship problems?	Yes	No	Unsure
10. Any other issues you notice?	Yes	No	Unsure

If you answered "yes" to any of these questions, Creating Change may be helpful to you. You can also apply what you learn in Creating Change to other issues in your life.

✧ Think about what *change* means to you. What are you hoping to change?

_____

_____

_____

(cont.)

HANDOUT 1 *(p. 4 of 5)*   Introduction

WHAT TO EXPECT AT SESSIONS

What Is the Session Format?

Each treatment session is structured to make the most of the time available.

1. **Check-in.** At the start of each session, you'll be asked five questions: "How are you feeling?," "What good coping have you done?," "Any substance use or other unsafe behavior?," "Did you complete your commitment?," and "Community resource update?" Some of these terms may be unfamiliar to you, but they will become clear.
2. **Handout.** You will be given a written sheet with the main points of the topic.
3. **Discussion.** Most of the session will be devoted to the session topic and how it relates to your life. Some topics will also have exercises to try. Your participation is always voluntary.
4. **Check-out.** At the end of the session, you'll be asked four questions: "Name one thing you got out of today's session," "Any problems with the session?," "What is your new commitment? (optional homework)," and "What community resource will you call?"

Will I Be Asked to Talk about My Trauma or Addiction?

You may choose to talk about these, but it will always be at your own pace and only what you want to share. It's your treatment and your recovery.

What If I Miss a Session?

You can rejoin at any time. Please try, however, to attend all sessions so that you can get the most from the treatment.

Will Anyone Be Asked to Leave Creating Change?

You won't be asked to leave unless the treatment appears to have a major negative impact on you, or unless you present a serious danger to staff or other clients (e.g., threatening assault, selling drugs onsite). The counselor will do what's needed to keep everyone safe.

What If I Have Concerns about the Treatment or Counselor?

Be direct and honest with your counselor. This helps get your needs met and improves the treatment for others. You can also speak with the counselor's supervisor. (And, although rare, if there is a serious ethical or legal concern, consult with outside authorities if needed.)

WHO DEVELOPED CREATING CHANGE?

Creating Change was developed by Lisa M. Najavits, PhD. She also developed Seeking Safety, a present-focused coping skills model that has become the most widely used and evidence-based counseling approach for trauma and addiction.

Dr. Najavits is Adjunct Professor at the University of Massachusetts Chan Medical School and Director of Treatment Innovations. She was on the faculty of Harvard Medical School (McLean Hospital) for 25 years and Boston University School of Medicine (VA Boston) for 12 years. Dr. Najavits is author of over 200 professional publications, as well as the books *Finding Your Best Self: Recovery from Addiction, Trauma, or Both* (2019); *Seeking Safety* (2002); and *A Woman's Addiction Workbook* (2002). She served as president of the Society of Addiction Psychology of the American Psychological Association and

(cont.)

HANDOUT 1 *(p. 5 of 5)*   Introduction

has consulted widely on public health efforts in addictions and trauma, nationally and internationally, including to the Substance Abuse and Mental Health Services Administration, the National Institutes of Health, the United Nations, and the U.S. Surgeon General. Dr. Najavits has received awards including the Betty Ford Award of the Addiction Medical Education and Research Association; the Emerging Leadership Award of the American Psychological Association Committee on Women; the Early Career Contribution Award of the Society for Psychotherapy Research; the Young Professional Award of the International Society for Traumatic Stress Studies; and the Barnard College Distinguished Alumna Award. She is a licensed psychologist in Massachusetts and conducts a counseling practice. She received her doctorate in clinical psychology from Vanderbilt University and bachelor's degree with honors from Barnard College (Columbia University).

WHO IS THE COUNSELOR?

[If you choose to, add below information about yourself as the counselor after deleting this sentence.]

HANDOUT 2 — Introduction

Practical Information about Your Treatment

✏️ **Counselor** name: _____

🗓️ **Schedule** of sessions: _____

📍 **Location** of sessions: _____

📱 **If you can't attend a session or need to reach the counselor for nonemergency reasons,** please use the following phone number or email: _____

EMERGENCY PROCEDURES

It is extremely important to reach out for help in an emergency!

✸ **What's an emergency?** Any situation in which you are in serious danger (suicide, physical harm to you or others) or have any extreme symptoms that need immediate psychiatric help (severe hallucinations, mental breakdown, etc.).

✸ **Emergency plan.** Specify as many options below as possible.

1. **Who you'll contact** (partner, friend, family, sponsor, counselor, doctor, crisis line, etc.).

Name and relationship to you	Phone number and/or email
Example: Carmina (my AA sponsor)	
1.	
2.	
3.	
4.	

2. **Where you'll go** (emergency room, clinic, shelter, friend's place, etc.) and list the address and contact information for each.

Location	Phone number and/or email	Address
Example: emergency room		
1.		
2.		
3.		
4.		

(cont.)

From *Creating Change* by Lisa M. Najavits. Copyright © 2024 Lisa M. Najavits. Published by The Guilford Press. Permission to photocopy this material, or to download and print additional copies (*www.guilford.com/najavits3-materials*), is granted to purchasers of this book for use with your own clients or patients; see copyright page for details.

HANDOUT 2 *(p. 2 of 2)* Introduction

    3. **Any other emergency procedures?**

_____

_____

_____

OTHER IMPORTANT SITUATIONS

If you feel in danger of addictive behavior or self-harm, contact:

✦ Supportive person 1: (name and phone number or email): _____

_____

✦ Supportive person 2: (name and phone number or email): _____

_____

✦ Supportive person 3: (name and phone number or email): _____

_____

✦ Helplines/crisis lines (phone numbers): _____

_____

✦ 12-step sponsor (name and phone number or email): _____

_____

Rehearse ahead. Do a trial run with any of the people listed. Rehearse what you'll say and what the other person will say. Be sure to let the person know in advance how best to help you.

I will do my best to stay safe and agree to all of the above safety procedures.

Client signature: _____ Date: _____

Witness signature (counselor): _____ Date: _____

HANDOUT 3 — Introduction

Creating Change Treatment Agreement

To promote positive change, we agree on the following.

CLIENT AGREEMENT

For individual or group sessions

- I'll try my best to recover, including reading session materials, completing *commitments* between sessions, and reaching out for all help available to me.
- I know I'm always welcome back, even if I relapse.
- I recognize that the more I put into treatment, the more I'll get out of it.
- I understand that I may feel worse before I feel better but should return to treatment no matter what.
- I'm aware that everything said in treatment will be strictly confidential. However, there are some scenarios where the counselor is legally obligated to release records: (1) if I'm in serious danger of harming myself or others; (2) if child or elder abuse becomes known; or (3) if a court demands the counselor's records.
- I understand that it's my choice what to reveal about my past; I can say, "I prefer not to talk about it" at any time.
- I'll strive to be totally honest with the counselor about my addictive behavior, my safety (including self-harm, suicidal impulses, and danger to others), and any negative reactions I have to the treatment or the counselor.
- I'll be on time for sessions and will leave a message if I need to cancel.
- If I arrive to a session intoxicated, I'm aware the session won't be held. I'll be escorted to a safe place until I can return home or will be sent home with a friend or in a taxi.
- In an emergency, I'll follow the written emergency instructions I've been given.
- I understand that buying, selling, or using substances with another client, or alone anywhere in or near this treatment office, is a serious danger and may lead to termination from this treatment.

For group sessions

- I'll strive to create an atmosphere of mutual respect (e.g., no interrupting others, no physical contact between group members).
- I'll maintain confidentiality. What anyone says in the session stays in the session.
- If I become aware that someone expresses a safety threat (e.g., suicide plan, intent to harm someone, offering substances), I'll report that to the counselor for the sake of all involved.
- I'm aware that contact with group members outside of sessions is discouraged so as to protect clients' boundaries, unless the counselor has stated some other policy in advance.
- I'll honor my own and others' recovery path. I'll try to respond with compassion.

(cont.)

From *Creating Change* by Lisa M. Najavits. Copyright © 2024 Lisa M. Najavits. Published by The Guilford Press. Permission to photocopy this material, or to download and print additional copies (*www.guilford.com/najavits3-materials*), is granted to purchasers of this book for use with your own clients or patients; see copyright page for details.

HANDOUT 3 *(p. 2 of 2)* — Introduction

Additional agreements. Your counselor may have additional treatment policies (e.g., missed sessions, addictive behavior limits, client contact outside of sessions, urine/breathalyzer testing, safety plan. If so, list them here or attach them to this handout.

_____
_____
_____
_____

COUNSELOR AGREEMENT

- I'll abide by ethical and legal counseling standards.
- I'll respect clients' right to decide what they want to share.
- I'll do my best to provide high-quality care.
- I'll keep what's said in sessions confidential except for team communications and reporting requirements relevant to clients' care.

Client signature: _____ Date: _____

Counselor signature: _____ Date: _____

Ideas for a Commitment

Commit to one action that will move your life forward!
It can be anything you feel will help you, or you can try one of the ideas below.
Keeping your commitment is a way of respecting, honoring, and caring for yourself.

✦ Option 1. Begin an *insight journal* to list what you learn as you go through Creating Change.

✦ Option 2. Tell a trusted person how you want to change. Be specific. Ask for feedback, if desired.

✦ Option 3. Decrease or stop one current unsafe behavior. What would it be?

✦ Option 4. Create a recovery scrapbook either online or hard copy—add writing, drawings, quotes, songs, poems, and any other inspiration that keeps you motivated.

Create Change

SUMMARY

This topic is central to Creating Change. It offers a list of over 70 past-focused skills that can be used throughout treatment, as well as an exploration of *how* people change.

ORIENTATION

Today's topic conveys a core concept of this model: Coming to terms with the past is a highly creative enterprise. There's no formula, no lock-step sequence that leads to enduring change. Rather, people construct their own unique ways.

Yet many clients have misconceptions about how change happens, believing it should be easier than it is, or the opposite, thinking it's hopeless ("I'll always be this way"). They typically haven't had strong role models to demonstrate how to make progress in healthy ways and so tend to fall back on old ways that keep them stuck. Trauma and addiction can become an unending cycle.

Handout 1 provides a list of Creating Change skills—there are myriad ways to change one's relationship with the past. Some skills relate more to addiction, others to trauma; some reinforce self-compassion, others accountability; some address clients' inner world, others their relationships. The following examples give a sense of the range.

¤ *Own your part*	But without blame.
¤ *Notice impossible choices*	There truly may have been no good options.
¤ *Repair when possible*	Do what you can to make it better now.
¤ *Notice how you tried to say "Help!"*	You may not have had words so it showed up in symptoms or behaviors.
¤ *Be kind to others who suffer*	But stay focused on your recovery, too.

Having a list reinforces the idea that it's about experimentation: If one way doesn't work, try another. It invigorates the process by giving clients a wide array of ideas to spark off of, while also encouraging them to share their own methods. It's formatted to serve as a reference throughout treatment, such as via posting on the wall. They may see new ideas to try each time. For counselors who are familiar with the list of safe coping skills in Seeking Safety, the Creating Change skills serve a similar purpose but are focused on overcoming the past rather than improving coping in the present.

Handout 2 helps clients notice patterns when they've tried to make important changes in their lives. It offers education about the psychology of how people get themselves to change. We go into the idea that resistance to change and mixed feelings are to be expected. Rather than signs of failure, they're a predictable part of the path. Different change trajectories are described, such as *incremental* (slow, up and down) versus *quantum* (instant, permanent). The handout also has practical strategies such as the 30-second rule and how to overcome negativity bias. It's validating for clients to understand that everyone has challenges when trying to change.

Your Emotional Reactions

A classic framework for change in the addiction field is *stages of change*. It identifies five levels of client readiness: *precontemplation, contemplation, preparation, action,* and *maintenance* (Prochaska et al., 1992). Counselors typically find clients in the early stages the most challenging ("I'm worried this client will die of an overdose"; "That client keeps no-showing sessions"). They may also unconsciously take on clients' apathy and give up on them. At the other end of the spectrum, clients who make progress evoke warm pride and satisfaction. The challenge is how to maintain connection with clients no matter what stage they're in (DiClemente & Crisafulli, 2022). This is especially true for past-focused work, which can take a long time. Sometimes there's pressure to move clients more quickly than they can go, whether from external agency or insurance demands or your own internal drive to help them recover. Today's topic is an opportunity to let clients choose their level—there are a wide range of skills, some more difficult than others. Whatever clients are drawn to is typically what they're ready for. Allowing gentle pacing will, paradoxically, help them gain greater ability to change. As Herman wrote, "The survivor must be the author and arbiter of her own recovery" (1992, p. 133).

Acknowledgments

The session quotation is from Estés (1992, p. 21). In Handout 1, the quote at the top is often misattributed to Charles Darwin but is a paraphrase from Megginson (1963); quantum change is described in Miller and C'de Baca (2001); the negativity bias is described in Cacioppo, Cacioppo, and Gollan (2014); the many ways to create change are adapted from Najavits, *Finding Your Best Self* (2019).

PREPARING FOR THE SESSION

If desired, you can photocopy the list of Creating Change skills in a larger size to post on the wall so it will be visible to clients throughout the treatment.

SESSION FORMAT

1. ***Check-in*** (up to 5 minutes per client). See Chapter 3.
2. ***Quotation*** (briefly). See page 113. Link the quotation to the session. For example, *"The quote—and today's topic—is about the idea that there are various paths ("doors") that will help you find a way forward in life."*
3. ***Handouts*** (relate the topic to clients' lives; in-depth, most of the session):
    a. Ask clients to look through the handouts:
       Handout 1: **Creating Change Skills**
       Handout 2: **How Change Happens**
    b. Help clients relate the topic to current and specific problems in their lives. See "Session Content" (below) and Chapter 3 for suggestions.
4. ***Check-out*** (briefly). See Chapter 3.

Create Change

SESSION CONTENT

Goals

☐ Explore the list of Creating Change skills.
☐ Help clients identify specific skills they want to try and reinforce those they're already doing.
☐ Discuss the psychology of how change happens.

Ways to Relate the Material to Clients' Lives

★ *Try various ways to cover Handout 1 (Creating Change Skills).* Here are some options.

1. *Mark the list.* Go over the instructions at the top of the handout. Clients can mark the skills they already do, want to try, or have questions about.

2. *"Point to a skill" game.* This can be done in individual or group treatment. With eyes closed, a client randomly points to any skill on the list, then reads it aloud and briefly discusses it. For example, a client lands on "Hear the messages in your behavior" and talks briefly about how her opioid use was a way to feel good when everything felt awful after trauma. If clients land on a skill that doesn't work for them, they can close their eyes and find another. In group, clients take turns, each choosing a new skill when it's their turn.

3. *Discuss what it means to them.* Clients can choose a skill and identify how it relates to their life. If done in group, let clients respond to each other and share on the same skill so that each skill becomes a dialogue among group members.

4. *Teams (for groups).* Clients break into teams. They get about 20 minutes to give specific examples of the skills. For example, for "Listen to your body," they could write, "When I feel my heart racing, I know it's a sign that I'm triggered." They can go in any order on the sheet.

5. *Brainstorm how to use the skills in the week ahead.* This can include discussion of how to bring the skills alive by writing about them or using other expressive methods. You can also address practical strategies, such as carrying the list in one's wallet or keeping a copy on a phone or tablet.

Note: Emphasize that what works for one person may not work for another (clients are each on their own path). And choosing a skill depends on the context. "Let yourself cry" may be good in a counseling session but not in the workplace, for example.

★ *Encourage sharing about Handout 2 (How Change Happens).* Clients can choose a question to answer aloud. Help them draw insight from past experiences of trying to make changes in their life. Focus on being optimistic yet realistic about what it takes to change.

★ *Relate the topic to trauma and addiction.* The concept of change is broad and can relate to all sorts of changes clients want to make (career, leisure activities, diet and exercise, parenting, etc.). Any changes can be productive to discuss but also keep a strong focus on trauma and addiction (sustaining substance abstinence, processing past trauma, etc.).

★ *Discussion*
- "What do you want to change?"
- "Why do you think this treatment is called *creating* change? What is *creative* about the change process?"
- "What did you learn growing up about how people change (or don't)?"
- "Any examples of change that you're especially proud of?"
- "What's been most challenging for you about trying to change?"
- "Do trauma or addiction ever *increase* your motivation to change (e.g., hitting bottom)?"
- "What inspires you to change (e.g., your children, belief in yourself, spirituality)?"

Suggestions

✦ ***Provide reassurance.*** Clients may have numerous failed attempts at change, such as relapses and missed goals. Help them understand they can become better at it by trying new methods (Handout 1) and understanding the psychology of change (Handout 2). Offer hopeful statements such as "You can make changes now; it's never too late." Praise them for skills they're already using and changes they've already made.

✦ ***Emphasize creativity.*** Encourage clients to bring a creative spirit to the work by brainstorming ideas, being open-minded, and experimenting with new approaches. This book's title, *Creating Change*, reflects the link between creativity and healing (which is described briefly in the topic "Introduction," Handout 1).

✦ ***Reinforce being conscious of choices.*** When people are under stress—and both addiction and trauma are highly stressful—it brings out impulsive decisions. The Creating Change skills can help them actively consider their choices in a planful way.

✦ ***Highlight that trauma and addiction can create positive or negative change.*** Their negative impact is clear. But they can also be a catalyst for positive change: increased empathy for others, a new sense of purpose in life, substance abstinence, and posttraumatic growth (see the topic "Growth" for more on the latter). It's helpful for clients to understand that trauma and addiction are not always negative when it comes to change.

✦ ***Return to the Creating Change skills list at future sessions.*** Have printed copies on hand, or post it on the wall so it's visible throughout treatment. Guide clients back to it at times. Different skills take on new meaning at different times.

✦ ***Note that today's session is not for exploring detailed narratives of the past.*** It's designed to build a strong foundation that will help clients in other sessions.

Tough Cases

* "I can change for a while but then always slip backward."
* "My partner needs to change, not me."
* "I've been told I should love myself just as I am."
* "I don't think anyone ever really changes."
* "I'll never get over my trauma/addiction."

Quotation

"The doors to the world of the . . . Self are few but precious. If you have a deep scar, that is a door, if you have an old, old story, that is a door. If you love the sky and the water . . . that is a door. If you yearn for a deeper life, a full life, a sane life, that is a door."

~ Clarissa Pinkola Estés, 20th-century Native American/Latin American author

HANDOUT 1

Creating Change Skills

You can come to terms with your past. This list of over 70 skills offers many options. Choose what works for you. Return to the list as you continue in recovery. Different skills take on new meaning at different times. Put the list in your wallet, mobile phone, or on your refrigerator door. Keep it present.

★ *Optional: Put a star (★) next to ones you want to try; a question mark (?) next to any you don't understand; and a check (✓) next to those you already do.*

Honor your survival	You did a lot of things right to be here today. Name some
Break the silence	Silencing is often part of trauma and addiction
Sit with a feeling	Something good can come of it
Take the long road	It takes time to heal
Listen to your body	It reveals a lot about your past
Write an imaginary letter to the world	What do you want others to understand about you?
Be kind to others who suffer	But stay focused on your recovery, too
Believe yourself	. . . if it's a respectful view of you
Don't believe yourself	. . . if it's a disrespectful view of you

(cont.)

From *Creating Change* by Lisa M. Najavits. Copyright © 2024 Lisa M. Najavits. Published by The Guilford Press. Permission to photocopy this material is granted to purchasers of this book for use with your own clients or patients; see copyright page for details.

HANDOUT 1 *(p. 2 of 4)*   Create Change

Talk to your younger self	What comfort can you offer?
Don't delay healing	The right time is now
Own your part	But without blame
Peel a layer	Then another, and another, and another
Let yourself get angry	At injustice and betrayal
Pace yourself	Sometimes *slower is faster*
Repair when possible	Do what you can to make it better now
Notice impossible choices	There truly may have been no good options
Be the hero of your story	How did you beat the odds, gain allies, overcome pain?
Imagine what change would look like	What would be different if you were at peace with your past?
Hear the messages in your behavior	What we don't talk out, we act out
Let yourself cry	It cleanses losses, pain, and shame
Accept uncertainty	It's part of the process
Strive to meet unmet needs	Give yourself now what you lacked then; nurturing, rest, choices, compassion
Notice how you tried to say "Help!"	You may not have had words so it became symptoms or behaviors
View a scene from your past with new eyes	What would a compassionate bystander see?
Choose healing methods	Counseling . . . self-help . . . peer support . . . medication . . . cultural practices
Be vulnerable	"Weakness" is strength when sharing with good people
Notice who you become under stress	Those patterns may be rooted in trauma
Experience your inner self	Without substances or other addictive behavior
Notice the good, too	Who helped? What went right?
See addiction for what it is	A way to feel more? to feel less? to fit in? to cope? self-medication?
See trauma for what it is	Wrong place, wrong time? People who didn't protect you? Family history?
It's OK to have regrets	Just don't stay stuck in shame

(cont.)

HANDOUT 1 (p. 3 of 4)　　　　　　　　　　　　　　　　　　　　　　　　　　　Create Change

Widen the lens	Notice how your past was shaped by family, peers, community, and culture
Share a secret	With someone safe
Let go	Do you need to let go of shame? over-attachment? an illusion?
Take it on	Do you need to increase acceptance? compassion? accountability?
Tell your story	To safe people, at a pace that works for you
Notice how you tried to get love	Was it healthy or unhealthy (giving too much, controlling, pretending)?
Respect how you responded during trauma	*Fight, flight, freeze,* or *appease*—you did your best at the time
Find good people	Who care and want to understand
Identify illusions	Denial, fantasy, magical thinking—below illusions there's often deep sorrow
Give yourself credit	You did the best you could with the tools you had
Prioritize recovery	Make time in your day for healing
Forgive yourself	For what you wish you did or didn't do
Become a detective	Explore who, what, when, where, and why
Don't take it out on others	Pain needs help; lashing out prevents healing
Gain wisdom	"If you lose, don't lose the lesson"
Notice how the past shows up	In your body, thoughts, feelings, spirit
Remember you don't *have to* forgive a perpetrator	It's a choice, not a requirement
Notice what's missing	What are you afraid to look at?
Let people know what you want	Guidance . . . comfort . . . feedback . . . a shoulder to cry on
Recognize growth	Notice strengths and wisdom you gained
Understand trauma roles	*Victim, perpetrator, bystander,* and *rescuer*
Balance past and present	Explore the past but also keep up with today
Identify who was and wasn't there for you	Who were your real supports?
Don't feel you have to justify your pain	If you feel it, it matters

(cont.)

115

HANDOUT 1 *(p. 4 of 4)*   Create Change

Choose messages you want to keep	Let go of those that don't serve you
Allow memories to emerge	Don't force them
Find ways to transform the past	Try service to others, spirituality, creative arts
Value yourself	Even if others didn't, you can
Observe how you relate	To people, food, money, substances, your body
Create a larger identity	Beyond trauma and addiction
Express it	In words, music, or art—discover new insights
Notice what moves you	It may link to important parts of your past
Experiment with trust	Build it slowly for a strong foundation
Watch for power dynamics that repeat the past	For example, speaking versus staying silent
Trust your truth	And let it evolve as you grow
Protect yourself—but not too much	Self-protection is good but not if it's isolation and avoidance
Love the child you were	That child deserves understanding
Compare *then* versus *now*	What's better and what still needs work?
Discover the connection	How did trauma and addiction impact each other across your life?
Notice fantasies	Do you wish for revenge? apologies? These are clues to your past
Know that it can get better	Recovery is possible, no matter what
Welcome all sides of yourself	The loving side, the angry side, the weak side, the playful side
Go beyond	Each generation can progress further

✧ **Other skills you've discovered?**

_____

_____

_____

HANDOUT 2 — Create Change

How Change Happens

"It is not the strongest of the species that survives, nor the most intelligent. It is the one most adaptable to change."

~ANONYMOUS

How do people change? This is one of the most important questions in recovery. Here are 10 key ideas.

◇ *Mark any that are relevant to you.*

1. Change is both easier and harder than it seems. Many people are either overconfident (think it's easier than it really is) or underconfident (think it's harder than it really is). Both can lead to giving up—the overconfident when they hit the wall of reality ("Yikes, this is too hard"), the underconfident before starting ("I'm not capable"). Change is possible if you learn to stay with the process, no matter what.

◇ Do you view change as easy or hard?

2. It typically takes 30 days to create a new habit. Try a new behavior daily for a month so it becomes more automatic. It also helps to let others know your goal so they can encourage you. Keep in mind that for long-standing issues the key is to *maintain* the change the month after, and the one after that, and so on.

◇ Is there a new habit you want to start?

3. There are many ways to create change. Some people change via relationships (counseling, peer supports); others via solitary learning (reading, videos). Some do well with physically based change (medication, exercise); others through spirituality. Some use creative arts; others find that a new job or volunteer work helps them. Experiment to discover what works for you.

◇ Which ways do you want to try?

4. It's normal to resist change. This typically shows up as procrastination, avoidance (finding reasons not to do what's needed), minimal effort, or giving up when you hit an obstacle. It happens to everyone, even if they really want to change. You may not notice you're resisting, but it shows up in your behavior. It can be overcome with preparation and support.

◇ Do you ever resist change? What does that look like?

5. Change can be quantum *(instant, permanent)* or steady *(slow, up and down)*. Both have lasting impact, but quantum change is rarer. An example is the alcoholic who suddenly, like a lightning bolt, finds God and gives up drinking forever. The key is to keep striving for change no matter how it occurs—fast or slow.

◇ Do your changes tend to be fast or slow?

(cont.)

From *Creating Change* by Lisa M. Najavits. Copyright © 2024 Lisa M. Najavits. Published by The Guilford Press. Permission to photocopy this material is granted to purchasers of this book for use with your own clients or patients; see copyright page for details.

HANDOUT 2 *(p. 2 of 2)*   Create Change

6. *Mixed feelings are common.* Change can feel hopeful, exciting, tense, fearful, guilty, conflicted, and much more. It rarely feels all good, all the time. Whatever the mix, don't wait for it to feel right. Take steps toward change now.

✧ Do you find yourself delaying change until it feels good?

7. *Change means a leap into the unknown.* It's human nature to be comfortable with what's familiar. So even if it's for a better future, change brings surprising reactions. People who grew up with violence may find safe people and situations boring or unappealing at first.

✧ What will help you not fall back into unhealthy patterns?

8. *It's important to overcome the brain's* negativity bias. People are hardwired to notice what's wrong more than what's right. This *negativity bias* helped the species survive in the wild. It thus requires extra effort to notice positives, such as changes you've already made. You did some things right to have survived trauma and addiction, for example.

✧ What changes are you proud of?

9. *Trauma and addiction impact change.* Sometimes they inspire change—they motivate you to escape adversity and build a new life. But they can also keep you stuck. You may feel you're abandoning your family if you move on. You may believe you're unworthy of a better life. You may think others don't believe in you because of your past. You may have had too much change and disruption already and are afraid to make new changes.

✧ How do trauma/addiction impact your ability to change?

10. *Many factors promote change, not just your own effort.* Change is often viewed as an individual responsibility ("Just try harder"). But it's more complex. It also relates to messages you learned growing up in your family and community; and opportunities such as education, finances, and other supports.

✧ What factors outside of you helped or hindered change?

Ideas for a Commitment

Commit to one action that will move your life forward!
It can be anything you feel will help you, or you can try one of the ideas below.
Keeping your commitment is a way of respecting, honoring, and caring for yourself.

- Option 1. Talk to a few people who have made a positive change. Ask how they did it.

- Option 2. Close your eyes, put your finger anywhere on Handout 2, then open your eyes and read the skill. Write about how it applies to you.

- Option 3. List three changes you want to make *in the next year*. Then next to each, list one action you can take *in the next week* to move it forward.

- Option 4. Write about this quote from Handout 1. What does it mean to you?

   "It is not the strongest of the species that survives, nor the most intelligent. It is the one that is most adaptable to change."

Trust versus Doubt

SUMMARY

Today's topic focuses on concerns that clients may have about treatment and recovery ("It's too hard," "I don't want pity," etc.). This exploration is framed in terms of *trust versus doubt*, which is a core theme in trauma and addiction. Also, clients are given a list of free national helplines they can contact for support.

ORIENTATION

It's natural for clients to have doubts about treatment and recovery. In today's topic, these can be aired, launching a conversation that continues throughout the work.

To help clients identify their concerns, Handout 1 has a list of typical doubts, such as "I'm too far gone" or "I should know how to do this." It then offers alternatives to help rethink the doubts. Some of these alternative perspectives may be surprising to clients, especially if they grew up in families and communities with inaccurate information about emotional health. This is sadly common. For example, clients may believe, "Time heals all wounds" or "Needing treatment means I'm weak." Trauma and addiction can become chronic when clients don't have the opportunity to learn how to work through pain and grow emotionally.

At a deeper level, clients' concerns may reflect trust issues that are common in trauma and addiction. They may instinctively distrust people, even those trying to help, due to harm from others in the past. Thus, clients' doubts are not simply "cognitive errors" to be restructured but rather understandable and legitimate experiences that create a filter based on their reality.

One of the earliest psychologists to write about trust versus doubt was Erikson, whose book *Childhood and Society* in 1950 identified it as the central task in early childhood development. In families with neglect or abuse, the child learns not to trust, not to hope, and not to rely on others to meet their needs. Erikson's work has inspired applications in adult mental health recovery, such as an article by Vogel-Scibilia et al., who are mental health consumers with serious mental illness. They identify two key tasks related to trust versus doubt in psychiatric recovery: helping clients (1) accept their diagnoses and (2) trust in the possibility of recovery. They write, "Recovery is a mind-state . . . [that] involves empowering oneself to live well" (2009, p. 412).

Today's topic encourages clients to balance growth, such as engaging in Creating Change, while also recognizing they may need to take it slow to build trust. It helps to remind them that they will be sharing only what they choose to and that they won't be pressured to continue in treatment beyond what's right for them. The list of helplines in Handout 2 empowers them to gain

Trust versus Doubt

additional support as needed. They can return to it throughout treatment. The goal is to build a success experience that honors their history while not being trapped by it.

Your Emotional Reactions

One of the most common challenges in treating people with trauma and addiction is concern about them worsening. Increased addiction, self-harm or harm to others, dropping out of treatment—the list goes on and on (Najavits, 2002b). Trust versus doubt is thus an issue for counselors as well as clients. There are no easy answers; it's not possible to know in advance how any particular client will do. Keep monitoring clients' progress and adjust as you go. (See the section "Watch for Progress and Worsening" in Chapter 3 for more on this.) The key is to manage anxiety about clients while also responding to real issues that need to be addressed, such as referral to additional treatments. Also remember that Creating Change takes a gentle approach to exploring the past, so there's quite a lot of built-in safety by having clients only go as deep as they're ready for.

Acknowledgments

The session quotation is from the video *James Baldwin: The Price of the Ticket* (Thompson, 1990). In Handout 1, the quotation from the trauma survivor is from Raphael (2003, p. 47).

SESSION FORMAT

1. *Check-in* (per Chapter 3).
2. *Quotation.* See page 124. Link the quotation to the session topic—for example, *"The quote encourages being open to growth, saying "yes" to new possibilities. Today we'll talk about changes you'd like to make."*
3. *Handouts* (relate the topic to clients' lives):
    Handout 1: **Trust versus Doubt**
    Handout 2: **Supportive Helplines**
4. *Check-out* (per Chapter 3).

SESSION CONTENT

Goals

☐ Identify concerns clients may have about treatment or recovery.
☐ Offer alternative perspectives to help them move forward.
☐ Validate *trust* as a major issue in trauma and addiction.
☐ Explore free national helplines to support clients outside of sessions.

Ways to Relate the Material to Clients' Lives

★ *Try a debate exercise (Handout 1).* If you're conducting group treatment, you can ask two clients to try this. For individual treatment, you would play one side and the client the other. A client chooses a doubt in Handout 1 to work on. One person role-plays the doubting voice and the other the trusting voice, then they switch roles. Emphasize that a debate brings out different perspectives and flexible thinking.

★ *Elicit additional concerns (Handout 1).* Ask questions such as "What doubts do you have?"; "Do you notice any feelings as you read this handout?" The more clients voice their specific beliefs, the more useful the session will be.

★ *Imagine.* Help clients envision the good that can come from exploring their past. What would it be like not to carry secrets or guilt? How would they feel with sustained sobriety? Emphasizing the positive is not about negating their genuine concerns but helps move beyond fears that may be holding them back.

★ *Take into account clients' prior treatments.* Clients' doubts may be based in part on prior experiences sharing about their past as part of treatment or AA. Help them identify what worked and what didn't. Sometimes it's a timing issue or the fit between them and the treatment model or provider.

★ *Identify supportive helplines to try (Handout 2).* Have clients identify which ones they're willing to try and under what circumstances (e.g., when having a flashback or urge to drink). Role-play if needed. Encourage them to practice contacting one helpline this week.

★ *Validate that it takes courage to reach out for help.* Emphasize that regardless of the outcome, the effort is valuable and usually leads to growth.

★ *Discussion*
  - "Why is it hard to trust if you have a history of trauma or addiction?"
  - "If a doubt comes up, do you try to counter it?"
  - "Any concerns about Creating Change in particular?"
  - "Do any helplines on Handout 2 appeal to you?"
  - "Do you know of any additional helplines that aren't on Handout 2?"

Suggestions

✦ *Adjust treatment plans if there are genuine, serious concerns about client safety.* For most clients, doubts about treatment are based on general fears rather than current realities. But for a few, the concerns may be serious enough to suggest delaying past-focused counseling. For example, clients who are currently highly suicidal (not just having thoughts but also intent and plan) would be better served by starting with present-focused trauma/addiction treatment. See the extra topic "Recovery Strengths and Challenges," which explores readiness for Creating Change.

✦ *Stay realistic about trust.* Handout 1 is about helping clients engage in treatment and recovery. It's not encouraging blind trust in general. Some clients have been too trusting of unsafe people and situations. Various other topics in Creating Change explore relationships, where such issues can be addressed.

✦ *Provide education.* Some points in Handout 1 may be new and even a bit controversial for some clients, such as the idea that it's better to work on both trauma and addiction than just one or the other. Offer additional educational materials as needed, such as from the internet and Seeking Safety.

✦ *As you get to know clients, watch for them under- or overestimating the work.* Some think the work is easier than it is (*under*estimating its impact). They share too much too soon or have difficulty pacing it ("It's easy, let's get on with it"). Others fear it excessively (*over*estimating it), believing they aren't strong enough to do it. As the treatment unfolds over future sessions, help them notice these tendencies.

✦ *In group treatment, discuss concerns about trusting other group members.* Clients may fear that other group members will judge them, betray their confidence, or not be able to relate to them. Open discussion is important as clients may have experienced these issues in prior groups. The Treatment Agreement in the "Introduction" topic can be helpful to review if needed.

✦ *Add additional resources to Handout 2.* Local resources can be especially helpful.

Tough Cases

* "How will this help me stay sober?"
* "How do I know I can trust you?"
* "What if I start talking about the past and can't handle it?"
* "This is for wimps—boo-hoo and all that."
* "I just don't like counseling; it never helps."

Quotation

"The trick is to say 'yes' to life."

~ JAMES BALDWIN, 20th-century African American writer

HANDOUT 1

Trust versus Doubt

It's natural to have questions and doubts as you begin counseling. It may be difficult to trust that recovery is possible or that counseling will make a difference.

One gift of recovery is greater trust— n yourself, recovery, relationships, and the future.

★ *Circle any statements below that are true for you, on each side: trust/doubt. Put a question mark (?) next to any you don't understand. There are no right or wrong answers—just notice where you are right now. The pages that follow describe the beliefs in more detail.*

✗ Doubt	versus	✦ Trust
1. "I'm too far gone."		"Recovery is possible, no matter what."
2. "Facing the past is too hard."		"I can go at my own pace and get support."
3. "I'm crazy, weak."		"I lived through a lot and need help sorting it out."
4. "I don't want pity."		"I deserve compassion."
5. "If I start to cry, I'll never stop."		"I can learn to move through emotional pain."
6. "It's best to forget the past. Time heals all wounds."		"Healing occurs with active effort."
7. "I should focus just on addiction [or just on trauma]."		"If I have addiction and trauma, it's best to work on both together."
8. "It's not fair. I shouldn't have to do this work."		"I'll be stronger and better if I do this work, even if it's not fair."
9. "If I talk about trauma or addiction, it's like it's happening all over again."		"Talking with safe people helps."
10. "If I recover, it means the trauma didn't matter."		"Recovery means I'm honoring my survival."
11. "I should know how to do this."		"I need to be patient with myself; I can learn."
12. "I don't want to tell my story."		"I can share only what I want, when I want."

Others? List here: _____ Others? List here: _____

(cont.)

From *Creating Change* by Lisa M. Najavits. Copyright © 2024 Lisa M. Najavits. Published by The Guilford Press. Permission to photocopy this material is granted to purchasers of this book for use with your own clients or patients; see copyright page for details.

HANDOUT 1 *(p. 2 of 3)*   Trust versus Doubt

EXPLORE

1. ✘ ***Doubt:*** *"I'm too far gone."*
   You may have struggled so long with trauma or addiction that you feel hopeless about getting better: "Nothing will work"; "I can't picture life without addiction"; "Don't waste your time on me." You may have been through treatment already but still have major problems. Yet recovery is *always* possible, no matter what. You may need to try different types of help, or sometimes it's a timing issue. Keep trying, and it *will* click eventually.

   ✦ ***Trust:*** "Recovery is possible, no matter what."

2. ✘ ***Doubt:*** *"Facing the past is too hard."*
   One trauma survivor said, "If I dared, dared for a moment to let myself know, feel what had really happened, my heart would burst, my head would explode." It's common to fear that you won't be able to tolerate the feelings and memories. But you can pace yourself, sharing as much or little as you choose. You can take it one session at a time and see how it goes. One client who completed Creating Change said, "Facing the past was far less painful than the depression, the suicidal thoughts, the constant need to be drinking or drugging and the feeling that I was never safe. It was better for me to face the ghosts of my past than to stay stuck with the ghosts of the present."

   ✦ ***Trust:*** "I can go at my own pace and get support."

3. ✘ ***Doubt:*** *"I'm crazy, weak."*
   There's a saying in trauma recovery: Rather than asking, "What's wrong with you?" ask, "What happened to you?" The same is true for addiction. Rather than self-blame, seek to understand how your history led to where you are now. It's not just you, but also family history, culture, genes, peers, and media influences. As you continue in recovery, you'll discover a new, more complete story that's not simply about your flaws.

   ✦ ***Trust:*** "I lived through a lot and need help sorting it out."

4. ✘ ***Doubt:*** *"I don't want pity."*
   Counseling isn't about pity, feeling sorry for yourself, or making excuses. It's about compassion, which means giving yourself credit for surviving while also being responsible and self-aware in the present. Self-pity is about staying stuck while compassion is about growth.

   ✦ ***Trust:*** "I deserve compassion."

5. ✘ ***Doubt:*** *"If I start to cry, I'll never stop."*
   If you've held on to emotional pain for a long time, it may seem that letting yourself cry will open floodgates you can't close. But pain comes in waves, not a continuous flood. "No feeling is final." You can learn to move through it and will be rewarded with greater insight, joy, and the richness of living life fully.

   ✦ ***Trust:*** "I can learn to move through emotional pain."

6. ✘ ***Doubt:*** *"It's best to forget the past. Time heals all wounds."*
   Time alone doesn't heal major trauma or addiction. Once they've taken root, they typically persist, and often get worse, unless there's a strong effort to break the cycle. Recovery occurs with active effort and good treatment—not just time.

   ✦ ***Trust:*** "Healing occurs with active effort."

(cont.)

HANDOUT 1 *(p. 3 of 3)*   Trust versus Doubt

7. ✘ **Doubt**: *"I should focus just on addiction [or just on trauma]."*
   It's highly recommended to work on both at the same time if you have both. Improvement in one helps the other, too, in an upward spiral. In older times, the idea was to focus only on the addiction ("Get sober for a year, then deal with trauma"), or only on trauma ("Healing trauma will resolve the addiction"). But it's now understood that if you have both, you need help for both.

   ✦ **Trust**: *"If I have addiction and trauma, it's best to work on both together."*

8. ✘ **Doubt**: *"It's not fair. I shouldn't have to do this work."*
   One trauma survivor said, "Why do I have to do this? She gets off scot-free and I spend the rest of my life focusing on what she did." It's understandable to resent the unfairness, to feel cheated and angry. But it helps to remember that you're doing recovery for *you*. And many people say that although they never wished for trauma or addiction, recovery gave them a profound appreciation for life they wouldn't have had otherwise.

   ✦ **Trust**: *"I'll be stronger and better if I do this work, even if it's not fair."*

9. ✘ **Doubt**: *"If I talk about trauma or addiction, it's like it's happening all over again."*
   One client said, "I spent my whole life trying to get away from memories. Why go into them now? It was bad enough the first time." It's true that simply remembering trauma or addiction isn't enough. *Working through* is the goal, transforming your relationship to them.

   ✦ **Trust**: *"Talking with safe people helps."*

10. ✘ **Doubt**: *"If I recover, it means the trauma didn't matter."*
    Some people believe moving forward is a betrayal. It means the perpetrator wins ("He was right; it didn't matter what he did to me"). Or they feel they're abandoning those left behind ("I survived but my combat buddy didn't, so what right do I have to a good life?"). They think getting better means the trauma wasn't really so bad. But none of these is true. Getting better is just that: It's valuing your life and the better future you have the right to create.

    ✦ **Trust**: *"Recovery means I'm honoring my survival."*

11. ✘ **Doubt**: *"I should know how to do this."*
    You may be impatient, wanting to move quickly to make up for lost time. "Why can't I stop using?" and "I should be over my trauma already." Just as the body heals at its own pace after injury, emotional healing goes at its own pace too. You may never have learned how to deal with feelings. You may have had poor role models in the past. Keep learning and doing all you can toward recovery. It will come.

    ✦ **Trust**: *"I need to be patient with myself; I can learn."*

12. ✘ **Doubt**: *"I don't want to tell my story."*
    Talking about the past can be done by sharing small pieces, at whatever pace you choose. It's always up to you. Both trauma and addiction erode personal power, and recovery helps restore it. You should never feel pressured into revealing more than you want to. In Creating Change, there are opportunities to share but never a requirement to do so.

    ✦ **Trust**: *"I can share only what I want, when I want."*

➢ **Any other doubts or trust you want to explore?**

_____

_____

HANDOUT 2   Trust versus Doubt

Supportive Helplines

Need some extra support? Remember it's a strength to reach out for help! Here are some national, free, reputable helplines for immediate assistance.

★ *Circle any that appeal to you. Keep this list on hand throughout treatment.*

- **211**
  Dial 211 for referrals to supportive services such as food and clothing banks, rent/utility assistance, work and transportation, family and school resources, and treatment. It's like dialing 911 except it's for human services.
- **Crisis Text Line**
  Text "HOME" to 741741
  crisistextline.org
- **Disaster Distress Helpline**
  800-985-5990
  samhsa.gov/find-help/disaster-distress-helpline
- **Domestic Violence Hotline**
  800-799-7233
  thehotline.org
- **Find Help (local resources such as housing, food pantries, transit)**
  findhelp.org
- **Find Treatment (Substance Abuse and Mental Health Services Administration)**
  findtreatment.gov
- **LGBT National Hotline**
  888-843-4564
  lgbthotline.org
- **National Alliance on Mental Illness HelpLine**
  800-950-6264
  nami.org/help
- **National Child Abuse Hotline**
  800-422-4453
  childhelphotline.org
- **National Eating Disorders Association Hotline**
  800-931-2237
  nationaleatingdisorders.org/help-support/contact-helpline
- **National Human Trafficking Hotline**
  888-373-7888
  humantraffickinghotline.org
- **National Runaway Safeline**
  800-786-2929
  1800runaway.org
- **National Sexual Assault Hotline**
  800-656-4673
  rainn.org
- **National Suicide Prevention Hotline**
  988 or 800-273-8255
  988lifeline.org
- **National Treatment Hotline for Mental Health/Substance Abuse**
  800-662-4357
  samhsa.gov/find-help/national-helpline
- **Parent Stress Line**
  800-632-8188
  parentshelpingparents.org/stressline
- **Partnership to End Addiction**
  Text "Connect" to 55753
  drugfree.org
- **Veterans Crisis Hotline**
  800-273-8255
  veteranscrisisline.net

Also:
- See *https://screening.mentalhealthamerica.net/screening-tools* for free, valid, anonymous online assessments you can take to identify and learn about mental health issues.
- Various free supports offer regular meetings, such as *aa.org, al-anon.org, alateen.org, smartrecovery.org, refugerecovery.org, nami.org*.

From *Creating Change* by Lisa M. Najavits. Copyright © 2024 Lisa M. Najavits. Published by The Guilford Press. Permission to photocopy this material, or to download and print additional copies (*www.guilford.com/najavits3-materials*), is granted to purchasers of this book for use with your own clients or patients; see copyright page for details.

Ideas for a Commitment

Commit to one action that will move your life forward!
It can be anything you feel will help you, or you can try one of the ideas below.
Keeping your commitment is a way of respecting, honoring, and caring for yourself.

✦ Option 1. Ask a trusted person to record supportive messages on your phone that you can play when you start to doubt yourself.

✦ Option 2. Try contacting a helpline in Handout 2 this week.

✦ Option 3. Write about *trust versus doubt* in your life. Do you have trust issues? When did they begin? Is it hard for you to trust yourself? other people? your recovery?

✦ Option 4. Choose a *trust* or a *doubt* in Handout 1 and explore it in more detail (by writing, drawing, music, collage, etc.).

Honor Your Survival

SUMMARY

In this topic, clients identify traumas and other painful events they experienced. They're encouraged to honor their survival and to understand that recovery is possible. They can also explore factors that impact recovery (e.g., isolation vs. the presence of supportive people).

ORIENTATION

To honor survival of trauma is not a small thing. It's a poignant awareness that goes beyond acknowledging the simple fact of physical survival. It's about having respect and even awe for the strength it took to endure, to just make it through. Too often clients feel degraded by their traumas—damaged, broken, weak. Taking pride in their survival is one step toward offsetting those feelings and serves as the focus of today's first handout.

In the second handout, clients are asked to identify traumas and other adverse events that continue to hold emotional pain for them, which in later sessions they can talk about in more detail. The traumas they name may be physical incidents that meet the formal definition of trauma in the DSM-5-TR but also a broader array that includes losses and nonphysical events, such as discrimination and emotional abuse.

Note that this is the first topic in Creating Change in which clients reveal their traumas, and it's intentionally designed to allow them to "dip a toe in the water" rather than diving in fully. Trust grows slowly and the hope is that they will have a validating experience that motivates increasing vulnerability over time. One counselor describes a client who "didn't think anyone could handle the truth. She believed if she told me what she'd really been through, I'd be crying so hard I wouldn't be able to stand it. She wanted to protect me from her story. It was important for her to learn that professional secret keepers, like myself, hear similar stories often. She'd stayed hidden and stuck for years. Slowly, ever so slowly, she was able to talk about her past."

The third handout addresses the context of trauma, which is often as or more important than the trauma itself. An example of a positive factor is the perpetrator being held accountable. Negative factors include humiliation and betrayal. Clients can explore how such factors played a role in helping or impeding their recovery. One said, "If only I had had someone to talk to after I was molested at 10, I wouldn't have become an addict." Many of the context factors also apply to addiction.

In sum, today's topic begins the exploration of trauma and other adverse events in ways that build a sense of dignity in clients' survival, rather than the shame and blame that too often add to the burden of recovery (Israel et al., 2022). It also allows for increasing alliance with you (and among group members in group treatment) by moving into emotionally vulnerable territory.

Your Emotional Reactions

Clients are often highly sensitive to counselors' reactions when trauma is revealed. They may fear that you don't really want to know what happened, just like people in the past who negated it. They may believe they'll be judged for what they did or didn't do. How you show up emotionally during the session, the presence and kindness conveyed, speak volumes. The work requires some level of vulnerability by the counselor as well as by clients—to truly hear, feel, and empathize with the suffering they lived. With large caseloads year in and year out, hearing too much awful trauma, there may be some amount of numbing within the counselor. The theme of honoring what clients survived can help recenter the work in a sense of reverence and depth of emotion. It's a privilege to do trauma counseling—not necessarily easy, but a privilege.

Acknowledgments

The session quotation is cited in van der Kolk (2014, p. 112). In the section "What Makes Recovery Harder" in Handout 3, "having to stay strong" and "questions and uncertainty" are adapted from Lazare (1979, as described in Rando, 1993, p. 134).

SESSION FORMAT

1. *Check-in* (per Chapter 3).
2. *Quotation.* Link the quotation to the session topic—for example, *"Today we'll talk about honoring your survival of difficult life experiences. The quote beautifully conveys that people do it in their own way, using whatever is available to them."*
3. *Handouts* (relate the topic to clients' lives):
    Handout 1: **Honor Your Survival**
    Handout 2: **What You Lived Through**
    Handout 3: **Context That Helped or Harmed**
4. *Check-out* (per Chapter 3).

SESSION CONTENT

Goals

- ☐ Encourage clients to honor their survival thus far.
- ☐ Identify traumas and other experiences that still hold emotional pain for them.
- ☐ Explore trauma context factors that helped or hindered recovery.
- ☐ Convey optimism that recovery is possible.

Ways to Relate the Material to Clients' Lives

★ ***Help clients appreciate the fact that they survived trauma (Handout 1).*** Handout 1 is very short, and it can be moving to have clients read it aloud (almost like a poem), taking turns if in group treatment. After that they could choose one item on the list and identify what it means to them or an example from their life that illustrates it.

★ ***Focus on events that are currently distressing (Handout 2).*** Clients may have had a lot of traumas, but some may not need clinical attention now. In Handout 2, they can identify events that are still upsetting, which they can address in more detail in future sessions. If needed, clarify what it means to have a trauma that "still bothers you now." You can say simply, "This means that you still think about it a lot or feel triggered when reminded of it." If needed, you can also refer to more detailed trauma symptoms such as flashbacks and nightmares.

★ *Draw clients' attention to events that are less commonly identified in trauma lists (Handout 2).* Trauma has become a widely known concept in many service systems and the media. Many clients are already aware of their traumas. Highlight other adverse events in this handout that are not on standard trauma measures, such as "stressful caretaking," "loss of innocence," and "historical trauma." (Keep in mind that these would fit the broader SAMHSA definition of trauma but not the narrower DSM-5-TR definition that is used for a diagnosis of PTSD. See Appendix A, "Key Terms," online (*www.guilford.com/najavits3-materials*) for more on these.

★ *Educate about trauma symptoms as needed.* Giving language to symptoms can be very healing and help validate clients' experience. As clients work on the handouts, they may mention trauma problems without recognizing them as symptoms. Educate as needed. If a client says, "I went through a sexual assault, but I don't remember most of it," you could mention that dissociation and blackouts sometimes occur during trauma, for example.

★ *Discussion*
- "How does it feel to honor your survival?"
- "What are you most proud of in your survival?"
- "Do you believe you can heal from trauma?"
- "How does your trauma relate to your addiction?"
- "What do you notice in your body when we talk about trauma?"
- "Why is the context of trauma so important?"

Suggestions

✦ *In group treatment, encourage mutual support but not comparison of suffering.* Clients generally offer support to other clients, but they may also engage in comparisons. Some convey they had it worse ("You think that's bad? Well, I went through . . . "). Others minimize their experiences ("She went through so much more. Maybe I don't belong in this treatment"). Emphasize that all pain is real and important. Each client has a unique story and comparisons don't promote recovery. The goal is compassion toward self and others.

✦ *Don't go into detailed trauma narratives in today's topic.* There will be time for that in future sessions. The goal now is to share about trauma in a more limited way. The client is still building trust with you (and other clients, if it's a group); and each session allows for greater vulnerability. So too if strong emotions arise, validate these but don't explore them in detail at this point. Offer kind responses, for example, "I really hope this treatment will help you with that," rather than "Say more about what you're feeling." If needed, use grounding to bring down intense emotions.

✦ *Encourage poignant awareness.* All three handouts are intended to evoke emotion, not just facts. For example, with Handout 1, offer deep respect for clients' survival. "It's amazing you got through all that"; "You must have had such inner strength to have survived."

✦ *Convey optimism about the future.* Emphasize hope and the importance of working hard on recovery to make the future better than the past.

✦ *Emphasize that trauma also leads to growth.* Future topics will address this more, but it's helpful to mention that trauma can lead to *posttraumatic growth* (positive transformation such as greater appreciation for life, other people, and personal strengths).

✦ *Observe how clients respond to Handout 3.* Some may be so "hungry" for validation of their pain that they mark off only negatives. It's best just to observe such patterns rather than trying to balance them by asking clients to focus on positives, too. As they continue in treatment, they can gain additional perspectives.

Tough Cases

* "This list of traumas is depressing."
* "How will this help my addiction?"
* "How many traumas have you had?"
* "Nothing bothers me; I'm numb."
* "I can't change the past. My life is ruined."
* "This makes me feel like hurting myself."

Quotation

"Every life is a piece of art, put together with all means available."

~ Pierre Janet, 19th-century French psychiatrist

HANDOUT 1

Honor Your Survival

★ *Circle any that are meaningful for you.*

- You are here today and that's an achievement.
    Honor your strength.
- Only you know what it took for you to make it through.
    Honor what you know.
- Whatever happened in the past, the future is yours to create.
    Honor your future.
- Emotional pain can heal.
    Honor your ability to grow.
- Everyone makes good and poor choices.
    Honor that you are human.
- You may have suffered many losses.
    Honor what you still have.
- Your body helped you survive.
    Honor your body.
- There are some good people.
    Honor the people who helped.
- You are not alone in recovery.
    Honor other survivors.
- Where there's life, there's hope.
    Honor your life.

Add your own:
- _____
    Honor _____ .

From *Creating Change* by Lisa M. Najavits. Copyright © 2024 Lisa M. Najavits. Published by The Guilford Press. Permission to photocopy this material is granted to purchasers of this book for use with your own clients or patients; see copyright page for details.

HANDOUT 2 — Honor Your Survival

What You Lived Through

In this handout, you can identify your difficult life events. Some may be in the past, others may be current.

★ *If you had more than one of the same type (e.g., two major accidents), fill out the columns below for the one that still upsets you the most.*

Losses	Mark (✓) any you experienced	Does it still upset you? Yes/No	If yes, how upsetting is it? 1 (a little) to 10 (extremely)
1. **Loss of someone close** (children taken away; family member dies or goes to prison)			
2. **Loss of health** (injury, disability, chronic pain)			
3. **Loss of reputation** (public shaming, scandal)			
4. **Loss of community** (orphaned, foster care, being a refugee, etc.)			
5. **Loss of who you hoped to become** (lost opportunities, feeling life is ruined)			
6. **Loss of ideals** (such as trust, justice, safety, sense of purpose, innocence, hope)			
7. **Loss of independence** (aging, jail, hospitalization, etc.)			
8. **Loss of important part of your life** (job or income, pet, home, substance or other addictive behavior)			
9. **Other loss:**			
Physical harm by others			
1. **Sexual abuse or assault** (rape, molestation, unwanted sexual touching)			
2. **Physical assault** (hit, beaten, attacked, shot)			
3. **Physical neglect** (lack of food, shelter, etc.)			
4. **Community violence** (gang violence, riots, school shootings, police/citizen clashes, terrorism, etc.)			
5. **Crime** (mugged, shot, kidnapped, carjacked, stalked, home invasion, arson, etc.)			
6. **War** (as a civilian or as military)			
7. **Other physical harm by others:**			

(cont.)

From *Creating Change* by Lisa M. Najavits. Copyright © 2024 Lisa M. Najavits. Published by The Guilford Press. Permission to photocopy this material is granted to purchasers of this book for use with your own clients or patients; see copyright page for details.

HANDOUT 2 *(p. 2 of 2)*   Honor Your Survival

Losses	✓	Yes/No	1–10
Physical harm from accidents or natural events			
1. **Major accident** (car, airplane, workplace, chemical spill, explosion, medical accident, nuclear disaster)			
2. **Natural disaster** (hurricane, tornado, avalanche, flood, famine, fire)			
3. **Severe or life-threatening illness or injury** (cancer, loss of limb, etc.)			
4. **Physical trauma as part of your work** (e.g., police, firefighter)			
5. **Animal attack** (e.g., mountain lion)			
6. **Other accident or natural event:**			
Other distressing events			
1. **Your addiction** (substance, gambling, shopping, food, TV, sex, internet, pornography, etc.)			
2. **Addiction in people close to you** (any type, per row above, or serious impact such as witnessing overdose, gambling, bankruptcy)			
3. **Forced to inflict physical harm** (you had to harm a person or animal, against your will)			
4. **Historical trauma** (genocide, slavery, concentration camp, or other culture-based violence)			
5. **Severe poverty** (lack of food, homelessness)			
6. **Mental illness** (addiction, depression, anxiety disorder, bipolar disorder, psychosis, etc.)			
7. **Serious relationship problems** (constant fighting, major betrayal, no friends or family, painful divorce)			
8. **Emotional abuse, bullying, or harassment** (put down, teased, humiliated, coerced, controlled)			
9. **Stressful caretaking** (sick or elderly relative, special needs child)			
10. **Major injustice** (wrongly sent to prison; discrimination based on race/ethnicity, gender, age, religion, or disability)			
11. **Abandonment** (caretaker left without warning; lack of rescue during disaster, etc.)			
12. **Other upsetting event:**			

❖ **A Better Future**

You can make the future better than the past. Each session of Creating Change offers a different way to do that.

HANDOUT 3   Honor Your Survival

Context That Helped or Harmed

Why do some people recover sooner than others from trauma or addiction? This handout explores factors that impact recovery—it's not just what happened to you but also the context.

★ **Mark any that were true for you.** *For multiple events, you can summarize across them or complete the handout multiple times.*

1. WHAT MAKES RECOVERY EASIER

___ ***Ability to speak about it.*** Even just one trusted person to confide in can make a difference.

___ ***Justice.*** The perpetrator is held accountable through the justice system or informal methods such as family or community supporting the victim rather than the perpetrator.

___ ***Doing well beforehand.*** You have more strength to draw on if you were already functioning well (holding a job, good social network, healthy).

___ ***Time to process.*** This means having time to sort through your feelings about what happened.

___ ***Public validation,*** such as sympathetic media coverage; memorials, awards, holidays (e.g., Veterans Day); or financial compensation.

___ ***Physical help,*** such as being provided with first aid, food, or shelter; or a bystander who intervenes.

___ ***Treatment.*** Getting help soon after trauma or addiction makes it easier to recover.

___ ***Ability to escape.*** The opportunity to flee can prevent worse harm.

___ ***Adult age.*** Adults are more able to cope and get help than children.

___ ***A one-time event.*** A single incident is usually easier than multiple ones.

___ ***Sense of meaning.*** In trauma, it helps if it was part of a larger purpose (e.g., saving someone or an important military mission).

___ ***Emotional support.*** Words of comfort make you feel less alone.

___ ***An impersonal event*** (not caused by people) versus *interpersonal* (people caused it). For example, a hurricane is usually easier than bullying or abuse.

___ ***Resources.*** Money, a safe community, access to health care and other important resources make it easier to cope.

___ ***Other positive factors?***

_____

_____

2. WHAT MAKES RECOVERY HARDER

___ ***Not being believed.*** "You're making that up" or "It wasn't so bad." This can be devastating when it's from parents, police, doctors, or others who are supposed to care for you.

___ ***Blame.*** You blame yourself or others blame you unfairly. At a community level, it may involve shunning or "canceling" you.

(cont.)

From *Creating Change* by Lisa M. Najavits. Copyright © 2024 Lisa M. Najavits. Published by The Guilford Press. Permission to photocopy this material is granted to purchasers of this book for use with your own clients or patients; see copyright page for details.

HANDOUT 3 *(p. 2 of 2)* Honor Your Survival

___ ***Isolation.*** Feeling alone during or after trauma or addiction increases the pain. You may doubt yourself and find it hard to get help.

___ ***Having to stay strong*** can mean you never get to heal or take care of your needs. This often occurs among first responders (police, fire, first aid), military, and in some families.

___ ***Physically damaging.*** Trauma or addiction that causes direct physical injury or intrusion is typically more distressing (e.g., sexual assault, overdose).

___ ***Normalized.*** Trauma or addiction may be so pervasive that it seems normal to you. It's "how things are" (in gangs, dangerous neighborhoods, some families).

___ ***Questions or uncertainty.*** It's harder amid important unknowns (e.g., not understanding why a loved one committed suicide or being unable to reach family during a disaster).

___ ***Humiliation.*** This means being debased, degraded, called names, or forced into sexual acts that felt shameful to you.

___ ***Taboo.*** Some events are so socially unacceptable that they're usually hidden and denied (e.g., incest, some addictions).

___ ***Hurting others.*** Harming others can leave you with intense inner conflict (e.g., wartime atrocities or forced to hurt a person or animal as part of abuse).

___ ***Being targeted.*** This means singled out for harm. One child may be abused while others aren't. Hate crimes target particular groups. You may also be targeted if you speak out or are perceived as a threat.

___ ***Unwanted pleasure.*** If positive feelings are part of trauma, it can be confusing. You may have felt aroused during sexual assault. In war, there may be guilt about sadistic pleasure in killing. Abuse victims may feel love for the perpetrator.

___ ***Moral injury*** means your ethics were violated as part of the event. Betrayal, corruption, or being forced to do things against your conscience adds greater injury to trauma.

___ ***Anticipation of harm.*** Knowing that trauma will occur creates intense stress.

___ ***Involving substances.*** If trauma occurs amid substance use, it can evoke negative reactions ("Well, you shouldn't have been drinking").

___ ***Other negative factors?***

_____

_____

✧ Reflections

- Did you have more positive or negative factors?
- Can you feel compassion toward yourself?
- Any new insights about what you went through?
- What feelings arose with this handout?

Honor Your Survival

Ideas for a Commitment

Commit to one action that will move your life forward!
It can be anything you feel will help you, or you can try one of the ideas below.
Keeping your commitment is a way of respecting, honoring, and caring for yourself.

- Option 1. What advice would you give to someone who experienced trauma or addiction? Write about that.

- Option 2. Do something meaningful this week to honor your trauma or addiction survival. Visit a comforting place (e.g., mountains or beach). Or volunteer your time to help other survivors.

- Option 3. What does *recovery* mean to you? What would it look like? Write or use art, music, video, collage, or other forms of expression.

- Option 4. Do you have a child who's been through trauma? Find help by searching online for "advice for parents of traumatized children" and "treatment for traumatized children." See also the "Families and Caregivers" section at *www.nctsn.org* (National Child Traumatic Stress Network).

Relationship Patterns

SUMMARY

In this topic, clients deepen awareness of how they relate. They explore healthy and unhealthy relationship patterns and share relationship wisdom they've acquired.

ORIENTATION

How clients relate—to others, to themselves, and also to material things such as substances, food, and money—is a mirror of who they are inside. Relationships are where the impact of trauma and addiction is sometimes seen most clearly but can also be a source of their greatest healing. This double-edged quality—relationships can drag clients down or raise them up—makes relationships one of the most potent forces in illness and recovery.

This topic offers several ways to explore relationships. Handout 1 identifies healthy relationship patterns (e.g., *more joy than pain*; *shared power*) and unhealthy relationship patterns (e.g., *isolation*; *giving too much*). Handout 2 offers relationship wisdom, such as "Conflicts are part of relationships; how they're resolved is what matters." The overarching goal is to help clients understand how current relationship patterns have origins in the past, arising from trauma, addiction, childhood messages, and key people in their lives. They adapted as best as they could, even if those adaptations later created new problems. "Personality will grow around adversity the way tree roots will grow around a rock, shaping itself in response to the immovable" (Febos, 2022).

Most clients endured serious relationship deficits growing up. Indeed, family history is one of the strongest predictors of who develops trauma symptoms and addiction, based on a mix of social and genetic factors. It's useful to remember, however, that this understanding is quite recent. For most of human history, trauma symptoms and addiction (even when not named as such) have been understood primarily as moral failure, character flaws, individual weakness, or even possession by "the devil." It's a major advance to understand them as illnesses, caused in part by harmful relationships.

Brown and Lewis observed,

The alcoholic family is now recognized as one of chaos (covert or overt), inconsistency, unpredictability, blurring of boundaries, unclear roles, arbitrariness, changing logic, and perhaps violence and incest. The "everyday" experience is one of chronic trauma, which becomes the context of "normal" family life. Episodes of "acute" trauma, such as marital affairs, acts of humiliation, physical and emotional abandonment, and violence, punctuate the normalized high level of tension. (1995, p. 285)

Even clients who first experience trauma and addiction in adulthood typically manifest relationship problems just due to the impact of those events.

There are many types of relationship issues. For some clients, their most important relationship may be to a substance of choice or a drug dealer. Others have no one they're close to or, the opposite, dive too quickly into intense relationships that fail. Some repeatedly get hurt or hurt others. The list goes on. Yet it's just as important to recognize relationship strengths that clients show—healthy relationship patterns and wisdom they have acquired; thus, the handouts also address these.

In sum, recovery provides an opportunity to relate in new ways that can help to "correct" the past.

Your Emotional Reactions

Observe clients' style of relating and notice what it evokes in you. Is the client trusting? Scared? Annoying? Engaging? Open? Shut down? In return, are you sympathetic? Frustrated? Angry? Bored? Kind? The relationship in the room presents an opportunity for clients to try out new ways of relating in a safe environment. Gently provide feedback, when relevant, to help clients understand the relationship dynamics you observe. It can be an important channel for growth if communicated with compassion. At the same time, take stock of your own relationship issues. A good step is to explore today's handouts in relation to your own life and identify how your relationship dynamics, both positive and negative, show up in interactions with clients. See Chapter 4 for more on this.

Acknowledgments

The session quotation is widely attributed to Virginia Satir. The quotation in Ideas for a Commitment is from Mister Rogers (2013, p. 96).

SESSION FORMAT

1. *Check-in* (per Chapter 3).
2. *Quotation.* Link the quotation to the session topic—for example, *"The quote emphasizes that relationships can be a healing force. Today, we'll talk about relationship patterns, both healthy and unhealthy."*
3. *Handouts* (relate the topic to clients' lives):
    Handout 1: **Relationship Patterns**
    Handout 2: **Relationship Wisdom**
4. *Check-out* (per Chapter 3).

SESSION CONTENT

Goals

- ☐ Use a relationship inventory to identify healthy versus unhealthy ways of relating.
- ☐ Identify how clients' relationship patterns changed over time.
- ☐ Explore how trauma and addiction impact relationships.
- ☐ Share relationship wisdom.

Ways to Relate the Material to Clients' Lives

★ ***Help clients identify their strengths and challenges in relationships (Handout 1).*** It's a long handout and there are different ways to approach it. You can have clients fill out just the first five in each section (Part I, Part II). If you're conducting group treatment, you could take turns reading one aloud, and then discuss it, then go to the next. Whatever method you choose it's recommended to have clients do the rating for past and present on each row to bring out how they've changed (which may be for better or worse).

★ ***Share relationship wisdom (Handout 2).*** The handout offers key points. You can have clients mark it up per the instructions at the top of the page. Also, invite them to share their own hard-won lessons about relationships.

★ ***Elicit specific examples.*** The handouts can launch a discussion of real-life relationship examples that clients want to address. If clients focus on a current relationship issue, try to connect it to their past—what were the origins of the dilemma?

★ ***Link relationship issues to trauma/addiction.*** Clients may be highly aware of a relationship problem yet not relate it back to trauma or addiction. Help them "connect the dots" when relevant to do so. For example, "Did your addiction have an impact on that relationship?," "Did your trauma lead to that belief?"

★ ***Guide clients to experiment with new relationship strategies.*** This can improve their current relationships and also deepen understanding of long-standing relationship patterns. As German psychologist Kurt Lewin said, "If you want truly to understand something, try to change it" (per Tolman, 1996, p. 31).

★ ***Discussion***
- "What would others say about what it's like to be in a relationship with you?"
- "Who are the most important influences (positive/negative) on your relationship patterns?"
- "How do you feel as you read the handouts?"
- "How has trauma affected your relationships?"
- "How has addiction affected your relationships?"
- "How have you changed in your approach to relationships?"
- "Are some types of relationships more difficult for you than others (boss/colleague/friend/partner/family)?"

Suggestions

✦ ***Explore relationships broadly.*** In addition to people, ask clients how they relate to: *themselves* (kindly or harshly); *possessions* (e.g., attitude toward money); *a higher power* (if they have one); *pets* (some clients feel closer to pets than to people); their *community*; their *addiction*; and the *environment*, for example.

✦ ***Encourage a balanced view.*** It's important to recognize that most relationships are not all good or all bad. Help clients sort through their dilemmas realistically (e.g., when to stay or leave, how to create more closeness, love/hate for an abusive family member).

✦ ***Try perspective taking.*** Have clients imagine what a relationship feels like not just from their point of view, but also the other person's, and perhaps an imaginary observer. (However, don't ask them to take the point of view of a trauma perpetrator, as that can invalidate their trauma experience.)

✦ ***Consider sharing observations about your relationship with the client.*** This can be immensely helpful if done with sensitivity and tact, pointing out both healthy and unhealthy aspects. This is typically best addressed in individual treatment but, depending on the group, could also be relevant in that modality.

Tough Cases

* "I'll never trust men after what they did to me."
* "When I take Ecstasy, I really like people."
* "I'm better off alone."
* "I had sex with my previous therapist."
* "I can't help flying into a rage."
* "I hate my daughter."
* "People will hurt you if you let them."

Relationship Patterns

Quotation

"We need 4 hugs a day for survival. We need 8 hugs a day for maintenance. We need 12 hugs a day for growth."

~ VIRGINIA SATIR, 20th-century American author
and developer of family therapy

HANDOUT 1

Relationship Patterns

What are your relationship patterns in the past and present?

There are two sections in this table: *healthy* and *unhealthy*. In recovery, the healthy outweigh the unhealthy.

★ *Rate each item from 0 (not at all) to 3 (greatly). The goal is awareness, without judgment or blame.*

0	1	2	3
Not at all	A little	Moderately	Greatly

Note: Relationships between adults have different dynamics and responsibilities than an adult to a child. It's never the case that a child who is abused was "relating badly" or in any way responsible for the abuse. Even in adult relationships, you may not always be able to get out of a toxic relationship.

PART I: *HEALTHY* RELATIONSHIP PATTERNS

Pattern	Description	True for you in the past? 0–3	True for you now? 0–3
1. More joy than pain	Close relationships have both. But a relationship must bring more joy than pain or it isn't healthy.		
2. Real conversations	Rather than small talk, clichés, or avoidance, there's honesty about important topics. The content may differ—what you discuss with your boss is different than with a partner. But you can talk about what matters.		
3. Shared power	Each person is respected and plays a part in decisions and ideas. Even with an imbalance of power (boss/worker, parent/child), there's valuing of the other's perspective.		
4. "Open eyes"	This means seeing people reasonably clearly. In contrast, unhealthy relationships have major distortions (seeing others as better or worse than they really are).		

(cont.)

From *Creating Change* by Lisa M. Najavits. Copyright © 2024 Lisa M. Najavits. Published by The Guilford Press. Permission to photocopy this material is granted to purchasers of this book for use with your own clients or patients; see copyright page for details

HANDOUT 1 *(p. 2 of 4)*   Relationship Patterns

Pattern	Description	True for you in the past? 0–3	True for you now? 0–3
5. *Noticing the good*	Some relationships start out well but then get mired in criticism and constant attempts to change the other. What's good gets lost amid the judgments. Unless the main feeling is appreciation, the relationship deteriorates.		
6. *Acceptance*	Everyone has flaws and vulnerabilities. In healthy relationships, you can be open about them and there's an attitude of acceptance (except for violence or other serious destruction).		
7. *Ebb and flow*	You can weather the natural ups and downs of relationships. There's closeness and also time apart.		
8. *Ability to resolve conflicts*	Conflicts aren't ignored or seen as a threat but understood as a normal part of relationships. They're addressed respectfully and some resolution is achieved, even if imperfect.		
9. *Give-and-take*	Everyone's needs are addressed rather than rigid roles of "giver" or "taker" (one person getting all the attention, care, or money). It's not about keeping score, but there's balance over the long term.		
10. *Positive energy*	There's a sense of spark and enjoyment of the other—rather than neutral (no feeling) or negative (angry, mean).		
11. *Loyalty when it matters*	In tough times, you're there for each other. It doesn't mean being a martyr to another's pain, but you show up rather than abandoning or rejecting.		
12. *Trust*	Trust is the foundation: acting honorably and, if a rift occurs, owning it and aiming to correct it. Lies, cheating, betrayal, or using people destroys trust.		
13. *Nourished by time and attention*	Good relationships require contact though the amount will depend on how close the person is. They fade if there's too little time and attention.		
14. *Love*	Genuine love is a desire to give to others, empathy, and wanting what's best for them, while still maintaining boundaries and a strong sense of self.		
Other healthy patterns:	_____ _____ _____		

(cont.)

HANDOUT 1 *(p. 3 of 4)*   Relationship Patterns

PART II: *UNHEALTHY* RELATIONSHIP PATTERNS

Pattern	Description	True for you in the past? 0–3	True for you now? 0–3
1. *Fantasy relationships*	If you felt unloved, you may have developed fantasy relationships to make up for that. One client said, "I'd watch *Mr. Rogers* on TV and pretend he was my father because my real father was abusing me."		
2. *Outside looking in*	Feeling like an outsider—apart, alone—is a core theme in trauma and addiction. You may feel less than, ignored, or freakish.		
3. *Relationship addiction*	This includes sex addiction, love addiction (also called codependency), and the inability to be alone. These may be a distraction from pain you're afraid to feel.		
4. *Constant conflict*	Conflicts (verbal or physical) can become a way of life. It may be a replay of past trauma or part of addiction (e.g., drunk rage). Whatever the reason, the relationship doesn't feel real unless there's arguing or drama.		
5. *Enmeshment*	This means overinvolvement, lack of independence. Boundaries are overstepped, there may be excessive guilt, overprotection, and messages that hold you back (don't move away, don't trust outside the family, don't go to treatment).		
6. *Highly critical*	You can end up disliked if you excessively criticize or show contempt. Underneath, it usually means you feel bad about yourself.		
7. *Clinging*	You have such a deep wish for connection that you smother people with your needs, not giving the other person space. You may stay too long in a relationship that isn't working.		
8. *Push–pull*	One person pursues, the other retreats, over and over. There's never a consistently safe, stable relationship. This pattern is also called approach/avoidance. It's typically based in insecure attachment growing up.		
9. *Giving too much*	You give all to others, but your own needs aren't addressed enough. There may be compulsive caregiving and lack of balance (e.g., too many gifts; too much self-blame). This typically comes from growing up with deprivation or neglect—deep down, you yearn for someone to care for you.		

(cont.)

HANDOUT 1 *(p. 4 of 4)*   Relationship Patterns

Pattern	Description	True for you **in the past?** 0–3	True for you **now?** 0–3
10. *Taking too much*	If you grew up around people who didn't value relationships, you may believe it's "everyone for themselves." You may take whatever you can get, rather than a having loving sense of care and reciprocity with others.		
11. *Attraction to unhealthy people*	You may be so used to being around people who are unsafe that you feel naturally drawn to them. Safe people may seem boring.		
12. *Taking it out on others*	If life has been too hard for too long, you may lash out or harm people. You may not care who you hurt (lying, cheating, using people). These patterns can also occur in active addiction.		
13. *Isolation*	You may have given up on relationships, viewing them as a source of pain or threat, or less compelling than your addiction. You may have *commitment phobia* (inability to develop sustained emotional intimacy).		
Other unhealthy patterns:	_____ _____ _____		

✧ Reflections

When you look at your most important patterns (healthy/unhealthy):

- When did they begin?
- Who did you learn them from (e.g., parents, siblings, partner)?
- Which has changed the most over time?
- How do they relate to your trauma?
- How do they relate to your addiction?
- Which ones do you most want to change?

HANDOUT 2　　　　　　　　　　　　　　　　　　　　　　　　　Relationship Patterns

Relationship Wisdom

Relationship wisdom is hard-earned if you've had trauma or addiction. You may have grown up with negative relationships or no one to teach you.

★ *Circle any you'd like to discuss. Star (★) any you want to work on.*

- The greatest closeness comes from opening up about real issues.
- Accept with grace that some people won't like you.
- As you get better, your relationships will get better, too.
- It's useful to find out how people who are trustworthy perceive you.
- Know when to leave.
- Enjoy people and use things, not vice versa.
- You can't control someone's behavior, but you can control your response to it.
- *Solitude* (time alone) is good; *isolation* (lack of relationships) is not.
- You may have the best intentions yet still hurt or offend people.
- You'll become like the people you spend time with, so choose wisely.
- Work on your relationship with yourself as much as you work on other relationships.
- If you cling too closely, relationships die.
- Your parents couldn't teach you what they didn't know.
- How you relate to substances, food, money, and time may mirror how you relate to people.
- Give a little more than you get.
- Conflicts are part of relationships; how they're resolved is what matters.
- Love is always worthwhile, but not easy.
- Too much criticism erodes a relationship.
- All types of relationships matter (people, community, the environment, higher power, etc.).
- *Others?* _____

✧ Reflections

- How does trauma play a role in what you learned/didn't learn about relationships?
- How does addiction play a role in what you learned/didn't learn about relationships?

From *Creating Change* by Lisa M. Najavits. Copyright © 2024 Lisa M. Najavits. Published by The Guilford Press. Permission to photocopy this material is granted to purchasers of this book for use with your own clients or patients; see copyright page for details.

Relationship Patterns

Ideas for a Commitment

Commit to one action that will move your life forward!
It can be anything you feel will help you, or you can try one of the ideas below.
Keeping your commitment is a way of respecting, honoring, and caring for yourself.

✦ Option 1. Write about this quotation from Mister Rogers, the children's TV show host.

   "I don't think anyone can grow unless he's loved exactly as he is now, appreciated for what he is rather than what he will be."

✦ Option 2. Ask a trustworthy person what's it like to be in a relationship with you. Ask about both the joys and challenges.

✦ Option 3. Describe the relationships that bring out your best. Be as broad as you choose—relationships can mean people, but also your relationship with your work, sports, pets, hobbies, food, exercise, art, religion.

✦ Option 4. If you believe in a higher power, how has your relationship to it changed during recovery? Write or use artwork to explore that.

✦ Option 5. Write about your relationship with yourself—harsh? kind? nurturing? indulgent?—and how it impacts your relationship with others.

Why Addiction?

SUMMARY

This topic helps clients reflect on why they became addicted, taking a nonjudgmental approach that explores various factors, including trauma. They can share pieces of their addiction story and identify the impact of addiction on their life. Positive aspects—insights and recovery successes—are also emphasized. For clients without addiction, parts of the topic can be applied to mental health issues.

ORIENTATION

Junk is not just a habit. It is a way of life. When you give up junk, you give up a way of life.
~WILLIAM S. BURROUGHS, *Junkie*

He hands the pipe to me. . . . He lights the white rocks at the end of the pipe and I draw. A dreamy warm smoke fills my lungs and goes immediately to a place inside of me that I have been unable to reach my entire life. The taste is both chemical and slightly sweet. . . . This is perfect. Nothing can compare to this. It is instant and it is profound. This is what has been missing from me my entire life.
~AUGUSTEN BURROUGHS, *Dry*

The power of addiction and the need to grieve it have been emphasized throughout the history of addiction treatment (White, 1998). It's not enough to give up the behavior; clients also need to face what it did to their lives—the intense preoccupation; losses and destruction; damage to the body; missed opportunities; wasted years; diminished joy and purpose; and sometimes devastating harm to their family. At its worst, there are awful stories of what people did in active addiction: killing innocent people while driving drunk, violent assaults, and even selling their children. One client never forgave himself after his younger brother was killed by a drug dealer instead of him in a case of mistaken identity.

But addictive behavior may also have protected the client. Clients often say that without substances, for example, they couldn't have survived trauma. It helped them to tolerate abuse they couldn't escape, get to sleep, or prevent suicide. Giving it up may feel like losing their only comfort. It's often described as their most important relationship, like a best friend or lover.

Today's topic takes the long view of addiction. There are four handouts, each an exercise to help clients see their history of addiction in a new light. Handout 1 addresses how trauma plays a role in addiction. Addiction may have been a cry for help or a way to hide after trauma, for example. Handout 2 encourages clients to share part of their addiction history and recovery. In Handout 3, they identify an important addiction event, such as a major relapse or hitting bottom, and compare how they perceived it at the time versus now. Events that seemed bad at the time may have led to something good and vice versa. Finally, Handout 4 explores circumstances, as children and adults, that may have impacted the development of their addiction.

Such exploration is never about rationalizing or excusing addictive behavior, but rather understanding it more deeply. Making peace with their past lets clients move beyond the judgments, by themselves and others, that so often accompany addiction. Clients can develop a narrative that's larger than just their own errors and weaknesses, although those, too, are part of the story. There are many angles to explore, including their resilience and what they did right at times. The hope is that this whole-picture approach will reinforce their resolve to continue on the hard path of recovery.

If clients don't have addiction, they can apply today's topic to mental health issues. However, also keep a broad addiction focus—not just substances but also behaviors. Clients sometimes don't recognize they have a behavioral addiction, especially as most are not listed in DSM-5-TR (e.g., gaming, sex, shopping addictions). The Excessive Behavior Scale (Handout 4 of the extra topic "Understanding Trauma and Addiction") provides a way to screen for these.

If clients don't agree with the term *addiction*, you can substitute *compulsive behavior*, *excessive behavior*, or *problem behavior* and encourage them to apply today's topic to that.

The primary goal is greater understanding of why clients became addicted and how it has affected their life. Yet some clients may also need basic addiction education and referrals; guidance on that is provided later in this topic.

Your Emotional Reactions

Clients with addiction can evoke intense feelings in counselors. These are usually described in negative terms—frustration, anger, burnout, cynicism, and power struggles (Imhof et al., 1983). However, equally important are positive feelings: empathy for their suffering; admiration for their resilience; protectiveness; and identification if addiction has touched your own life in some way. To increase positive reactions, consider attending AA speaker meetings to hear amazing stories of recovery in raw, direct ways. You can attend without having an addiction problem yourself. Some clinicians even attend Al-Anon to obtain support when feeling burned out in their work.

Acknowledgments

In the "Orientation" section on the previous page, the quotation from Augusten Burroughs is from *Dry* (2003, p. 270) and the quotation from William Burroughs (originally published under the pseudonym William Lee) is from White (1996, p. 1). The session quotation is from Lewis (1980, p. 84). The Handout 1 quotations are from Mate (2022) and Mattiessen (2023, p. 46). On the Commitment page, the link in option 3 is Twombly (2021).

PREPARING FOR THE SESSION

Optional: Provide colored pens for Handout 4.

Why Addiction? 151

SESSION FORMAT

1. *Check-in* (up to 5 minutes per client). See Chapter 3.
2. *Quotation* (briefly). See page 154. Link the quotation to the session. For example, *"The quote encourages curiosity about why people become addicted. Today we'll explore that in a compassionate way."*
3. *Handouts* (relate the topic to clients' lives; in-depth, most of the session):
   a. Ask clients to look through the handouts:
   Handout 1: **The Tangled Web of Addiction and Trauma**
   Handout 2: **20 Questions: Tell Part of Your Addiction Story**
   Handout 3: **Then versus Now**
   Handout 4: **Lifetime Advantages and Disadvantages**
   b. Help clients relate the topic to current and specific problems in their lives. See "Session Content" (below) and Chapter 3 for suggestions.
4. *Check-out* (briefly). See Chapter 3.

SESSION CONTENT

Goals

☐ Discuss how trauma plays a role in addiction.
☐ Encourage clients to share important parts of their addiction history and recovery.
☐ Try an exercise to see how time changes the perception of key addiction events.
☐ Explore advantages and disadvantages in life that impact the development of addiction.

Ways to Relate the Material to Clients' Lives

★ ***Guide clients to discuss how trauma and addiction were linked in their lives (Handout 1).*** After they mark handout items that are true for them, you can ask questions such as "When did you first notice the connection between trauma and addiction in your life?," "Which ones on the list are most important for you?," "Are any on the list new to you?," "Is there an example you'd like to share?"

★ ***Let clients share part of their addiction story (Handout 2).*** See the topic "Tell Your Story" for suggestions on how to structure the sharing in both individual versus group modality (e.g., for groups, how much time each person shares, how other clients can best provide feedback). Handout 2 is organized into chapters of the person's addiction story as a way to let clients focus on any phase of their addiction. And they can choose a question to focus on, with some questions being more challenging than others. If clients don't have addiction, they can choose questions that relate to their mental health issues or make up a question they'd like to answer. However, if clients start to describe "war stories" or highly triggering addiction details, redirect them to keep the group safe.

★ ***Discuss how time can change the perception of addiction events (Handout 3).*** Negative addiction events may ultimately bring gifts of recovery. Hitting bottom, health and legal problems, and losses due to addiction can become turning points, such as entering treatment for the first time or finding the motivation to reduce addictive behavior. But there's no one interpretation. It's important to honor clients' perceptions. Some events may still hold emotional pain or be perceived negatively. No matter what they glean from the events, taking a "then versus now" perspective deepens their ability to learn from experiences and, hopefully, reinforces their commitment to recovery. *Note:* This handout could be used for mental health events if the client doesn't have addiction.

★ ***Have clients identify life circumstances that played a role in the development of their addiction (Handout 4).*** Handout 4 provides a worksheet on *advantages* versus *disadvantages* in various categories. It can help clients understand why they developed addiction, moving beyond self-blame (or blame by others) to offer a broader context of life circumstances. Another way to frame disadvantages is *unmet needs* that created vulnerabilty. It's important to emphasize, however, that the development of addiction is complex and rooted in genetic and other factors that go beyond Handout 4. Also, help clients understand that advantages/disadvantages are not simply financial; wealthy people too can have significant disadvantages, as defined on Handout 4. *Note:* This handout can also be used for mental health issues.

★ *Discussion*
- "How can looking back on your addiction history help your recovery?"
- "What aspect of your addiction history feels most important to share?"
- "How are trauma and addiction linked in your life?"
- "What disadvantages in life contributed to the development of your addiction?"
- "What advantages in life helped protect you?"
- "Has your view of your addiction changed over time?"
- "What feelings come up as you work on this topic?"

Suggestions

✦ *If clients don't have addiction, help them apply the material to mental health issues.* As noted in the previous section, some of the handouts can be applied to mental health issues. Clients can ignore the term *addiction* in those handouts if needed. But also be sure that all clients have been screened for addiction, including behavioral addictions, as some may have an addiction and not know it.

✦ *Help clients move beyond a judgmental view of their addiction.* All of the handouts are, in different ways, designed to help clients understand the many forces that played a role in the development of their addiction. They still need to own mistakes they made but are more likely to do so if they can tell their story with compassion rather than superficial judgment.

✦ *Strive for poignant emotion rather than intellectual awareness.* Both are important, but the hope is that clients will feel a deep resonance with the material. Moreover, positive as well as negative feelings can be evoked—love, attachment, appreciation (for themselves and supportive others) as well as shame, guilt, anger, and sadness.

✦ *Vary your approach based on severity of addiction.* Some clients have chronic and severe problems; others have brief and mild problems. Allow multiple sessions as needed. Also use whatever term fits for the client. *Addiction* may be too strong a term for someone with a mild problem or for people in the precontemplation stage of change (Prochaska et al., 1992). Per earlier in this chapter, terms such as *problem behavior, compulsive behavior,* or *excessive behavior* are fine to use.

✦ *Provide practical help for addiction.* Today's topic focuses on clients' history rather than basic addiction education, assessment, and referrals. However, attend to those as needed.

1. *Offer additional topics if clients lack basic knowledge.* The extra topic "Understanding Trauma and Addiction" describes what addiction is. If you're familiar with Seeking Safety, pertinent topics from that model include "When Substances Control You," "Coping with Triggers," and "Recovery Thinking." Motivational Interviewing is also helpful, especially for clients new to addiction treatment or who have an addiction but don't yet recognize it as such (Miller & Rollnick, 1991).
2. *Refer clients to additional help.* Clients typically need multiple supports such as 12-step groups and medication consultation. The Seeking Safety topics "Introduction to Treatment/Case Management" and "Community Resources" provide guidance on engaging clients in outside help.
3. *See the section "Best Practices in Addiction Treatment" in Chapter 4.* It addresses key aspects of

care, such as ensuring that clients have a written plan for reducing addiction, and signs of worsening that need attention.

Tough Cases

- "I think the reason I got addicted is God is punishing me."
- "I already know my trauma and addiction are connected. What now?"
- "A lot of people have disadvantages and don't get addicted."
- "I'm afraid bad memories will come up if I stay sober."
- "People have said I'm addicted to drama and chaos—is that a thing?"
- "I've been addicted so long I doubt I can stop."

Why Addiction?

Quotation

"If drugs are the answer, what's the question?"

~Anonymous

HANDOUT 1

The Tangled Web of Addiction and Trauma

"The question is not why the addiction but why the pain?"
~Gabor Maté, MD

"[Alcohol was the] magical elixir that helped me feel comfortable in the world, a sensation for which I would eventually sacrifice almost anything."
~Luke Matthiessen, *First Light*

❖ **When most people focus on addiction, they notice the harm it causes:** failed relationships, jobs lost, legal and medical problems, time and money wasted.

 ◆ What are the main *harms* your addiction has caused you or others? List up to four.

 1. _____
 2. _____
 3. _____
 4. _____

Notice how you feel after listing those—sad? distressed? guilty?

❖ **Now add trauma into the picture . . .**

 ◆ Mark any below that are true for you. And then notice how it makes you feel—does it soften your heart?

 Note: Addictive behavior can be replaced with *problem* (or *compulsive* or *excessive*) behavior if you don't have an addiction.

 ___ *Addictive behavior* can be **a way to survive trauma**. Some people say that substances, for example, were the only way they knew to tolerate intolerable situations. Alcohol numbed them or pills gave them energy. It bought them another day, over and over. It may have saved them from suicide or violence.

(cont.)

From *Creating Change* by Lisa M. Najavits. Copyright © 2024 Lisa M. Najavits. Published by The Guilford Press. Permission to photocopy this material is granted to purchasers of this book for use with your own clients or patients; see copyright page for details.

HANDOUT 1 *(p. 2 of 2)*   Why Addiction?

___ *Addictive behavior can be **a cry for help after trauma**.* It's a way to say, "I'm hurt, I need help, I don't know what to do." It says, "Now do you see the damage?" You may not have words for the trauma, but the addiction says it for you.

___ *Addictive behavior can be **self-medication for trauma**.* Substances, food, and other addictions can be a way to manage trauma symptoms such as flashbacks, nightmares, rage, and panic. People reach for comfort when in distress.

___ *Addictive behavior can **feel like an important relationship when trauma made you feel alone**.* Some people describe it as a best friend, lover, or companion. It offers solace and predictability when people don't provide them.

___ *Addictive behavior can be **part of the trauma itself**.* A trauma perpetrator may have coerced you into substance use, for example, to get you to engage in sexual acts or violence that you didn't want to do.

___ *Addictive behavior can **set you up for trauma**.* It makes you vulnerable to unsafe people and situations such as being assaulted while intoxicated or involved in crime related to gambling.

___ *Addictive behavior can be **an attempt to work through trauma**.* Some people use substances to access feelings that are blocked. Or some types of sex can reenact trauma, but now you feel you're in control rather than the perpetrator.

___ *Addictive behavior can be **a way to hide**.* You may hate yourself due to trauma. The addictive behavior lets you not be you for a while.

___ *Addictive behavior can **give a sense of purpose**.* Trauma can make life feel meaningless, eroding your sense of self. Addiction focuses your time and energy, giving a sense of purpose even if it's a self-destructive one.

___ *Addictive behavior can **appear to give what trauma took away**.* Trauma makes you feel powerless, but gambling makes you feel big and important. Trauma makes you feel dead inside, but substances, food, pornography, or spending makes you feel alive.

___ *Addictive behavior can be **self-punishment**.* Severe, repeated trauma can make pain so familiar that you turn against yourself. Food or use of drug needles can become forms of self-punishment. Self-harm such as cutting can become addictive.

___ Any others?

_____

_____

❖ **Recovery**

The reasons listed in this handout don't justify continuing addictive behavior. But understanding the link between trauma and addiction offers compassion that can aid your recovery. Just as trauma and addiction develop together, they also heal together.

HANDOUT 2　　　　　　　　　　　　　　　　　　　　　　　　　　　　　　　　　　Why Addiction?

20 Questions: Tell Part of Your Addiction Story

Whatever stage you're at in recovery, it helps to share your story (or parts of it), to not be alone with it.
If you don't have an addiction, you could focus on any *compulsive behavior* you may have—a behavior you can't control, such as excessive eating, internet use, pornography, work, or gambling.

The challenge is to be honest with yourself and maintain balance—neither beating yourself up ("It's all my fault") nor totally defensive ("I've never done anything wrong"). You may have had real strength at times and poor judgment other times.

★ *Choose one or more of these questions that are meaningful or "hold energy" for you. The term* behavior *refers to the addiction or other compulsive behavior you choose to focus on.*

Chapter I: How It Began
1. Was there an important person who made the behavior seem OK?
2. Was the behavior a way to cope with trauma?
3. What do you know now about the behavior that you didn't know then?
4. What were you like before the behavior became a problem?
5. Why do you think the behavior became a problem for you?

Chapter II: From Casual to Problem Use
6. When did you first think you had a problem?
7. Did anyone express concern or try to help you with it?
8. How did you explain your increasing usage to yourself? to others?
9. How did it feel to admit you had a problem?
10. Do you think you have an addiction now?

Chapter III: What It's Like
11. What is one thing the behavior gave you and one thing it cost you?
12. Are there secrets about the behavior you haven't shared?
13. What would you want people to understand about your problem behavior?
14. What is most difficult for you about the behavior?
15. How do the behavior and your trauma impact each other?

Chapter IV: Your Recovery
16. What choices did you make that launched your recovery?
17. What is hardest about reducing or giving up the behavior?
18. What help do you most need for it now?
19. What are you most proud of in your recovery?
20. Are you more motivated to work on the behavior or on trauma?

Or make up question(s) you'd like to answer:

_____

_____

From *Creating Change* by Lisa M. Najavits. Copyright © 2024 Lisa M. Najavits. Published by The Guilford Press. Permission to photocopy this material is granted to purchasers of this book for use with your own clients or patients; see copyright page for details.

HANDOUT 3   Why Addiction?

Then versus Now

This exercise explores how time can change your view of addiction events. What seemed bad may turn out to be good, and vice versa.

★ *Choose an important addiction event. Describe how you viewed it then* versus *how you view it now.*

Step 1: Addiction event (choose one)

- First time using
- Binge incident
- Blackout incident
- Relapse
- Hit bottom
- Legal problem
- Health problem
- Major loss due to addiction (e.g., person, job, home, money)
- Someone noticed you had a problem
- You noticed you had a problem
- Started treatment
- Dropped out of treatment
- Other addiction event _____

If you want, describe it briefly here:

Step 2: How did you view it then?

Step 3: How do you view it now?

◆ Reflections

- Has time changed your view of the event?
- How did the event impact your recovery?
- How did the event change you as a person?
- Any surprises in what the event revealed?
- Did trauma have any impact on the event or what it means to you?

From *Creating Change* by Lisa M. Najavits. Copyright © 2024 Lisa M. Najavits. Published by The Guilford Press. Permission to photocopy this material is granted to purchasers of this book for use with your own clients or patients; see copyright page for details.

HANDOUT 4   Why Addiction?

Lifetime Advantages and Disadvantages

This exercise explores what you were up against, which may help explain your addiction and/or other mental health issues. There are many causes, but environment plays a role just as much as genetics (biology).

The more *disadvantages* you had in the domains below, the more likely you were to develop problems. In contrast, *advantages* helped protect you.

★ *Rate each section on the scale below, with one rating for childhood and one for adulthood. Add notes if you want to.*

0	1	2	3	4
Strong disadvantages				**Strong advantages**

1. Physical

***Physical* advantages:** good health . . . housing . . . enough money . . . quality health care . . . attractive . . . athletic . . . healthy lifestyle (exercise, diet)

***Physical* disadvantages:** poor health (chronic or serious illness or injury) . . . lack of money for food, clothes, shelter . . . having to sell your body (prostitution or damaging physical work) . . . physical neglect . . . incarceration . . . homelessness

Your physical ratings (use scale above): **As a child:** _____ **As an adult:** _____

Notes:

2. Social

***Social* advantages:** people loved you . . . took care of you . . . supported your interests . . . positive role models . . . sense of community . . . people encouraged recovery

***Social* disadvantages:** isolation/loneliness . . . low/rigid social class (unable to advance) . . . lack of respect (put down, devalued) . . . abandoned . . . ignored . . . people encouraged addiction

Your social ratings (use scale above): **As a child:** _____ **As an adult:** _____

Notes:

3. Sense of purpose

***Sense of purpose* advantages:** people around you had a positive mission . . . idealism . . . optimism . . . positive habits . . . spirituality

***Sense of purpose* disadvantages:** people around you lacked goals or had negative ones (promoted violence, disrespect) . . . life seen as meaningless . . . hopeless . . . objects valued over people . . . bias

Your sense of purpose ratings (use scale above): **As a child:** _____ **As an adult:** _____

Notes:

(cont.)

From *Creating Change* by Lisa M. Najavits. Copyright © 2024 Lisa M. Najavits. Published by The Guilford Press. Permission to photocopy this material is granted to purchasers of this book for use with your own clients or patients; see copyright page for details.

HANDOUT 4 *(p. 2 of 2)* — Why Addiction?

4. Opportunity

Opportunity advantages: strong schooling . . . career options . . . support and help

Opportunity disadvantages: limited education or poor-quality schools . . . low-paying jobs . . . lack of mentorship and guidance

Your opportunity ratings (use scale above): **As a child:** _____ **As an adult:** _____

Notes:

5. Emotional

Emotional advantages: encouraged to express yourself . . . taught about feelings . . . people around you resolved conflicts respectfully . . . compassion . . . access to mental health care

Emotional disadvantages: told you don't have a right to feel what you feel . . . mocked for emotions . . . chronic stress . . . lack of guidance on feelings . . . people around you were extreme (numb or explosive) . . . emotional abuse . . . family addiction or mental illness . . . cut off from feelings (numb, detached)

Your emotional ratings (use scale above): **As a child:** _____ **As an adult:** _____

Notes:

6. Cultural

Cultural advantages: positive traditions (e.g., rituals, foods) . . . a sense of belonging based on culture and community . . . media that promoted a positive lifestyle . . . your culture was valued by those in power . . . positive cultural beliefs

Cultural disadvantages: cultural beliefs that kept you stuck . . . stigma or bias against your culture . . . challenges preserving your culture . . . media influences that encouraged addiction or violence

Your cultural ratings (use scale above): **As a child:** _____ **As an adult:** _____

Notes:

SCORING

Total your score for *childhood* and *adulthood* separately. The maximum possible is 24 for each. Lower scores indicate greater vulnerability for addiction.

- ◊ What is your *childhood* score? _____
- ◊ What is your *adulthood* score? _____

✧ Reflections

- What advantages are you most grateful for?
- What disadvantages had the most impact on your addiction?
- Was your childhood or adulthood score higher?
- What can you do now to best meet your needs?
- What can others do now to help meet your needs?
- Any insights based on this exercise? Any feelings that arose?

Ideas for a Commitment

Commit to one action that will move your life forward!
It can be anything you feel will help you, or you can try one of the ideas below.
Keeping your commitment is a way of respecting, honoring, and caring for yourself.

✦ Option 1. If a genie granted you a magic wish to go back in time, what is one thing you would do differently to change your addiction history? Write about that.

✦ Option 2. Creative writing: Take the quotation from today's topic and imagine it's the title of a story. Write the rest of the story.

✦ Option 3. Read the article below about the deep generosity of one alcoholic to another. Describe how it relates to your addiction and/or recovery.

www.nytimes.com/2021/01/08/well/family/alcoholic-babysitter-sobriety.html

✦ Option 4. Choose a question in Handout 2. Express your answer in writing, art, music, photos, video, or collage.

✦ Option 5. Look at Handout 4. Take an action step in the week ahead to improve your life in any of the categories listed.

Respect Your Defenses

SUMMARY

This topic explores *emotional defenses* as necessary self-protection that helped clients survive trauma and addiction. They're encouraged to respect defenses for having helped them in the past, but which may be good to change now as part of recovery. Examples of defenses are "overendurance," "isolation," and "looking for love in all the wrong places."

ORIENTATION

"I had justified lying so often that it became almost noble to lie."

"I look good on the outside but am bleeding to death on the inside."

The concept of defenses originated in psychodynamic therapies and is convergent with other theoretical orientations such as the behavioral concept of conditioned responses and the cognitive concept of schemas (deeply rooted assumptions that have persistent expression in both thinking and behavior). The term *defenses* is used in this topic as it vividly conveys the basic idea: Clients have developed ways of protecting themselves that have become too rigid—a sort of emotional armor.

Defenses are overarching patterns that go beyond the list of symptoms of particular disorders. Clients with the same disorders, such as PTSD or substance use disorder, may have very different defense styles. One client turns to isolation when under stress; another turns to physical expression of emotional pain. In part, this may be due to additional disorders that are so common with this comorbidity, including personality disorders. But defenses also arise based on a complex mix of culture, history, and biology.

In today's topic, Handout 1 provides general information about defenses and Handout 2 offers a list of typical defenses in trauma and addiction. There's no one list of defenses in the field, so the goal here was to create a list with memorable names and clear descriptions. It's lengthy so that all clients, even the most defensive, can find something that fits for them. It gives language for a conversation about styles of reacting that can serve throughout the treatment. Proactively working on defenses offers a way to more easily address them if they become activated later. This is especially important for past-focused treatment, which is more likely to arouse defenses than a present-focused model such as Seeking Safety. Indeed, it's important to normalize that defensive reactions arise even in treatments that are highly successful. As Chu states, "Even in the hands of experienced therapists . . . difficulties cannot always be avoided or circumvented. In fact, the nature of successful treatment of [trauma] survivors demands that therapists become involved and fully appreciate the dilemmas and psychological pain that patients experience" (1992, p. 368).

Throughout, clients are encouraged to *respect* their defenses. All defenses can be understood as a response to painful feelings and realities. Defenses allowed them to survive. One client said, " drank so I wouldn't kill myself." While trying to change these patterns, clients can come to appreciate that the defenses may have been the best they could do at the time and perhaps saved them from worse outcomes. They're not wrong or bad for having them but now can choose healthier ways of responding.

An honest discussion of defenses also recognizes the "dark side" of trauma and addiction. Some clients were not just victims, but perpetrators. Some have lied, stolen, cheated, abandoned their children, used others for sex or money, or assaulted people. It's important for counselors and clients to address these behaviors when they're present, rather than perpetuating a one-sided, sentimental view of such clients as wholly victims. Clients themselves often appreciate an unvarnished view of the truth. One client said, "I got tired of counselors telling me what a good person I was. I stole, I started a fire on purpose, I hit my kids just 'cause I was annoyed, and I got busted several times. I wasn't all that great a person at times." In today's topic and throughout treatment, the idea is to hold on to all realities, both beautiful and ugly.

Your Emotional Reactions

When counselors feel frustrated or hopeless about a client, it's understandable that their own defenses may become activated. Ironically, teaching about *defenses* can become a way of expressing negative feelings to the client, even if unintended. For example, "This one on the handout, *'losing steam,'* happens with you a lot. You don't seem to want to get better." Instead of this harsh style, a counselor who isn't frustrated might say, "Do you think this one, *'losing steam,'* is true for you? If life has been really hard, you may feel hopeless that anything can get better." This gentle questioning approach has a very different feel and is more likely to help the client face the truth. In short, when broaching a topic as sensitive as defenses, do it with a clear head and heart. Clients with trauma and addiction often evoke intense reactions and it's normal to feel a wide range of feelings. Stay aware of your own defenses so they don't get taken out on the client.

Acknowledgments

The session quotation is from Rogers (1995, p. 17). In Handout 2, the term *myths and rules* is from Catherall (1997), and the term *looping* is from EMDR (Shapiro, 1995).

SESSION FORMAT

1. *Check-in* (per Chapter 3).
2. *Quotation.* Link the quotation to the session topic—for example, *"Today we'll be talking about survival strategies you developed. Try to bring a deep sense of acceptance toward yourself as we look at them."*
3. *Handouts* (relate the topic to clients' lives):
    Handout 1: **Emotional Defenses**
    Handout 2: **Ways of Surviving**
4. *Check-out* (per Chapter 3).

SESSION CONTENT

Goals

☐ Introduce the concept of *defenses* as a necessary survival mechanism.
☐ Describe emotional defenses that are common in trauma and addiction.

Respect Your Defenses

☐ Help clients identify one or more defenses they use.
☐ Explore how to shift from an unhealthy defense to a healing alternative.

Ways to Relate the Material to Clients' Lives

★ *Discuss key points about psychological defenses (Handout 1).* You can make it interactive by asking questions (e.g., "Is it possible for a person to have no defenses?"). You can also ask clients to identify parts of the handout that are new or surprising to them.

★ *Identify real-life examples of defenses in Handout 2.* Clients can choose a defense in the handout and give an example from their own life. For *isolation*, examples might be:
- "I take my phone off the hook."
- "Sometimes I don't go outside for days."
- "I don't have any close friends."
- "I get high alone and watch movies all day."

For groups, you can also do a brainstorming exercise in which you (or a group member) names a defense and then members name an example from their life, if they relate to it. If you do the latter, make clear that (1) it's voluntary and (2) they aren't allowed to give examples about other group members as that could be hurtful and destructive.

★ *Explore feelings.* Ask clients to notice their feelings when they read the left versus right side of the page in Handout 2 (*defenses* vs. *healing alternatives*). Exploring feelings moves beyond just an intellectual level.

★ *Relate defenses to trauma and addiction.* Validate that their defenses may have been the best option they had under difficult circumstances. Even defenses that seem destructive, such as *walking into harm's way*, were a response to pain (e.g., harm came to seem normal to them).

★ *Ask clients about the origins of their defenses.* Which family members or peers influenced them? Why do they think they turned to some defenses over others?

★ *Ask clients to imagine letting go of a defense.* "What would happen if you were to stop _____ (e.g., perfectionism)?" This helps them become more aware of why they have the defense.

★ *Role-play.* The client chooses a *defense* from Handout 2 and speaks from the point of view of that defense. You play the *healing alternative* and offer therapeutic responses. If you have time, switch sides and try it again (you play the defense, the client plays the healing alternative).

★ *Discussion*
- "What are your typical ways of protecting yourself emotionally?"
- "Why is it important to respect your defenses?"
- "How are defenses related to trauma/addiction?"
- "When you're under stress, what defenses are most likely to arise?"
- "Do you think defense styles run in families?"
- "How does culture impact defenses?"
- "Do you give yourself credit for surviving trauma/addiction?"

Suggestions

✦ *Watch clients' reactions closely.* Defenses are difficult to admit. It requires honesty and vulnerability. If clients are too detached or intellectualized, or the opposite, too upset, this provides important information to adjust the level of the discussion.

✦ *Expect resistance.* You are able to see defenses that clients can't yet see in themselves. It's a sensitive subject and likely to evoke shame and other difficult feelings. Don't push them to acknowledge the defenses—they may not be ready to face certain truths yet. Respecting defenses is the counselor's job as well as clients'.

+ *Pace the work.* The handouts are long. It's usually too much for a single session, both in the amount of content and in emotional impact. Have clients go over small sections or skim the whole and then focus on one or two areas.

+ *Notice differences among defenses.* Some reflect too much self-protection, such as *isolation* and *avoidance*. Others reflect too little, such as *walking into harm's way* and *too much too soon*.

+ *Offer realistic expectations.* Clients can gradually replace defenses with new approaches. But it's unrealistic to wipe out a defense quickly. As Rothschild states, "Regard defenses as resources. Never 'get rid' of coping strategies/defenses; instead, create more choices" (2000, p. 90).

+ *Distinguish* **defenses** *from* **character defects.** The latter term is used in 12-step groups. Although there's some overlap in these concepts, in general, defenses can be considered a response to an emotional wound, whereas character defects are personal shortcomings (impatience, arrogance, enviousness, jealousy, messiness, etc.). *Defense* may be easier for clients to hear and might be considered more trauma-informed. But 12-step groups are enormously helpful to many clients, and it's essential to respect their concepts and language while also reinterpreting them from a trauma lens (Marich, 2012).

Tough Cases

* "I don't have any defenses."
* "I'm going to tell my boss about his defenses."
* "In my culture, we hide feelings. Are you saying that's wrong?"
* "This makes me feel bad about myself."
* "This is BS. I just need everyone to stop hassling me."

Respect Your Defenses

Quotation

"The curious paradox is that when I accept myself just as I am, then I can change."

~ CARL ROGERS, 20th-century American psychologist

HANDOUT 1

Emotional Defenses

Humans and animals are built to survive. They'll naturally try to defend themselves to protect against pain, attack, and threat.

◇ **When you think of the word *defense*, what comes to mind?**

- A military
- A boundary
- A fort
- A wall
- A weapon
- A moat
- An escape
- Others? _____

A defense is a *survival strategy*—it's an attempt to keep you (or a country) safe.

Emotional defenses are as important as physical ones. They protect against psychological danger.

- If people around you are untrustworthy, *isolation* may become your defense.
- If painful feelings are too intense, *numbing* may become your defense.

***Everyone* has defenses.** They're only a problem if they're too extreme, too frequent, or too rigid (preventing growth).

In trauma and addiction, you needed defenses to survive. They may have helped you to:

protect from further harm . . . keep going . . . forget the past . . . tolerate pain you couldn't escape . . . feel connected to others . . . have moments of good feeling . . . save someone else

Defenses are usually unconscious. They're automatic, not willful.

(cont.)

From *Creating Change* by Lisa M. Najavits. Copyright © 2024 Lisa M. Najavits. Published by The Guilford Press. Permission to photocopy this material is granted to purchasers of this book for use with your own clients or patients; see copyright page for details.

HANDOUT 1 *(p. 2 of 2)*   Respect Your Defenses

Become aware of your defenses. Listen at a deep level, not judging or blaming. Every defense says something about what you experienced.

There are many types of defenses. See Handout 2 for examples.

Defenses are sometimes "asleep" and sometimes "awake." On a good day, your defenses may not kick into gear. On a bad day, they can take over. They tend to activate if you're stressed. The letters "HALT" are good to remember—**H**ungry, **A**ngry, **L**onely, **T**ired—these can trigger your defenses.

Respect your defenses for having protected you. If you grew up in a violent home, staying silent may have been a wise choice, for example. But you can try new approaches now. There's a saying, "What got you here won't get you there." Some defenses may no longer be healthy for you; they may get in the way of recovery.

Culture impacts defenses. You may have learned to "keep a stiff upper lip" or "not air dirty laundry in public." Your culture may emphasize physical rather than emotional pain (tiredness rather than depression).

HANDOUT 2

Ways of Surviving

Be proud that you survived trauma and addiction. But also take stock of the costs of survival. This table describes emotional defenses you may have developed (left column) and healthier options to try now (right column).

★ *Rate yourself on each defense below from 0% (not at all) to 100% (greatly).*

Emotional defense	Definition	Why it makes sense	Examples	Rate (0–100%)	Healing alternative
Shrinking (too small)	You go underground, hide, and try to stay invisible and out of the way.	You made yourself small to survive. It wasn't safe to say what you really thought or to be who you really were.	"I never get angry." "My mother was an alcoholic; I had to walk on eggshells or she'd fly into a rage."		**Learn who you are.** It takes time to grow into your full self after it's been pushed down for so long. Give yourself time; figure out what you like; experiment with expressing yourself.
Expanding (too big)	You don't show weakness. You fight to protect yourself.	You made yourself big to survive. "Kill or be killed."	"It's a jungle out there; you're on your own." "When I'm gambling I'm a big shot, king of the world."		**Let your guard down.** Earlier in life you did what you had to do, but now you can choose people and situations that let you relax.
Myths and rules	You want to control your behavior (or others') so you keep creating rules, but they don't actually work.	The situation has been out of control for a long time, but the rules create an illusion of control.	"If I do better, he won't hit me." "I drink beer instead of liquor, so I'm not an alcoholic."		**Face the truth.** However difficult, the truth is so much healthier than illusions that keep you stuck. Ask others for a reality check: Does what you're saying add up?

(cont.)

HANDOUT 2 (p. 2 of 5)

Respect Your Defenses

Emotional defense	Definition	Why it makes sense	Examples	Rate (0–100%)	Healing alternative
Too much too soon	You move too quickly and intensely (into relationships, jobs, etc.).	You may be so desperate for relief that you don't see the red flags. Or you may be addicted to adrenaline (quick-fix excitement).	"My counselor says I watch too many trauma movies. It's like picking at a scab." "I'm in love with a guy at detox. We're moving in together when we get out."		**Remember slower is faster.** It's understandable to want to make up for lost time after trauma and addiction. But real rewards come from pacing, planning, and patience.
Over-endurance	You're too good at tolerating pain. You tough it out, accepting discomfort longer than is healthy.	This allowed you to survive awful situations.	"After the child abuse I lived through, my partner beating me up seemed normal to me." "I'm a workaholic."		**Set limits.** The task is to set stronger boundaries within yourself and with others. Identify what you need and want, deep down. That may feel hard but brings growth.
Looking for love in all the wrong places	You escape inner emptiness by repeated attractions to untrustworthy people or superficial activities.	If you didn't get enough love growing up, you may be seeking it now in unhealthy ways.	"I know she's toxic, but I can't break up with her." "It's 'retail therapy.' I shop even though I can't afford it."		**Seek depth.** Learn how to develop real love through emotional intimacy, meaningful work, creativity, spirituality, and other deeper pursuits.
A secret life	You appear strong, you say you're fine. No one knows what's really going on.	Secrets are part of trauma and addiction, often from shame or guilt.	"I get straight A's in school but keep thinking of killing myself." "I can't tell my wife I gambled away our savings."		**Let someone know.** Find at least one safe person—a counselor, sponsor, friend—to open up to. Living a double life, pretending, keeps you stuck in the past.

(cont.)

Respect Your Defenses

HANDOUT 2 (p. 3 of 5)

Emotional defense	Definition	Why it makes sense	Examples	Rate (0–100%)	Healing alternative
Losing steam	You start and stop, don't finish tasks, give up too easily.	You may have grown up in a chaotic environment, lacking support. You lose faith in yourself and expect failure.	"I was criticized so much that I never feel good enough." "I can put together 6 months of sobriety but then relapse again."		**Navigate hope.** When you feel hopeless, explore what's underneath. Fear of not being good enough? Difficulty accepting where you're at in life? Not knowing how to set realistic goals? Ask others for support in those moments.
Walking into harm's way	You go into dangerous situations even when you don't have to.	Danger may feel normal if you lived with abuse or neglect. Or you may never have learned how to take care of yourself.	"I take risks like jogging alone at night. I don't know why." "I test myself by going into bars."		**Become conscious.** The first step is awareness. Get feedback from trustworthy people. Develop "radar" for unsafe people and situations. Acknowledge red flags as early as possible.
Turning against yourself or others	You act destructively out of desperation.	You've become so lost in weakness or pain that you become pure impulse at times.	"I didn't plan to hit him. It just happened." "I binge-eat when I feel rejected."		**Create a pause between feeling and action.** Identify consequences. Wait an hour; set a timer; sleep on it.
Looping	You stay stuck in a behavior or thought.	You go into overdrive trying to resolve an inner conflict you don't know how to resolve.	"I recheck my door locks over and over." "When I finish a drink, I'm already planning the next one."		**Shift.** Any way you can, draw away from the magnetic pull of looping. Use grounding, distraction, delay. Gain distance to gain perspective.
Isolation	You withdraw from the world, as self-protection.	It's natural to want to escape if you feel damaged or ashamed.	"Getting close means getting hurt." "I have to hide my addiction."		**Connect.** Learn how to find good people and build healthy relationships. Help from others enhances survival (humans are social in nature).

(cont.)

HANDOUT 2 (p. 4 of 5)

Respect Your Defenses

Emotional defense	Definition	Why it makes sense	Examples	Rate (0–100%)	Healing alternative
Ignoring your needs	Your needs come last; you may not even be aware of them anymore.	This often reflects neglect or dysfunction earlier in life.	"I was taught that I don't matter." "I make excuses for my partner when he's hung over and can't go to work."		**Turn the focus back to you.** Self-care isn't selfish. Keep practicing. And you may have to let go of relationships where your needs can't get met too.
Driven by feelings	Your feelings run the show. They lead you too quickly into action you later regret.	You didn't learn to manage your feelings, likely because people you grew up around didn't manage theirs.	"If my boyfriend distances, I panic and go overboard texting him." "If I can't sleep at night, I light a blunt."		**Sit with a feeling.** Do some grounding, then sit quietly for a few minutes, without judgment, and see if you notice deeper, vulnerable feelings below the surface. They will lead you to what you really need.
Perfectionism	Your standards for yourself (and others) are inhuman. You sacrifice health, relationships, and/or leisure.	You were emotionally wounded and never feel good enough.	"I constantly help other veterans, but it never feels like enough." "My track coach told me to take rest days, but I can't do it."		**Widen the lens.** Perfectionism is a narrowing of perspective. Regain perspective: Lower your effort to 90%; love yourself despite flaws; find new ways to spend your time.
Numbing	You're shut down, hollow, going through the motions.	Numbing protected you from feelings that were too intense.	"I'm like sand or cement. Life is drab. It passes me by." "I do coke to feel alive."		**Learn to feel.** You can learn it just like any other skill. As you do-paced and with support in counseling—the numbing goes down. Gray turns to color. The frozen pond melts.
Glorifying pain	Suffering becomes overvalued.	You romanticize suffering out of a wish to be noticed or admired.	"My trauma was worse than yours." "Addiction comes from my creative artist soul."		**Take pride in healthy goals.** Your suffering is real and important, but you can find other ways to be noticed.

(cont.)

HANDOUT 2 (p. 5 of 5)   Respect Your Defenses

Emotional defense	Definition	Why it makes sense	Examples	Rate (0–100%)	Healing alternative
Avoidance	You retreat from people, situations, or feelings that you need to face.	Life became too hard and you did all you could to get away from the pain.	"Even the simplest things are hard for me to start." "I can't handle life without using."		**Create a new habit.** Practice taking on what you need to do. It may feel like a leap, but it gets easier the more you do it. Learn the difference between self-protection that's *healthy* (pacing) versus *unhealthy* (avoidance).
Saving face	You want others to think well of you so you put forth a good story.	You felt misunderstood or disrespected in the past.	"She hit me, too, but I got blamed because I'm a man." "Urine tests make mistakes."		**Find genuine acceptance.** You're likely yearning for belonging and love. Get in touch with that. Admitting mistakes often makes others like you more.
Your body "speaks"	Emotional pain shows up as physical problems (nausea, racing heart, etc.).	Your emotional needs may have been ignored.	"When I talk about the assault, I get a headache." "My doctor says I take too many pain meds."		**Put it into words.** Find ways to express yourself in the language of feelings and thoughts. (Also be sure to see a doctor to identify actual medical problems.)

Others? Fill in the blanks.

Name	Definition	Why it makes sense	Examples	Rating	Healing alternative

Respect Your Defenses

Ideas for a Commitment

*Commit to one action that will move your life forward!
It can be anything you feel will help you, or you can try one of the ideas below.
Keeping your commitment is a way of respecting, honoring, and caring for yourself.*

✦ Option 1. Ask a trustworthy person to identify one of your emotional defenses, using Handout 2. Others can typically see your defenses more clearly.

✦ Option 2. Handout 1 says, "What got you here won't get you there." Write about what that means to you.

✦ Option 3. Choose a *healing alternative* in Handout 2 and do one thing this week to increase it.

✦ Option 4. Circle two or more of these words or phrases and write or draw about them, in any way you want.

> *self-protection   life   why   defense   healing   survival   trauma   addiction
> respect   reasons   heart   alone   hope   love   wish   if only   regret   future
> past   present   honesty   people   too much   too little   hate   inside
> outside   family*

Break the Silence

SUMMARY

Silencing is common in both trauma and addiction. In today's topic, clients can share a vulnerable truth about their past and identify what they'd like to hear back. There's also discussion of when it's safe or unsafe to break silences and how to share with people outside of treatment.

ORIENTATION

"Do you know what happens if you allege that a leader in a nationally recognized youth organization is a predator or that you believe your child has been molested? Do you think they would search for the truth? Do you think they would offer you empathy and act concerned or caring? You would be quite mistaken. They will do all they can to protect and elevate themselves and put you down."
　　　　　　　　　　　　　　　　　　　　~SHAWNA, mother of a child molested at a scouting camp

Silence is a core issue in trauma and addiction. In trauma, clients may have had no one trustworthy to talk to, or may have been threatened into silence by a perpetrator. In addiction, it's common to pretend everything is fine when it's actually falling apart. A culture of silence about trauma and addiction also occurs in institutions such as sports teams, the military, corporations, and religious organizations.

When no one acknowledges what's happening, clients doubt their own reality. Silence leads to terrible isolation that adds to the pain of trauma and addiction. Clients feel misunderstood, may question whether their suffering is real, and may never receive support. As Herman writes, "The conflict between the will to deny horrible events and the will to proclaim them aloud is the central dialectic of psychological trauma" (1992, p. 1).

Clients sometimes blame themselves for not speaking out sooner and, all too common, may be judged by others: "You should have told someone," "If you spoke up, maybe it wouldn't have gone on so long." It's essential to validate that, especially for trauma, staying silent was self-protection that may have saved clients from worse harm. In addiction, it's often part of the illness to deny how bad it is until enough consequences shatter the illusion of control, such as "hitting bottom."

Today's topic aims to shift away from silencing. There's education on silencing in trauma and addiction (Handout 1), and then an exercise for clients to share some aspect of their past (Handout 2). It may be a secret or vulnerable part of their history; it's anything they view as important to share. It may be something painful or could be something positive they're proud of. For the counselor, the exercise lets you observe how they respond: Do they choose to share? What feelings does the sharing evoke? It's a sampling of emotional intimacy that will be deepened in other Creating Change topics.

Just as important as the sharing is guidance on *how* to share, which is addressed in Handout 3. Clients can be harmed by spilling too much to people who are unsafe—people who betray their confidence or judge them harshly. Sharing shouldn't be approached naively.

The hope is that clients can experience how sharing personal experiences in the context of trusting relationships, such as counseling, can be a step toward healing. As one counselor said, "The goal is to move toward not fearing the secret and the pain behind it. Clients usually fear that something awful will happen if they reveal it. That's the power of keeping the secret. Once they tell and something awful does not happen, the secret loses its power and they feel more powerful. Nothing is worse than feeling powerless over your life and emotions, to feel that the power is elsewhere. It is immobilizing and depressing. So doing something different, such as talking, is crucial."

Even clients who have been in treatment for a while usually have important layers they haven't revealed yet. If trauma or addiction symptoms are present, secrets and silence are not far behind. One client said, "No matter what people say, there are always some parts they couldn't ever tell."

Your Emotional Reactions

When silencing is part of clients' history, it may be something they enact with others, including you. They may say, "Please don't tell my psychiatrist I relapsed" or "If you report missed sessions to my probation officer, I'll get in trouble." There can be a strong pull to empathize with them and become a party to silencing. It helps to remember that a team approach is the healthiest one, where all providers know what's going on. If you feel pressured to keep a secret from another provider, seek supervision or a trusted colleague so that you're not alone with it and can get an outside perspective.

Acknowledgments

The quotation in the "Orientation" section on the previous page is from Kelly (2020). The session quotation is from Milosz (1980). The quotation in Handout 1 is from Crawford (2020).

SESSION FORMAT

1. *Check-in* (per Chapter 3).
2. *Quotation.* Link the quotation to the session topic—for example, *"To break a long-held silence takes courage. Today we'll talk about silencing in trauma and addiction and how to overcome that."*
3. *Handouts* (relate the topic to clients' lives):
    Handout 1: **Silencing in Trauma and Addiction**
    Handout 2: **Feeling Heard**
    Handout 3: **Sharing Outside of Treatment**
4. *Check-out* (per Chapter 3).

SESSION CONTENT

Goals

- ☐ Explore silencing as a core theme in trauma and addiction.
- ☐ Try an exercise on sharing about the past.
- ☐ Discuss how it feels to share and hear sharing by others.
- ☐ Identify how sharing about the past can strengthen recovery.
- ☐ Offer guidance on how to share outside of treatment in healthy ways.

Ways to Relate the Material to Clients' Lives

★ *Explore clients' experiences of silencing (Handout 1).* Emphasize that it made sense to keep secrets in the past. In trauma, staying silent was often an intelligent survival strategy to protect against further harm, or may have been a physical freeze response that was out of the person's control. In addiction, it's the nature of the illness to hide or deny it. Ensure that clients don't feel blamed or judged for staying silent in the past. It's also worth mentioning that everyone keeps secrets at times. It becomes a problem when it causes dysfunction or reinforces shame. Help them see the toll that silencing takes and why they may want to break silences now.

★ *Try an exercise on sharing (Handout 2).* The exercise is straightforward in *individual treatment*: The client looks through the handout and shares as desired. You'll likely have time to cover several items and can process how it feels for the client to share.

Group treatment requires more structure to balance time and promote positive interaction. The following method is suggested for groups.

1. *Set the framework.* Briefly reinforce the bullet points at the top of Handout 3. Also tell clients how long each person will have so they won't feel cut off when you go to the next client. It's suggested that each gets up to 3 minutes to speak, followed by about 2 minutes of supportive feedback from the group; then the next client goes, and so on. Adjust the timing based on group size and your sense of their capacity for sharing and listening but choose an amount that keeps it from becoming a long narrative. Use a mobile phone timer that everyone can hear and include a 1-minute advance bell. If a client uses less time, that's OK, but if a share starts to go too long, limit it in a kind way, emphasizing the need to balance among members. If you conduct large groups, allow more than one session so everyone can share. *Note*: Some counselors like a shorter approach than this method. You could tell clients they can speak one sentence from Handout 2, rather than a specific number of minutes.

2. *Give clients a few minutes to silently work on filling out Part I in Handout 2.* They can do this even if they choose not to share aloud. Here are examples of content (and clients could speak a bit longer on each): "I'm proud of surviving my childhood. I ended up an alcoholic but just to stay alive was a victory. . . . " "My husband doesn't know I had an abortion after incest. He wouldn't understand and I never told him. . . . "

3. *Encourage supportive group feedback.* After each client shares, offer brief validation and invite group members to do so as well, using Part II in Handout 2 as a guide. Examples of feedback are "You were so strong to move out of that toxic environment" and "Now I understand why you turned to pills and how tough that was for you." Not all group members need to respond, and timewise it's best to allow a few responses and then move to the next share. If a client provides feedback that is not consistent with the guidelines in Handout 2, gently bring it back to that.

★ *Explore sharing outside of treatment (Handout 3).* This handout helps clients expand their sharing, with careful attention to doing it in healthy ways to create a successful experience. The handout can launch a discussion and possibly a role-play for clients to test what the interaction would sound like.

★ *Discussion*
- "Why are silence and secrets so common in trauma and addiction?"
- "What makes it hard to break through silence?"
- "What does 'culture of silence' mean?"
- " 'You're only as sick as your secrets'—what does this AA phrase mean?"
- "How might your recovery be enhanced if you opened up more?"
- "How would it feel to share a vulnerable personal truth?"
- "How can you tell if someone is safe to share with?"
- "How is sharing different for trauma than addiction?"

Suggestions

+ ***Validate clients who choose not to share.*** Reassure them that they're making a positive choice by being sensitive to their own needs. Let them know trust builds over time and they shouldn't feel pressured to share in or outside of treatment. If you have concerns that this is encouraging "avoidance," see Chapters 3 and 4 for more on that.

+ ***Encourage clients to offer their insights on breaking silence.*** They likely have wisdom on what works and what doesn't based on past attempts they've made.

+ ***Keep the focus.*** Today's topic is just "dipping a toe in the water" to briefly share something vulnerable and feel heard on that. Other topics in Creating Change delve into more detail (e.g., "Tell Your Story," "Deepen Your Story") and address interpersonal conflicts (e.g., "What You Want People to Understand").

+ ***Recognize that there are many reasons for breaking silence.*** Clients may have various motivations for sharing: to express feelings about what happened; to gain support from others; to feel the relief from not holding a secret; to seek forgiveness; to take legal action or obtain financial compensation; or perhaps to protect others from harm.

+ ***Help clients understand the difference between sharing their experience and betraying a confidence.*** Betraying a confidence means, for example, telling a secret that a friend asked them to keep confidential, outing someone's sexuality, or revealing confidential information such as what was discussed in group treatment. However, there are also situations where someone may ask clients to keep a secret that shouldn't be kept, such as a parent who sexually abuses a child and says, "Don't tell"; or a family member who enables addiction by saying that the client shouldn't talk about it. Allow clients to get feedback, if needed, if they're unclear whether it's a betrayal versus a healthy airing of a personal experience.

Tough Cases

* "Trusting people is too hard; I'd rather be alone."
* "I share all the time, but I'm still an addict."
* "Talking about silencing triggers me."
* "Someone in this group betrayed me; I don't feel safe sharing."
* "I need you to keep a secret from my probation officer."
* "I know I'll feel worse after sharing."

Break the Silence

Quotation

"In a room where people unanimously maintain a conspiracy of silence, one word of truth sounds like a pistol shot."

~ Czeslaw Milosz, 20th-century Polish poet

HANDOUT 1

Silencing in Trauma and Addiction

"It's so simple, what happened at St. Paul's [school]. It happens all the time, everywhere. First, they refused to believe me. Then they shamed me. Then they silenced me. So I've written what happened, exactly as I remember. . . . To go back to that girl leaving the boys' room on an October night, sneakers landing on the sandy path, and walk with her all the way home."

~Lacy Crawford, *Notes on a Silencing*

Did people doubt or ignore your trauma or addiction?	Yes / No / Maybe
Did you stay silent to protect yourself or others?	Yes / No / Maybe
Were you pressured not to tell?	Yes / No / Maybe

CULTURE OF SILENCE

The phrase *culture of silence* conveys how strong a force silencing can be. People may say, "Why didn't you speak up?" or "You should have told someone," not understanding that a family, community, or institution can create extraordinary pressure *not* to speak up. Silence may have been so automatic that you couldn't fully admit, even to yourself, what was happening.

In trauma, you may have felt that . . .

- You weren't believed.
- You didn't want to "rock the boat."
- You'd be harmed if you told.
- Your mind and body froze and you couldn't speak up.
- You were to blame, so didn't tell.
- You just wanted to move on and not talk.

(cont.)

From *Creating Change* by Lisa M. Najavits. Copyright © 2024 Lisa M. Najavits. Published by The Guilford Press. Permission to photocopy this material is granted to purchasers of this book for use with your own clients or patients; see copyright page for details.

HANDOUT 1 *(p. 2 of 2)* Break the Silence

In addiction, you may have . . .

- Felt too ashamed to tell anyone.
- Been part of a culture where addiction was invisible, ignored.
- Been in denial, unaware that you had a problem.
- Asked others to keep secrets so you could keep using.
- Not wanted to admit how bad it was.
- Hidden telltale signs to avoid being found out.

THE REWARDS OF BREAKING THE SILENCE

relief . . . staying true to yourself . . . a path forward . . . inner peace . . . personal power . . . closeness with others . . . distance from people who harmed you . . . acceptance

✧ Any other rewards? _____

_____

HANDOUT 2	Break the Silence

Feeling Heard

This exercise is voluntary. *If you choose to, fill out one option from Part I below to share aloud in the session.* The goal is to feel heard about something important in your past. There's no judgment or analysis, just support.

- Choose something about your past that matters, something that perhaps feels vulnerable.
- It can be positive or negative. Sharing something positive, such as what you're proud of, is just as important as sharing something negative.
- No one will see what you write.
- Don't share something that would betray a confidence you need to honor.
- In group counseling, everyone can share. Or you can say "pass" (not sharing) or "later" (you'd like the leader to come back to you). But please don't use the share to try to resolve a conflict with a group member.
- You can also request what you'd like to hear back (e.g., "I'd like to hear I'm a good person" or "I'd like a moment of silence, no words").
- If you need more space, continue on the back of the page.

PART I: IDEAS FOR YOUR SHARE

1. I never told anyone that _____
2. One of the hardest things I ever did was _____
3. To survive, I had to _____
4. I'm proud of _____
5. If only I had known _____
6. What I always wanted was _____
7. I want to be forgiven for _____
8. I'm ashamed that _____
9. My trauma made me _____
10. My addiction made me _____
11. I feel so [angry/guilty/secretly happy/humiliated/afraid/sad] about _____
12. I still can't figure out why _____
13. I may look strong now, but in the past _____
14. If I could go back in time, I would _____
15. No one around me knew that _____
16. I regret that _____

Or make up your own: _____

(cont.)

From *Creating Change* by Lisa M. Najavits. Copyright © 2024 Lisa M. Najavits. Published by The Guilford Press. Permission to photocopy this material is granted to purchasers of this book for use with your own clients or patients; see copyright page for details.

HANDOUT 2 *(p. 2 of 2)*   Break the Silence

PART II: GIVE SUPPORTIVE FEEDBACK TO OTHERS

Tips for feedback. Make it about them (don't bring it back to you). Be positive and kind. Be specific. Don't ask the person questions at this point. Here are examples.

- ❖ It was amazing how you _____
- ❖ You were so strong to _____
- ❖ I was moved when you said _____
- ❖ Now I understand why you _____
- ❖ I appreciate you for _____
- ❖ I believe you are _____

Or make up your own: _____

◆ Reflections

- How did you feel *before* sharing aloud?
- How do you feel *after* sharing aloud?
- If you heard others share (group treatment), what did you learn?

Give yourself credit for taking a risk to share.

HANDOUT 3 — Break the Silence

Sharing Outside of Treatment

It can be powerful and validating to share about your past with safe people outside of treatment, too.

Try these suggestions to help it go well.

- Choose a safe person (ask your counselor for feedback if needed).
- Ask if the person is open to you sharing (don't "truth bomb"). People may want to support you but are struggling themselves. It takes emotional energy to listen.
- If you don't know someone well, *start low and go slow*: Share a small thing, briefly, and not too often until you see trust building.
- Coordinate. Ask if it's a good time, say how much time you want, and what you want (e.g., "I'd like to tell you something important about my past" or "I'd like your advice").
- Make clear the sharing is not about the other person so that individual doesn't feel defensive. (This exercise is not designed to resolve a conflict with someone.)
- Only share when sober.
- Consider a role-play or talk it through in advance with a counselor or other helper.
- Plan what you'll do after, such as how to soothe yourself and get support if needed.
- Remember: It may feel difficult but gets easier with practice.

TRY IT OUT

❖ Is there some part of your past that you'd like to share?

➢ Who will you tell? _____

_____

➢ What do you want to share? _____

_____

➢ What can you do *before* to help it go well? _____

_____

➢ What can you do *during* to help it go well? _____

_____

➢ What can you do *after* that may help? _____

_____

From *Creating Change* by Lisa M. Najavits. Copyright © 2024 Lisa M. Najavits. Published by The Guilford Press. Permission to photocopy this material is granted to purchasers of this book for use with your own clients or patients; see copyright page for details.

Ideas for a Commitment

Commit to one action that will move your life forward!
It can be anything you feel will help you, or you can try one of the ideas below.
Keeping your commitment is a way of respecting, honoring, and caring for yourself.

- Option 1. Talk to people with solid recovery from trauma or addiction. Ask how they changed over time in their views of silence, secrets, and sharing.

- Option 2. Search online using the term *culture of silence*. What do you learn from that? Does it validate your experiences?

- Option 3. Fill in more rows in Handout 2. You can do it just for yourself or share what you write with safe people.

- Option 4. Write about a time that you felt truly heard. How did it help you? What made it a positive experience?

Darkness and Light

SUMMARY

Clients are guided to express the dark and light sides of their experience, both what is awful and what is beautiful. By expressing these extremes, they can be more in touch with themselves and learn to shift between these states in healthy ways.

ORIENTATION

Clients benefit from expressing what they feel inside however irrational or "crazy" it may seem. This is especially true for trauma and addiction, where clients' experiences have so often been extreme. One client said, "Professionals need to know how to deal with people's despair, fear, anxiety, grief, rage/anger, cutting, suicidal thoughts—not make them feel guilty for feeling it or respond with 'Oh, you shouldn't feel that way' " (Jennings & Ralph, 1997, p. 40).

Today's topic goes beyond facts and real events. Darkness and light can be a literal place but also a psychological place and metaphor for experiences. For example, "My dark place is where I beat myself up and want to hurt myself" or "My life has been like a prison cell, cold and alone." It's been suggested that dark and light are fundamental aspects of human experience, that we're hardwired to perceive in these terms (Palmer & Schloss, 2010). They're far-reaching—feelings, physical experiences, states of mind, and for some, a spiritual realm. The terms *darkness* and *light* are used because they are so visually and powerfully expressive but can be reworded to other terms if desired (see Handout 1 for examples).

Social psychology research has found that *negative* events, information, and self-image are much more powerful than positive ones. This appears to be an enduring characteristic of people (Baumeister, Bratslavsky, Finkenauer, & Vohs, 2001). Thus, it takes special effort to access the "light," and all the more so when people have trauma and addiction.

Several handouts are offered. Handout 1 provides key concepts about darkness and light (e.g., the idea that everyone has these sides, but in trauma and addiction they may be more intense. Handout 2 has exercises to help clients access their dark and light sides. Handout 3 suggests ways to shift between these states. The guiding principle is flexibility: learning to feel what's inside, being able to observe without acting on it, and gaining greater ability to alternate between dark and light as needed.

It may seem at first that staying on the "light" side is best, but this can be just as unhealthy as staying just on the "dark" side. Jung is one of the most important writers on this topic, recognizing the shadow side that's part of the human psyche yet often goes unacknowledged. As described by Zweig and Abrams: "The shadow goes by many familiar names: the disowned self, the lower self, the dark twin or brother in bible and myth, the double, repressed self, alter ego, id. When we come face-to-face with our darker side, we use metaphors to describe these shadow encounters: meeting our demons, wrestling with the devil, descent to the underworld, dark night of the soul, midlife crisis" (1991, p. 3).

This work is about deepening clients' self-awareness—understanding more about what moves and frightens them. Especially for chronic, severe trauma and addiction, clients need opportunities to learn who they are, which for a long time may have been clouded by their disorders.

Also, it's worth noting that today's topic relates to the concept of splitting yet is broader. *Splitting* in trauma and addiction refers to a psychological defense in which different sides of the self are compartmentalized (the young side, the angry side, the side that wants to use a substance, etc.). This is described in the topic "Integrating the Split Self" in *Seeking Safety* (Najavits, 2002c). Darkness and light go beyond splitting. They are central to human experience and exist in everyone regardless of psychological defenses.

Your Emotional Reactions

Exploring your own "darkness" and "light" heightens your ability to go there with clients. Try the exercises in Handout 2 for yourself. Notice how darkness and light tap the sometimes irrational, primitive parts of the self. Also watch for extreme views of clients—"angels who have been harmed" or "rotten scoundrels," that is, idealizing or devaluing. So, too, clients may project onto you extremes of all light (you're the best ever) or all darkness (you can do no right). Staying aware of extremes helps recognize the humble truth that everyone has both dark and light that emerge in different times and circumstances.

Acknowledgments

The session quotation is from Gide (1950/2011). The quotations at the start of Handout 1 are from Shay (1994, p. 33), Tolstoy (1867, part 12, Chapter 16), and Camus (1968, p. 169) and the Thistle quote is from McDermott (2021). In Handout 2, exercise 3 is partly adapted from Shapiro (1995).

SESSION FORMAT

1. *Check-in* (per Chapter 3).
2. *Quotation.* Link the quotation to the session topic—for example, *"Today's topic focuses on extremes of experience—what we'll call 'darkness and light.' The quotation conveys the importance of flexibility ('gray areas') and different perspectives."*
3. *Handouts* (relate the topic to clients' lives):
    Handout 1: **Darkness and Light**
    Handout 2: **Expression Exercises**
    Handout 3: **Build Flexibility**
4. *Check-out* (per Chapter 3).

SESSION CONTENT

Goals

☐ Explore the idea of darkness and light—the extreme, sometimes irrational sides of experience.
☐ Help clients put their dark and light sides into words.
☐ Practice shifting between darkness and light to aid recovery.

Darkness and Light

Ways to Relate the Material to Clients' Lives

★ *Help clients relate the concepts to their own life (Handout 1).* The handout has a lot of rich concepts and clients will differ in which are most meaningful to them. The key goal is to not remain abstract but rather help them see how it relates to their experiences and recovery.

★ *Try the exercises (Handout 2).* This handout is highly impressionistic—tapping senses and feelings rather than just intellectual awareness. Encourage clients to try exercises that appeal to them, letting go of those that don't. Let them know there are no right or wrong answers; the intent is to increase awareness. Doing the exercises aloud is helpful too.

★ *Brainstorm ways to shift (Handout 3).* Encourage clients to think of times they were able to move between darkness and light. What ways worked for them? What did they say to themselves? Did anyone help? Use Handout 3 to identify multiple methods. It can also become a commitment for today's session.

★ *Identify family-of-origin issues that relate to this topic.* Clients absorbed messages from their family about how to respond to internal experiences. They may have learned to hide what they were feeling, to numb it through substances, or to become aggressive or act out, for example.

★ *Teach grounding if needed.* Grounding is a key skill for shifting feelings and is mentioned in Handout 3. It may already be familiar to clients but, if not, teach it to them. Seeking Safety has a full chapter and exercise on grounding: "Detaching from Emotional Pain (Grounding)."

★ *Discussion*
- "Which side are you more in touch with—darkness or light?"
- "How would you describe what dark/light feel like for you?"
- "When you are in your dark/light place, where do you notice it in your body?"
- "What helps you shift from one to the other?"
- "What messages did you get growing up about expressing your feelings?"
- "How do trauma and addiction create more intense extremes?"
- "How much time are you in a moderate place ("gray") in which you're aware of both dark and light at once?"

Suggestions

✦ *Encourage clients to explore the "gray" as well as darkness and light.* It's good to notice the middle—moderate, midway between darkness and light. In this state, they're aware of both but neither fully dominates. Indeed, many healthy people experience this integrated state much of the time.

✦ *Validate clients' experience.* Clients may misinterpret today's topic to believe that it's asking them to erase the reality of pain or awful things they experienced. Trauma and addiction are horrific experiences, and the goal is not to pretend these are "light." Rather, it's about validating both: what's been good and what's been bad in their lives. Some clients may focus so much on negative experiences that they lose touch with what's positive (people who helped them, good times they've had, what they like about themselves). Remind them that the intent is to own all sides of their experience.

✦ *Watch for triggering.* Handout 2 may be triggering for some clients, such as those new to recovery. Use grounding as needed.

✦ *Keep expression within reasonable bounds.* Remind clients that they can express their extremes in words but not in actions such as throwing things. However, intense language and emotions are part of acceptable expression.

✦ *Provide guidance on opening up outside of counseling.* Clients may need help learning how to choose safe people to open up to, especially for dark feelings. For some clients, it may be best to keep expression just within the counseling setting for now.

Tough Cases

* "This sounds like all-or-none thinking."
* "Why would I want to talk about darkness? I've spent too much time there already."
* "Is this some sort of religious thing?"
* "When my dark side comes up, I want to hurt someone."
* "Isn't the goal to always stay in the light?"
* "I'm not able to move between dark and light. I'm always stuck in a negative place."

Quotation

"The color of truth is grey."

~ ANDRÉ GIDE, 19th-century French author

HANDOUT 1

Darkness and Light

People in successful recovery from trauma or addiction will tell you they've experienced extremes of both darkness and light, what is most awful and also most beautiful.

Darkness. The dark side of your experience may be a real or a psychological place: nighttime, a dark basement, a prison cell, an abyss, war, a black hole, hitting bottom, demons, the cold, a monster, dead inside.

Light. The light side of experience is described as sunlight, oneness, peace, recovery, victory, a higher power, the wise mind. It's calm awareness, healthy activity, positive connection, integration, joy.

Examples of *Darkness*

"A sense of pain sucking me in. A gravitational pull of my past. It wants me down, wants me to crash and burn, tells me I'm no good: 'You're fat, you're stupid, you have no life, look what you've done. It's horrible and it's too late.'"

~TRAUMA SURVIVOR

"I wanted to hide from the world and from my addictions, from all the mistakes and all the people that I'd hurt along the way. I just wanted to rot away and die."

~JESSE THISTLE (in McDermott, 2021)

Examples of *Light*

"In the depths of winter, I finally learned that within me there lay an invincible summer."

~ALBERT CAMUS, *Lyrical and Critical Essays*

"All, everything that I understand, I understand only because I love."

~LEO TOLSTOY, *War and Peace*

KEY POINTS

✦ **Everyone has their own version of darkness and light.** It's part of being human. Also, you may have different versions at different times. Darkness may feel "lost, sad, hopeless" at one point and "obsessed, craving, unable to relax" at another. The light takes different forms, too—perhaps calm when sitting quietly alone; energized when connecting with others.

(cont.)

From *Creating Change* by Lisa M. Najavits. Copyright © 2024 Lisa M. Najavits. Published by The Guilford Press. Permission to photocopy this material is granted to purchasers of this book for use with your own clients or patients; see copyright page for details.

HANDOUT 1 *(p. 2 of 2)*   Darkness and Light

✦ **Choose your own terms.** *Darkness* and *light* are often used, but you can choose words you prefer. See examples at the beginning of this handout.

✦ **If you were taught not to feel, this work may be especially important.** You may have received messages that it's bad to feel; that your feelings were a burden; or that it's only acceptable to express positives. You can learn a healthier approach now and become comfortable with the full range of your experience.

✦ **It may be biologically based.** Some experts believe that humans are hardwired to experience life in terms of these opposites of darkness and light.

✦ **Trauma and addiction make the darkness and light more intense.** They are extreme experiences so they take you to higher highs and lower lows. And having *both* trauma and addiction is more intense than either alone. The dark side may include hitting bottom, life-and-death struggles, despair, violence, and feeling haunted by disturbing memories. The light side may include appreciation for having survived, empathy for others who suffer, recovery, a sense of purpose, connection, and strong spirituality.

✦ **Darkness is not always "bad" and light is not always "good."** Your dark side can be a source of wisdom when it's processed and worked through. So too, expressing only your light side isn't genuine; one can't be positive and loving all the time. Both dark and light are part of human experience; it's about how you respond to each.

✦ **Learn to shift.** It's like learning any other skill; you can get better at accessing your darkness and light by choice.

✦ **It has a strong pull.** There's often a feeling of being drawn into it. When trauma or addiction are active, it's typically "darkness" that pulls you more, and in later recovery it's more your "light."

✦ **It's more than feelings.** It's also action, physical states, how you relate to yourself and others, spiritual sides, states of mind. It's the full range of experience.

✦ **If you aren't aware of your dark side, you're more likely to express it in action.** The person who "never feels angry" often acts angry (passive-aggressive or suddenly blowing up).

✦ **It can be healing to put it into words.** This is especially important for darkness—it helps to express what feels irrational or "crazy" as a way to move beyond it. If you speak about darkness, it loses some of its power.

✦ **There's also *gray*.** Healthy people typically spend a lot of their time in this integrated middle state: both broken and mending, not perfect but growing, aware of shortcomings and also strengths.

✦ **Darkness and light may represent people in your life,** such as a perpetrator who harmed you or a loving aunt who protected you. It's part of growing up to *internalize* important people, to carry their influence within. This doesn't mean you *become* them, though. You can choose how you want to be.

✦ **The goal isn't 50:50.** There's no perfect middle. Rather, it's dynamic—in and out of different states. Sometimes it helps to let yourself explore painful parts of your past; at other times, to focus on the light.

✦ **Make careful choices** on whether to act on darkness and light. Don't lash out with dark rage. Love, too, should not always be expressed. The more you're in touch with your full self, the more you can make healthy judgments about when to speak versus stay silent, when to act or not act.

HANDOUT 2   Darkness and Light

Expression Exercises

See if you can access the light, then darkness, then the light again, really feeling it. These exercises increase awareness and strengthen your ability to shift in and out by choice.

EXERCISE 1: PUT IT INTO WORDS

Light

★ *Glance at the list below. Circle at least five words that feel true for you when you're there. Does it put you in touch with your light side (healing, recovery, connection, etc.)?*

> hopeful aware conscious respectful mature wise clear grounded calm soothed focused balanced even quiet relaxed confident amused fun objective solid connected observant in the zone likable warm beautiful friendly helpful kind compassionate excited insightful knowledgeable safe active spiritual accepting reasonable serene appreciative interested awake lively attractive nurturing generous organized vibrant friendly sturdy body-aware humble secure attached loving easy-going attentive comforted part of things patient energized careful brave curious relaxed powerful good-natured humorous ambitious planful understanding practical honest enthusiastic responsible passionate empathic nonjudgmental unique hardworking creative competent playful fun polite normal attuned sensual positive outgoing honorable witty true committed goal-oriented sexual tolerant in touch trustworthy forgiving straightforward managing coping loyal intuitive thoughtful paced open embracing surviving thriving joyful peaceful bright determined sincere

Any others? _____

★ *Is there a specific memory that shifts you into those feelings? Describe it briefly on the back of the page or aloud. For example, "At my college graduation . . . "*

Darkness

★ *Glance at the list below. Circle at least five words that feel true for you when you're there. Does it help you access your dark side (trauma, addiction, etc.)?*

> betrayed upset wounded humiliated chaotic broken impulsive out of control afraid outraged freakish inhuman washed up panicky cruel immoral terrorized craving stuck dead enraged self-hating scared small young stressed tearful triggered ashamed abandoned nauseous lightheaded devalued addicted damaged pained despairing lonely bored burned out old lost used up narrow neglectful stupid out of my body isolated pathetic scapegoated pressured embarrassed ugly failed confused numb hurtful guilty bad lazy monstrous hateful spiteful brainwashed mournful rejected depriving deprived degraded cynical strange distrustful tortured dismissive empty burdened worn out exhausted paranoid corrupt perverted lost tense slutty tired distrustful fake

---

From *Creating Change* by Lisa M. Najavits. Copyright © 2024 Lisa M. Najavits. Published by The Guilford Press. Permission to photocopy this material is granted to purchasers of this book for use with your own clients or patients; see copyright page for details.

HANDOUT 2 (p. 2 of 3) Darkness and Light

> bitter fragmented damaged abnormal hidden perverted depressed excluded
> bizarre ugly avoidant racy spacy furious weak unforgiving intolerant irritated
> annoyed wicked distant dishonest manipulative vengeful jealous detached
> defeated inferior overwhelmed

Any others? _____

★ *Is there a specific memory that shifts you into those feelings? Describe it briefly on the back of the page or aloud. For example, "When I ran away from home at age 15 . . ."*
★ *Now try to access light feelings again by going back to the light words on the previous page.*

EXERCISE 2: NOTICE IMAGES

Sometimes there's a powerful image that evokes light or darkness.

Examples of Light

A colorful tapestry
A strong animal
A warm blanket
A beautiful day
A healer

★ *Describe your image. For example, "My image is a big silk tapestry with bold colors and a soft weave. The flaws in the fabric are part of the whole. It's like my addiction recovery: complex, rough at times, and colorful for sure."*

Examples of Darkness

A child crying
A forest at night
A lonely landscape
A corpse
An animal attacking

★ *Describe your image. For example, "A child crying reminds me of being 5 years old. When I cried, I was belittled. I shut down and felt alone. I still get those feeling even though I'm 37 now."*
★ *Now try going back to your light image.*

EXERCISE 3: RECOGNIZE WHO YOU TEND TO BECOME

What do darkness and light bring out in you?

★ *Circle any that are typical for you.*

Light

1. I see my part in things.
2. I'm patient with people.

(cont.)

HANDOUT 2 *(p. 3 of 3)*   Darkness and Light

3. I maintain sobriety.
4. I can concentrate on work.
5. I take things in stride.
6. I'm more fun.
7. I can have an impulse without acting on it.
8. I can express my needs.
9. I'm a good parent.
10. I see the good in others.
11. I set boundaries.
12. I plan for the future.
13. I'm capable of physical intimacy.
14. I'm kind to myself.

Others? _____

_____

Darkness

1. I get upset about small things.
2. I make poor choices.
3. I escape into _____ (substances, spending, porn, etc.).
4. I get involved with unsafe people.
5. I become overprotective of my kids.
6. I start fights.
7. I focus too much on work.
8. I lie a lot.
9. I harm myself (cutting, etc.).
10. I become afraid to leave the house.
11. I mooch off others.
12. I worry all the time.
13. I neglect my kids.
14. I hate myself.

Others? _____

_____

Who Influenced You?

★ *If you want, identify people from your past who most influenced your patterns above (parents, friends, a favorite teacher, religious figure, etc.). On any row above, list names that apply to that row.*

◇ Reflections

- Any new insights from these exercises?
- How well were you able to access the darkness/light?
- How can this topic help your recovery?

HANDOUT 3 — Darkness and Light

Build Flexibility

Do you tend to remain too much in the dark (unable to shift out) or too much in the light (afraid to see the pain or "ugliness" within)?

Like an athlete, try as many ways as possible to strengthen your flexibility so you can own your experience rather than it owning you.

★ *Circle any that you want to try.*

• *Talk yourself through it*

  I'm in my dark place again; I need to move to the light. I'm going to do what it takes to get there.

• *Use action*

  Take a walk, shower, light a candle, listen to music, change clothes—whatever gets you into a different state of mind.

• *Ask someone to help*

  Let a trusted person guide you.

• *Try grounding*

  It helps shift feelings. Learn about it online or from your counselor.

• *Write a letter to the other side*

  Create a dialogue between dark and light.

• *Observe patterns*

  What sets off your darkness and light?

• *Let yourself feel*

  Taking time to sit with a feeling can strengthen it.

• *Be kind to yourself*

  Gentleness can "open the door."

• *Other ways that work for you?*

_____

_____

From *Creating Change* by Lisa M. Najavits. Copyright © 2024 Lisa M. Najavits. Published by The Guilford Press. Permission to photocopy this material is granted to purchasers of this book for use with your own clients or patients; see copyright page for details.

Ideas for a Commitment

Commit to one action that will move your life forward!
It can be anything you feel will help you, or you can try one of the ideas below.
Keeping your commitment is a way of respecting, honoring, and caring for yourself.

✦ Option 1. "Actions speak louder than words." Write how have darkness and light have shown up in your actions.

✦ Option 2. Identify a time you experienced your light side and describe the following.

  ◆ What **words** you said to yourself _____

  ◆ What you felt in your **body** _____

  ◆ What **image** came to mind _____

  ◆ What your **feelings** were _____

  ◆ What your **thoughts** were _____

  ◆ Which **people** were around _____

✦ Option 3. Choose one of today's handouts and circle the main ideas that are helpful to you.

✦ Option 4. Read online about the concept of the *shadow self* advanced by Carl Jung, a famous 19th-century psychiatrist.

Emotions and Healing

SUMMARY

Emotions are central in trauma and addiction and also in recovery. In today's topic, clients learn about emotions and explore messages they got growing up (what feelings are acceptable, how conflicts are handled). There's also an exercise to shift feelings about a difficult past event.

ORIENTATION

An essential yet challenging aspect of recovery is how to deal with the feelings that arise. How people *feel* determines how they think, act, and relate.

Trauma and addiction can intensify feelings but also numb them, and some clients alternate between the two extremes. Many clients are so damaged by severe trauma and addiction that they don't even know what they feel. As one therapist describes it: "Most of my group members, over the 25 years that I have done this work, don't know how they feel about much. They were conditioned that their feelings didn't count and what others wanted was all that mattered. So they often don't know what they like or want or need. They feel guilty or selfish if they start to think about that. I always say that we make better decisions if we know what we feel. When clients don't know, it's upsetting to them, but there's no answer for how to feel—it develops as they do the work."

It helps to teach clients the difference between feelings and emotions. These are often used interchangeably but *feelings* are what is perceived, whereas *emotions* are the "raw data" below the surface and may not yet be conscious (Damasio, 2003). A client may say, "I'm not angry" yet her actions (passive-aggressive) and body (tension, heart rate) indicate the emotion of anger. This concept is clinically useful as clients often need to learn to recognize their true emotional reality. Yet the research literature shows many different terms (e.g., mood, affect) and no fully agreed-on definitions, so rather than getting caught up in language, the key goal is to encourage clients to better understand and express their emotional experiences. There may also be gender and cultural aspects that guide which emotions they acknowledge: "Boys don't cry, they get even"; and "Nice girls don't get angry."

To add to the mix, some feelings aren't productive in and of themselves, but rather targets to be reduced via effective treatment (e.g., paranoia, self-hatred, rage). No feeling is bad per se, and all feelings provide information that can deepen clients' awareness of what they've lived through and what they need. But clients need to discover what is and isn't healthy for them. Some feelings may be too frequent, too intense, or cause harm to themselves or others.

In today's topic, Handout 1 offers education about emotions, using a quiz format to create engagement. Handout 2 helps clients identify and evaluate emotion messages they absorbed growing up. Handout 3 is an exercise to shift perspective about a difficult event so as to access new feelings about it.

Emotions and Healing

In all, the goal is to help clients gain greater awareness of what they feel and why. These lessons have impact throughout Creating Change as emotions are at the heart of all the work. The hope is that feelings can become an ally in the healing process. As one client said, "I discovered that I could love even though so little love had been given to me."

Your Emotional Reactions

Your emotions are bound to be touched by the work. It can be painful to listen to how clients have been hurt. One counselor said, "On my worst days, the pervasiveness and horror of what I listen to in the experiences of trauma survivors colors my whole life and perceptions of others. I start to perceive 'yucky slime' on everything. I see every father with his child and interpret that he is abusing that child" (Jennings & Ralph, 1997, pp. 43–44). *Secondary traumatization* can occur (also known as *vicarious traumatization*), in which counselors develop symptoms that mirror PTSD after listening to a lot of disturbing material; they may experience hopelessness, nightmares, and intrusive thoughts (Pearlman & Saakvitne, 1995). Addiction, too, can evoke strong reactions (Najavits et al., 1995). Yet for both trauma and addiction, the range of emotions includes positive ones, too, such as gratification and excitement (Najavits, 2002b). Try taking a free, brief scale that helps identify how you're doing: the Professional Quality of Life Scale for health workers (Center for Victims of Torture, 2021), which has "strength" subscales (*compassion satisfaction, perceived support*) and "vulnerability" subscales (*burnout, secondary traumatic stress, moral distress*). You can complete it online or download it, with multiple languages available (*https://proqol.org/proqol-health-measure*).

Acknowledgments

The session quotation is from Dante's *Inferno*, canto 33 (Alighieri, 1321/1996). In Handout 1, the quote on chaos is from Bjornestad et al. (2019); the expression "put words between feelings and actions" is from Pearlman (2007); the 90-second rule is from Taylor (2021); and research on the length of emotions is from Verduyn and Lavrijsen (2015). In Handout 1, the four primary emotions are from Gu, Wang, Patel, Bourgeois, and Huang (2019). In Handout 3, the replay-the-scene exercise is adapted from exercise 35 at *www.addictions.com/blog/36-addiction-recovery-group-activities*. On the Commitment page, option 1 is a quotation from Black (2020).

SESSION FORMAT

1. *Check-in* (up to 5 minutes per client). See Chapter 3.
2. *Quotation* (briefly). See page 198. Link the quotation to the session. For example, *"The quote says we can become numb, like a stone, if we don't let ourselves grieve. Today we're going to focus on how emotions of all kinds are an essential part of recovery."*
3. *Handouts* (relate the topic to clients' lives; in-depth, most of the session):
   a. Ask clients to look through the handouts:
      Handout 1: **Emotions and Healing Quiz**
      Handout 2: **What Did You Learn about Feelings?**
      Handout 3: **Shift Your Emotional Perspective**
   b. Help clients relate the topic to current and specific problems in their lives. See "Session Content" (page 196) and Chapter 3 for suggestions.
4. *Check-out* (briefly). See Chapter 3.

SESSION CONTENT

Goals

☐ Discuss how emotions relate to healing from trauma and addiction.
☐ Explore messages about feelings that clients learned growing up.
☐ Invite clients to try an exercise on shifting their emotional perspective.
☐ Identify healthy approaches to emotion.

Ways to Relate the Material to Clients' Lives

★ *Use the quiz as a therapeutic game (Handout 1).* Start by handing clients just page 1 of the handout (the quiz questions) so they don't see the answers on the remaining pages. Then try one of these variations.

Option 1. In group treatment, create two or more teams. Each team gets 15 minutes to write down answers to as many questions as they can and then gets a point for each correct answer but with emphasis on understanding the ideas, not just on the points.

Option 2. In group or individual treatment, ask for any number from 1 to 15 (there are 15 questions). Read the corresponding question aloud. The goal is to answer the question correctly. In group, you can have clients take turns choosing a number; and the first person to raise a hand and answer it correctly gets a point.

For both options, to keep the exercise interactive as you go over the answers, you can ask a client to read aloud the answer from the handout and then ask, "Does that make sense?" "Any thoughts on that?"

★ *Explore childhood messages about emotions (Handout 2).* Note that half the messages in the handout are positive (a plus sign, +) and half are negative (a minus sign, –). This keeps a balanced view as most people had both positive and negative messages. Also, let clients know that while many messages were communicated in their family, they can broaden it to include messages from other influences such as peers, school, sports, religious education, culture, and jobs. Encourage them to share how the messages impact them now, and which messages they want to keep versus let go of.

★ *Try an exercise on shifting emotional perspective (Handout 3).* This exercise helps clients deepen their emotional awareness of a difficult past event. The two steps are described in the handout. Be sure to emphasize that the goal is not to shift from negative to positive feelings. Rather, it's to explore a past event in a new way, which can evoke emotions they may not have been aware of. There's an example at the bottom of the handout.

In individual treatment, the focus is just on one client, so the exercise is straightforward. But group treatment requires a bit more planning. A suggested method for groups is to ask for a volunteer who wants to go through the steps aloud, with you leading the exercise. Group members, as well as you, can help brainstorm on step 2 (generating "guidance, comfort, or knowledge"). This helps everyone participate and also broadens the possible perspectives. However, the client doing the exercise does not have to agree with the ideas being generated.

Note: When doing this exercise, depending on your sense of clients' capacities (current symptoms and functioning), you may want to suggest that they choose a moderately distressing event (between a 4 and a 7 on the 0–10 intensity scale in the exercise), rather than an intensely distressing event.

★ *Discussion*
  - "What do you wish someone had taught you about feelings?"
  - "What have you found helpful in dealing with feelings?"
  - "Do you use alcohol, drugs, or food to manage your feelings?"
  - "What feelings in *yourself* are most difficult to deal with?"
  - "What feelings in *other people* are most difficult to deal with?"

Emotions and Healing

- "How often are you unsure what you really feel?"
- "How often are your feelings out of control?"
- "How often do you feel joy?"
- "Do you lash out at others? If so, what triggers that?"

Suggestions

✦ ***Emphasize that all feelings are valid—but not all feelings are equal.*** It can help to give examples.

- "Have you ever been intoxicated and had a lot of intense feelings that went away after a few hours once you were sober (for example, anger, sadness, or paranoia)?"
- "When people have clinical depression, they may feel hopeless, but once they get on medication, that feeling goes down."
- "Do you ever get irritable because you're tired and then it goes away when you get some sleep?"

These examples highlight that some feelings are artifacts of altered states or moods and are not necessarily deep feelings that need to be processed. There's no hard-and-fast rule on which feelings are important to address, but it can help to guide clients toward more enduring emotions that need attention.

✦ ***If helpful, refer to the concept of*** **sides of the self.** Clients may be aware of particular feelings at one time but not another. This is common in trauma and addiction, called *splitting*. It's addressed in the topic "Knowing and Not Knowing" and also in detail in the Seeking Safety topic "Integrating the Split Self." There are also entire treatments that address this, such as Internal Family Systems therapy (IFS; Schwartz, 2013). In today's topic, it can be reassuring for clients to know that flipping between different feelings is common in trauma and addiction and that with recovery, integration occurs—the ability to hold on to multiple feelings at once.

✦ ***Convey that expression of feelings needs to stay safe.*** Clients can *talk* about any feelings but need to be mindful to not act them out in unsafe behavior such as substance use or harm to self or others. If a feeling becomes so strong that they can't contain an impulse, it's important to do grounding, ask for help, and use other safe coping skills.

✦ ***Steer clear of assumptions about the right way to feel.*** Some counselors hold strong beliefs that clients should express specific emotions. For example, "Clients need to express anger after trauma" or, the opposite, "Anger is a problem." Others believe sadness is essential and try to get clients to cry. And some counselors are uncomfortable with emotional intensity and try to reduce difficult feelings, rather than letting clients have an emotional experience. In short, there's no recipe for the order or types of emotions that need to be expressed. Clients differ in their ability to access emotion, express it, and tolerate it.

✦ ***Validate that research on emotions keeps evolving.*** For example, Handout 1 refers to four primary emotions (anger, sadness, joy, and fear), but some research suggests additional ones, too, such as excitement and trust. If clients debate particular aspects, try to steer back to what is clinically relevant—how it relates to their recovery.

Tough Cases

* "I don't feel anything."
* "I only feel normal when I'm high."
* "Ever since my trauma there's no joy."
* "I've hurt people and feel guilty about that."
* "I've had panic attacks for years. Nothing helps."
* "I feel anxious around you."

Emotions and Healing

Quotation

"I wept not, so to stone within I grew."

~ Dante Alighieri, 13th-century Italian poet

HANDOUT 1

Emotions and Healing Quiz

"I ran out of tears in the war."

"Recovery taught me what love is."

"I like chaos. I found it so boring when there was no action around me."

🍃

Dealing with feelings is a major challenge for everyone, but all the more so for people with trauma and addiction.

- Some want to feel *more*—they're numb or unaware of feelings.
- Others want to feel *less*—they're overwhelmed by feelings.

Learn all you can to support your recovery.

15 QUESTIONS ON EMOTION AND HEALING

✧ *Try answering the questions yourself before reading the answers that follow.*

1. What's the difference between *feelings* and *emotions*?
2. What does "feelings are not facts" mean?
3. Does it help to vent feelings?
4. What four emotions occur across cultures?
5. What's *toxic positivity*?
6. What's the 90-second rule?
7. "What we don't talk out, we act out"—what does this mean?
8. What's *splitting*? And the opposite of it?
9. Are triggers ever useful?
10. What's a *traumaversary*?
11. What's *expressing* versus *processing* feelings?
12. Is love essential for survival?
13. What are *primary* versus *secondary* emotions?
14. What's *addiction to pain*?
15. What are examples of *healthy* approaches to emotions?

(cont.)

From *Creating Change* by Lisa M. Najavits. Copyright © 2024 Lisa M. Najavits. Published by The Guilford Press. Permission to photocopy this material is granted to purchasers of this book for use with your own clients or patients; see copyright page for details.

HANDOUT 1 *(p. 2 of 3)*   Emotions and Healing

1. **What's the difference between *feelings* and *emotions*?**
   Feelings are what you're aware of. Emotions are below the surface; you may not be aware of them. You may say "I'm not angry," yet show signs of anger (annoyance, sarcasm, grudges, passive-aggressiveness). The goal is to become more and more aware of your real emotions.

2. **What does "feelings are not facts" mean?**
   Just because you *feel hopeless*, it doesn't mean there's no hope. Feelings are so powerful that they feel true. But if you can see the difference between facts and feelings, it opens up new worlds. Maybe it's a fact that you failed a test, but it doesn't mean you're doomed to fail forever, even if it feels that way.

3. **Does it help to vent feelings?**
   Yes and no. *Venting* means expressing your feelings about something distressing. It can help to rehash a difficult situation but can also lead to greater distress unless there's also soothing, feedback, and gaining new perspectives. Research shows that expression alone can increase distress. For example, yelling, swearing, posting angry social media messages, or punching a pillow just *fuel* anger.

4. **What four emotions occur across cultures?**
   Anger, sadness, joy, and fear ("mad, sad, glad, and scared") are the emotions that occur across cultures, according to research. But many more derive from these; you can find lists of emotions online. Notice what you're feeling and give language to it.

5. **What's *toxic positivity*?**
   It's important to recognize all emotions. The belief that one should stay positive all the time has been called *toxic positivity* because it's so unhealthy—for example, "Positive vibes only," "Delete negativity," "Don't worry, be happy," "Smile!," "Find the silver lining."

6. **What's the 90-second rule?**
   The brain's activation of a feeling lasts about 90 seconds, according to research. This means when anger washes over you, you can set a timer for 90 seconds to watch it go down. But some feelings last longer than others (e.g., sadness stays longer than boredom or fear). Research in this area is new, but the key takeaway is to discover for yourself how long particular feelings last by using a timer. This also helps with managing flashbacks, panic attacks, and cravings.

7. **"What we don't talk out, we act out"—what does this mean?**
   Emotions that aren't dealt with can show up in destructive behaviors ("acting out") such as cheating on a partner, self-harm, and causing fights. Unaddressed emotions can also show up as physical problems and illness. The solution? "Put words between feelings and action." Acknowledge your feelings and talk about them.

8. **What's *splitting*? And the opposite of it?**
   Trauma and addiction can be so emotionally overwhelming that part of you shuts down at times, leaving you aware of one side but not another. This is called *splitting*. For example, you flip between "I'm good/I'm bad"; or disown a side that feels unacceptable ("I'm never afraid"). The opposite is *integration*, meaning wholeness—being aware of all sides of yourself and able to respond to them

(cont.)

HANDOUT 1 *(p. 3 of 3)* — Emotions and Healing

9. **Are triggers ever useful?**
   A trigger is a strong painful emotional reaction. It's set off by something *small* that relates to something *big* from your past. A trigger can be a smell, sound, person, image, object, body sensation, or anything else. Your reaction is intense because it's really about something important in your past. The best immediate response is to do grounding to stay safe (distracting yourself from the trigger). But in the long term, exploring triggers can deepen your understanding of yourself and diminish their power over you.

10. **What's a *traumaversary*?**
    "Traumaversary" is a real thing. It refers to distress on the anniversary of a trauma. If someone you loved died in the spring, seeing spring flowers may bring grief again; or a February 8th car accident may upset you each year on that day until you've fully dealt with the trauma.

11. **What's *expressing* versus *processing* feelings?**
    Expressing feelings is called "catharsis." It means communicating intense feelings as you experience them. *Processing* feelings is called "working through" and goes beyond just expression. It's exploring feelings from new perspectives to gain insight and move forward ("I realized I did the best I could do under the circumstances"; "I don't have to tolerate bad relationships").

12. **Is love essential for survival?**
    Yes. Love (a deep, positive emotional connection) is one of the most important emotions. Humans are born needing love and without it they don't thrive. There are many ways to experience love, including people, God, nature, arts, and dedication to an important cause. But love can also be unhealthy if it's out of balance (giving all to others; stalking).

13. **What are *primary* versus *secondary* emotions?**
    A primary emotion is a direct, genuine reaction to something happening (someone breaks up with you and you feel sad). Secondary emotions are an emotional defense against the primary emotion. For example, instead of sadness you may feel anger because growing up you heard "It's weak to cry," so you can't let yourself feel the sadness (the primary emotion). Any emotion can be primary or secondary. Notice which emotions are easy or hard for you to let yourself feel.

14. **What's *addiction to pain*?**
    Addiction to pain isn't a formal diagnosis but is nonetheless real. You may be so used to emotional pain that you don't feel alive without it. So you keep tolerating pain even if you don't need to, or harm yourself, or keep sparking conflicts with others. All of these create an adrenaline rush—a chemical reward in the brain that keeps you going back. It's a convergence of trauma and addiction: It has the pain of trauma and the pattern of an addiction. *Note:* Addiction to pain is different than tolerating trauma you're unable to escape; a child who has to endure abuse is not "addicted to pain."

15. **What are examples of *healthy* approaches to emotions?**
    You acknowledge all feelings and have some ability to shift in and out of them—containing them at times and letting yourself experience them at other times. You learn from your feelings, respond to them, soothe them, and talk about them. You let yourself cry and are not numb. You feel love toward yourself and others in a balanced way. You don't stay stuck in unproductive feelings for long. Your actions are calm, planned, and rational rather than impulsive reactions to feelings.

◇ **Other key points about emotion that you want to share?**

_____
_____
_____

HANDOUT 2 — Emotions and Healing

What Did You Learn about Feelings?

As a child, you absorbed what you saw around you. Many messages about feelings are silent but powerful.

★ *Select one or more questions below to discuss.*

WHEN YOU WERE GROWING UP . . .

Note: "+" are positive examples; "−" are negative examples.

1. **Were all feelings respected?** How did your family/peers respond to each other's feelings?

    For example:
    + "We could talk openly about almost anything."
    − "If I felt bad, I was told I was being dramatic and to cut it out."

2. **How was love expressed?** Aloud ("I love you")? in action (buying a gift)? not at all?

    For example:
    + "My mother gave me big hugs."
    − "Showing affection was mocked."

3. **What were the "rules" about feelings?** Even if not said aloud, what did you learn?

    For example:
    + "It's healthy to cry."
    − "Pretend it's OK when it isn't."

4. **Was there anyone to share your feelings with?**

    For example:
    + "My sister and I were really close."
    − "I was totally alone. I'd go to my room until the feelings passed."

5. **What did you do to get love?** Achievement? people pleasing? humor?

    For example:
    + "I felt loved for who I was."
    − "I pretended to be perfect even though inside I was a mess."

6. **What's an important memory about feelings?**

    For example:
    + "When I got bullied, my mother advocated for me to switch schools."
    − "My brother committed suicide and no one talked about it."

(cont.)

From *Creating Change* by Lisa M. Najavits. Copyright © 2024 Lisa M. Najavits. Published by The Guilford Press. Permission to photocopy this material is granted to purchasers of this book for use with your own clients or patients; see copyright page for details.

HANDOUT 2 *(p. 2 of 2)*   Emotions and Healing

7. How were conflicts handled?

For example:
+ "We took turns stating our point of view."
− "My father would lash out; he could never be wrong."

8. Were there strong cultural beliefs about feelings?

For example:
+ "Being in harmony with others is valued."
− "Girls always have to be nice."

◇ **Other key messages?**

_____

_____

_____

◇ **Reflections**

- How did the messages impact how you respond to *yourself*?
- How did the messages impact your *relationships*?
- Which messages do you want to *hold on to*?
- Which messages do you want to *change*?

HANDOUT 3 — Emotions and Healing

Shift Your Emotional Perspective

Do you find it difficult to come to terms with an event in your past?

This exercise lets you see it in a new way. It doesn't mean you'll be happy about it, but you may be able to access new feelings that help you heal.

★ Do the exercise aloud or in writing. See the example at the end of the handout.

STEP 1: DESCRIBE A DIFFICULT PAST EVENT

Examples: ✘ "My overdose." ✘ "When I lost custody of my kids." ✘ "Getting fired."

    a. **Briefly describe what happened.** Aim for a paragraph or, if aloud, up to 3 minutes.

    b. **List your current feelings about it and intensity** from 0 (low) to 10 (high) [e.g., guilty = 7; embarrassed = 5].
-
-
-

STEP 2: IMAGINE THE HELP YOU WOULD HAVE WANTED

Examples: ✦ "Someone to ask me what was really going on." ✦ "A lawyer to help me sue him." ✦ "Someone to stand up for me." ✦ "Being accepted for who I was."

    a. **What would your past self have wanted at the time?** What guidance, comfort, or knowledge would have made a difference? Who would you have wanted by your side? Some people like to imagine a force or ally (a dragon, superhero, celebrity, or animal) that helps them through it.

    b. **Focus on this step 2 version and list your feelings about it now** and ratings from 0 (low) to 10 (high).
-
-
-

(cont.)

From *Creating Change* by Lisa M. Najavits. Copyright © 2024 Lisa M. Najavits. Published by The Guilford Press. Permission to photocopy this material is granted to purchasers of this book for use with your own clients or patients; see copyright page for details.

HANDOUT 3 *(p. 2 of 2)* • Emotions and Healing

✧ **Reflections (describe any insights here)**

_____
_____
_____

Notes

* Some people find that Step 2 brings up more vulnerable feelings or a sense of yearning, which helps them grieve, gain acceptance, or in other ways come to terms with the event.
* If your feelings stayed the same, that's OK; just notice what comes up for you.
* You can also try adding more help and comfort to Step 2.

EXAMPLE

Step 1: Describe a Difficult Past Event

a. *"I got arrested for driving drunk. I'd do anything to go back and change what happened. I couldn't drive for a year and lost my job. It's on social media and forever online."*

b. **List your current feelings about it and intensity** from 0 (low) to 10 (high)
- Humiliated = 10
- Ashamed = 10

Step 2: Imagine the Help You Would Have Wanted

a. *"I'm picturing my mother, who died 10 years ago, giving me a hug. She says, 'You could've died in that car but you're still alive, and that's what matters. Even though you made a mistake, don't waste more time blaming yourself.' She's right. I completed my jail sentence. I have to release myself from the regret and live life forward. I imagine her telling me I have a lot to live for, wanting me to be happy."*

b. **Focus on this Step 2 version and list your feelings about it now** and ratings from 0 (low) to 10 (high).
- Sad = 9
- Lonely = 8
- Ashamed = 3

✧ **Reflections (describe any insights here)**

"My eyes teared up writing that. I miss her so much. Whenever I made mistakes growing up, she still loved me. I don't have anyone in my life like that now. I think that's why I can't stop blaming myself. I'm lonely and get caught up in my own head. It makes me want to drink. I need to build new relationships. It was sad to do this exercise, but I see what I need to do."

Ideas for a Commitment

*Commit to one action that will move your life forward!
It can be anything you feel will help you, or you can try one of the ideas below.
Keeping your commitment is a way of respecting, honoring, and caring for yourself.*

- Option 1. Write about this:

    "The three unwritten rules in an alcoholic home are don't talk, don't trust, don't feel."

- Option 2. Create a list or scrapbook of joyful memories. It's a reminder that life has beauty and warmth, too.

- Option 3. If you're a parent, what messages about emotions do you want to communicate to your children? See Handout 2 for examples.

- Option 4. Ask people who know you what you're like when you're stressed versus relaxed.

- Option 5. Are any of the answers in Handout 1 surprising to you? Write about that.

Tell Your Story

SUMMARY

Clients have the opportunity to share part of their story of trauma and addiction. There are various options for sharing, empowering them to share at whatever level they feel ready for.

ORIENTATION

Telling one's story is part of most therapies, across theoretical orientations and types of treatment. It's prominent in trauma models and in addiction treatment, too, such as 12-step speaker meetings and writing an autobiography of addiction in rehabilitation programs.

Indeed, throughout history it's been part of human experience to overcome emotional pain by talking about the past. By nature, humans are storytellers, which serves a variety of functions—to entertain, amuse, inform, inspire, and, not least, to overcome suffering. In today's topic, telling one's story means, of course, telling the truth (not fiction).

During the session, clients can share part of their story if they choose to. They're guided to identify a part that still holds energy for them, that they want to reveal. Handout 1 offers suggestions for sharing as well as a framework of different types of stories such as *untold* stories and *unknown* stories (Griffin, Ledbetter, & Sparks, 2018). Handout 2 provides poignant questions to launch their share. Handout 3 has a timeline to identify important events in the past, both negative and positive. There's also a story card exercise for group modality that provides a structured way for clients to receive support from the group.

However, clients aren't asked to tell their whole story or to repeatedly retell the same narrative, in contrast to exposure-based therapies. In Creating Change, each session addresses a different aspect of their story; the narrative per se isn't the central focus. This approach worked well in our studies and clinical implementation projects, which typically focused on clients with complex trauma and chronic addiction. It helped them feel empowered to take control of their story and reduced a sense of being overwhelmed by the full narrative. On a practical level, the approach is feasible for group modality in terms of balancing time and clients' needs. It also helps clients recognize that telling their story is a long-term goal. In the session, they experience a sample of what it feels like; it's a template of the work rather than a promise of completion. They typically have so many adversities in their past that it's not realistic to view resolution as a near-term goal. It's a marathon rather than a sprint.

Note, too, that clients can select a *theme* rather than an *event* to talk about. Events occur at a point in time, such as "the night I got arrested for drunk driving" or "the time my uncle threatened me." Themes, in contrast, are broad patterns such as "Growing up, I had to pretend things

Tell Your Story

were OK" or "I've always felt like a bad person." Whatever they select, it can relate to trauma, addiction, or both.

One counselor beautifully describes what it's like.

"I don't believe people necessarily have to tell their story in detail. I believe they need to tell whatever they need to tell. Some want to share a lot and others not so much. It's the emotional content, not all the facts, that's important. They want us to truly understand what it was like for them. And I want them to feel supported and valued in the process—that this time the experience of telling is different than the other times when no one cared."

Your Emotional Reactions

It's essential to respect clients' version of the past, being careful not to impose your own view. It may feel tempting to state what was or was not important, to assume where the story is headed ("premature knowing"), or to decide the meaning of it (Pearlman & Saakvitne, 1995). "What seems like a minor detail to the therapist may be the most important aspect of the story to the patient. Conversely, an aspect of the story that the therapist finds intolerable may be of lesser significance to the patient" (Herman, 1992, p. 179). It's thus important to tolerate being uncertain; to ask open-ended questions (e.g., "What happened next?"); and to offer support rather than assumptions ("That sounds hard" rather than "You must have felt angry"). Clients are the authors of their story.

Acknowledgments

The session quotation is from Dinesen (interview with Mohn, 1957). In Handout 2, the framework comes from communications theory (specifically, *coordinated management of meaning theory* by Pearce and Cronen, as summarized in Griffin et al., 2018). The story card exercise has been used in various clinical settings, including with trauma survivors and older adults (and was suggested by Gabriella Grant, MA).

PREPARING FOR THE SESSION

If you're doing the story card exercise, prepare the materials ahead, per the instructions in the section "Ways to Relate the Material to Clients' Lives."

SESSION FORMAT

1. *Check-in* (per Chapter 3).
2. *Quotation.* Link the quotation to the session topic—for example, *"Today you'll have the opportunity to tell part of your story if you choose to. As the quote suggests, talking about the past can help overcome it."*
3. *Handouts* (relate the topic to clients' lives):
    Handout 1: **About Telling Your Story**
    Handout 2: **What Do You Want to Share?**
    Handout 3: **Timeline**
4. *Check-out* (per Chapter 3).

SESSION CONTENT

Goals

- ☐ Encourage clients to tell part of their story if they choose to.
- ☐ Offer suggestions on sharing.
- ☐ Explore poignant questions to access important parts of their story.
- ☐ Identify patterns of best and worst events on a timeline.

Ways to Relate the Material to Clients' Lives

★ ***Help clients know what to expect (Handout 1).*** Handout 1 provides information and you can add key points from the following list as well:
  a. Sharing is always optional. Say "pass" if desired.
  b. The goal is to work on part of their story; it won't be the whole story.
  c. Telling a part today paves the way for more in the future. It might take them months or years to fully tell their story.
  d. They can choose anything they're ready to share, small or large. There's no obligation to choose the worst event.
  e. They can choose anything related to trauma or addiction. It may be an actual event or a theme, such as loss of innocence or hope.
  f. It's not just facts, but also how they feel and the meaning it holds.
  g. They will have _____ minutes for their share and won't be interrupted. (Fill in the number of minutes based on your session length and whether it's individual or group modality. See the section "Suggestions" on the next page for allocating time in group.)
  h. After their share, they'll receive support.

★ ***Read aloud the guidelines for group modality to create a respectful process (Handout 1).*** These are listed at the end of Handout 1 and are important for ensuring a productive session. If a client doesn't abide by these guidelines, steer it back on track.

★ ***Let clients choose questions to answer in Handout 2.*** For group treatment, you can ask a client to choose a question to answer aloud and then others can answer that same question if they want to. Then another client picks a new question, and so on. This allows them to spontaneously share without having to select part of their story in advance. It also works in individual treatment, with the client choosing and answering several during the session.

★ ***Use the timeline as a structured, lighter method (Handout 3).*** The timeline can serve as a more contained way to have clients start telling their story. It is not as open-ended as Handouts 1 and 2. The timelines can also be helpful in other sessions of Creating Change; clients can return to some of these major events in the context of other topics.

★ ***Try a story card exercise.*** This is typically used in groups but can also be done in individual counseling.

- *Preparation (prior to the session).* Take a small box and put in words and images written or cut out from magazines, including trauma, addiction, and recovery themes (e.g., *survivor, friends, alcohol bottle, resilience, desperation, pills, growth, children, war, hope, broken, heal, family, school, playground, work, prayer, art, food, money, sex, body, gang*). Also have plain paper; pens; tape; a timer; and, if desired, art supplies such as stickers and glitter.
- *Step 1, in session.* Each client takes a blank sheet of paper and folds it in half. They then choose four to five words/images from the box that represent an important part of their story and tape them in a vertical row down one side of the paper. They can add their own drawings and words, as well as decorations if you have those, but their work still needs

Tell Your Story

to be limited to four to five words/images total. Allow about 10 minutes for them to do this and then the group comes together for sharing.

- *Step 2, in session.* Each client gets 5 minutes, using a timer, to show their story card and tell a bit about it, using the sequence of words/images to keep the narrative moving forward. After the client shares, the client's card is passed along to group members, who can write brief words of support on the other half of the paper. When it comes back around, the client can also write a brief note of support to self. Clients can keep their card as a reminder of the session and the support they received. If there's not enough time for each client, conduct additional sessions as needed.

★ *Explore what it means to tell one's story.* Guide clients to the first part of Handout 1 ("Many Possible Stories"). Ask them about their different types of stories—how much of their story have they told already? What's left to tell? Are there parts they're not ready for but want to tell in the future? Are there safe people they can open up to about their story? If they told their story before, how did it go? This type of dialogue moves the session away from sharing memories and instead addresses the broader concept of what it means to tell one's story and how to do it therapeutically.

★ *Balance time in group modality.* Individual treatment is easier as the focus is on one person. Group requires more planning. Consider a timed structure for sharing so that everyone who wants to tell part of their story gets a chance to do so. Let clients know your method at the start so they won't feel cut off during their share. Any of the following can be good choices, depending on group size and session length. Each has a different feel and somewhat different goal. Note that you may need two or more sessions for all clients to get a chance to share, depending on your group size.

- *Try the story card exercise described on page 208.* This keeps each share brief while also emphasizing support for each client.
- *Open share.* Decide on a time length (e.g., up to 5 minutes per client). Anywhere from 5 to 12 minutes is suggested.
- *Choose a question.* Each client chooses one question from Handout 2 to answer.
- *Choose a timeline event.* Each client talks about one aspect of the timeline for a specified number of minutes.

★ *Discussion*
- "What good can come from telling your story?"
- "What support would you like to hear when you share?"
- "Do any feelings come up when you look at the handouts?"
- "Do you have any concerns about telling part of your story today?"

Suggestions

✦ *Help clients address harm done to them but also, when relevant, harm they did to others.* Harm suffered by clients is usually what comes to mind when people think of telling their story. But harm they did is also powerful to address. A military veteran may feel inner conflict for having killed civilians. A father may feel regret for being an absent parent while in active addiction. Some clients may have committed awful crimes.

✦ *Preserve clients' emotional space.* Interrupting the client or putting the client's experience into your words disrupts the flow of emotion and memory, even if you mean well. Like a spool of yarn, let the yarn unravel fully, within the allotted time, rather than jumping in. See Chapter 4 for more.

✦ *Don't assume clients need to express intense emotions.* Today's topic may appear to resemble trauma treatments such as Exposure Therapy in which clients access strong feelings connected to their memories. In Creating Change, some clients may experience strong feelings but there isn't pressure to do so. See the section "Working with Emotion" in Chapter 3 for how emotions are addressed in this model.

✦ *Access the full range of experience, including positive aspects.* The handouts offer a broad range of prompts for sharing. Even in trauma and addiction, there are positive aspects such as insights gained and moments of heroism (e.g., protecting a sibling). But don't push clients to identify positives. Let them choose what to express without editorializing on what to focus on. Some may speak just about painful events; others may do a mix.

✦ *Be neutral about the accuracy of clients' stories.* The role of the counselor "is to be an open-minded, compassionate witness, not a detective" (Herman, 1992, p. 180). Rather than "Are you sure that really happened?," you can say, "I really hear you feel a lot of pain." Clients may be telling the truth as best as they can yet may not always be accurate on the facts. This is especially true for those who suffered early child abuse or blacked out from substances.

✦ *Stay aware of clients' needs.* This may seem obvious, but today's topic can evoke strong positions among counselors. At one end are counselors who so value exposure-based work that they may unintentionally pressure clients into telling more than they're ready for, without sufficiently adjusting to their pacing, choice, and readiness. Sometimes there's even a voyeurism in wanting to hear trauma or addiction details, to delve into the "muck." At the other end are counselors who hesitate to hear another painful narrative. They feel a need to protect themselves from clients' (and perhaps their own) upsetting material. The primary way out of these reactions is to stay centered in what clients need and want.

Tough Cases

* "The past is the past. No need to relive it."
* "I can't remember most of what happened."
* "I've told my story many times, and it doesn't help."
* "I've done some really bad things that I can't talk about."
* "If I talk about substance use, it makes me want to use."
* "How will I know when I'm over it?"
* "Will you call Child Protective Services if I tell you what happened to my kids?"
* "I told my doctor about my abuse and now he thinks my problems are all in my head."

Tell Your Story

Quotation

"All sorrows can be borne if you put them into a story or tell a story about them."

~ Isak Dinesen, 20th-century Danish writer

HANDOUT 1

About Telling Your Story

Today you can share an important part of your story of trauma, addiction, or recovery.

"Story" doesn't mean made up. It's telling the truth about what you lived. It's also called *autobiography*, *testimony*, or *narrative*.

MANY POSSIBLE STORIES

We all have . . .

- **Lived** stories—*what we directly experience*
- **Unknown** stories—*information that's missing*
- **Untold** stories—*what we choose not to say*
- **Unheard** stories—*what we say that isn't heard or acknowledged*
- **Untellable** stories—*stories that are forbidden or too painful for us to tell*
- **Told** stories—*what we have shared*

HOW TO SHARE

- It's your choice whether or not to share.
- Share only what you want.
- Accept feelings that arise.
- If you prefer, you can write it and read it aloud.
- After your share, you'll get support. Or you can also request a moment of silence or say what you'd like to hear back ("I'd like to hear that you believe me, that it wasn't my fault").
- You won't tell your full story today but can share more in other sessions.
- Tell any parts you choose—what it felt like, how it changed you, what you noticed in your body, and any other details.
- You can also share positive aspects, such as pride in your survival or people you're grateful for.
- After your share, give yourself credit for doing it. Also notice feelings, body sensations, and insights that arose.

For group treatment

- Your counselor will identify how much time each person has.
- If you're a listener, stay silent while others share. Afterward, provide brief positive support (don't give advice or relate it back to you). Each person's truth is to be honored.

From *Creating Change* by Lisa M. Najavits. Copyright © 2024 Lisa M. Najavits. Published by The Guilford Press. Permission to photocopy this material is granted to purchasers of this book for use with your own clients or patients; see copyright page for details.

HANDOUT 2   Tell Your Story

What Do You Want to Share?

Share part of your past that still holds energy for you—about your trauma, addiction, or recovery.

★ *Choose any questions that are meaningful to you.*

- What happened (specific events)?
- What do you wish had happened?
- Why do you think it happened to you?
- What are you proud of in how you handled it (e.g., strength, survival)?
- What do you know now that you didn't know then?
- What did you need that you didn't get?
- Who was/was not there for you?
- What do you feel in your body as you remember it?
- What would you say to your younger self if you could go back in time?
- What apology would you want to hear?
- How did people respond? (Blame? Comfort? Silence?)
- How were trauma and addiction connected?
- Did you try to help or protect others?
- Did you cause harm to others?
- What did you lose? What did you gain?
- How did it change your view of yourself? (Do you feel damaged? heroic?)
- What advice would you have for someone going through it?
- How did you feel when it happened (e.g., betrayed, shocked, empowered, compassionate)?
- What about it stays with you today?
- Are there aspects you're afraid to look at?
- Do you have regrets (what you wish you had or hadn't done)?
- Is there anything you're grateful for, such as someone who helped you?
- Did it change your core beliefs (e.g., trust, innocence, faith)?
- What would you want to say now to the person who hurt you?
- What lessons, positive or negative, did it leave you with?
- How did it impact your life (relationships/work/health/finances/opportunities)?
- Did it change how others view you? (Stigma? Respect?)
- How does it show up in your current behavior?
- Did you suffer deprivation (lack of food, shelter, treatment)?
- Do you feel guilt or shame?
- Is there something you don't forgive yourself for?
- What did you have to do to get through it?
- What was the worst part?
- What do you understand about it that others don't?
- Were you able to tell someone about it?
- Do different sides of you have different reactions to what happened?
- Any other aspects? _____

From *Creating Change* by Lisa M. Najavits. Copyright © 2024 Lisa M. Najavits. Published by The Guilford Press. Permission to photocopy this material is granted to purchasers of this book for use with your own clients or patients; see copyright page for details.

HANDOUT 3 Tell Your Story

Timeline

Timelines can offer new insights.

★ *For each timeline, you can list up to four events. If an event goes across years (e.g., emotional abuse), draw a squiggly line to indicate that. See the example at the end of this handout.*

You can use colors and add lines or other marks. Some people make this into an art project, such as collage. For more space, use larger sheets of paper.

∽ Up to four of *your best life events* ∾

Major joyful or growth events, such as graduation, marriage, entering treatment

Event #1. _____

Event #2. _____

Event #3. _____

Event #4. _____

Birth -- **Now**

♦ Up to four of *your worst life events* ♦

Trauma, onset of mental illness, emotional abuse, neglect, divorce, job loss

Event #1. _____

Event #2. _____

Event #3. _____

Event #4. _____

Birth -- **Now**

✶ Up to four *important addiction events* ✶

First use, age you became addicted, "hitting bottom," sobriety date, recovery attempts (can be any addiction, e.g., food, gambling, shopping)

Event #1. _____

Event #2. _____

Event #3. _____

Event #4. _____

Birth -- **Now**

(cont.)

From *Creating Change* by Lisa M. Najavits. Copyright © 2024 Lisa M. Najavits. Published by The Guilford Press. Permission to photocopy this material is granted to purchasers of this book for use with your own clients or patients; see copyright page for details.

HANDOUT 3 *(p. 2 of 2)* Tell Your Story

✧ Reflections

- Do you notice any patterns or messages when you look across your timelines?
- What feelings come up when you look at your timelines?
- Were there particular stages of your life that you coped better/worse?
- How did your trauma and addiction emerge over time—did one lead to the other?
- Did personal strengths have an impact?
- Did personal weaknesses have an impact?
- What can help you in the future?

EXAMPLE

❧ **Up to four of *your best life events*** ☙

Major joyful or growth events, such as graduation, marriage, entering treatment

Event #1. _Moved to my aunt's house, which got me away from my abusive father_

Event #2. _Met Carrie who later became my wife_

Event #3. _Won a basketball scholarship that got me into college_

Event #4. _My sobriety (I have 6 years)_

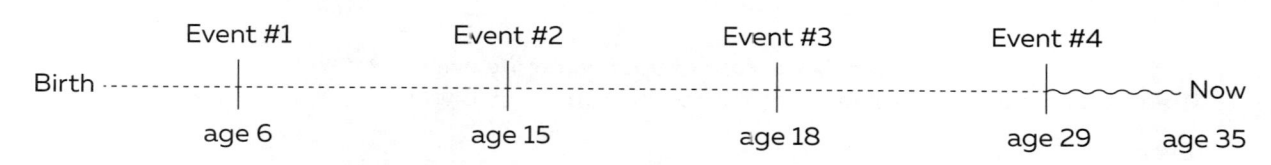

```
            Event #1          Event #2          Event #3          Event #4
Birth -------|-----------------|-----------------|-----------------|~~~~ Now
            age 6             age 15            age 18            age 29    age 35
```

Tell Your Story

Ideas for a Commitment

*Commit to one action that will move your life forward!
It can be anything you feel will help you, or you can try one of the ideas below.
Keeping your commitment is a way of respecting, honoring, and caring for yourself.*

- Option 1. Whose story of survival inspires you? It may be someone you know or a famous person. Write about that.

- Option 2. Create an imaginary timeline for the next 10 years. What *best events* do you hope for? What *worst events* are you afraid may happen?

- Option 3. Find something that symbolizes your resilience and bring it to the next session, such as a small object, photo, song, quotation, or anything else.

- Option 4. Find three to five photographs of key times in your life that tell part of your story.

Influences
Family, Community, Culture

SUMMARY

Trauma and addiction develop in a context beyond the individual—including family and social influences, culture, media, institutions, and societal responses. Today's topic explores how these wider circles of influence play a role, both positive and negative.

ORIENTATION

For humans the most dangerous power—and at the same time the power most able to confer heart-swelling beneficence—has always been other human beings acting together in a social institution.
~Jonathan Shay, *Achilles in Vietnam*

Society, in its many forms, has enormous power over the individual. When the "tribe" speaks—valuing and supporting or devaluing and rejecting—this becomes internalized at a deep level. Societal impact occurs all along the way: in the development of trauma and addiction, the response to these issues, and in recovery. Societal messages are expressed from the largest units (institutions, media, culture) to the smallest (neighborhoods and families).

There are heartbreaking stories of societal breakdown in relation to trauma and addiction: families that encourage children into prostitution and drugs; long waiting lists for addiction treatment; people with mental illness mistreated in institutional homes; backlash for reporting military sexual trauma; and negligent response to community disasters. Such failures create a major psychological burden for clients, who have not only trauma and addiction to overcome, but also betrayal by others. To be abandoned or scorned by people and institutions that are supposed to protect is devastating (Herman, 2023). Systems of care are not always caring.

Yet societal influences also save clients. Treatment, AA, or religion can be a turning point without which the client wouldn't be alive. Institutional actions such as arrests, mandated treatment, or loss of custody of children can start the healing process by helping clients finally face what they were doing. There's also been progress in addressing trauma and addiction systemically. Where these had so often been denied or ignored, there are now stronger protections (mandatory reporting of child and elder abuse; drunk driving penalties), more government programs, and specialized treatment. Institutions of all kinds now provide education on trauma and addiction, and *trauma-informed care* has become part of the treatment landscape. Humane treatment of trauma survivors has also improved with less use of isolation and physical and chemical restraint.

Societal impact is also expressed through culture, which is especially powerful because it's often unconscious. Culture arises from various characteristics (age, profession, social class, religion, nationality, geography, race/ethnicity, gender, etc.). Some cultures encourage substance use, while others are neutral or negative. Attitudes toward trauma also differ, with some traumas more "acceptable" than others. Natural disasters typically evoke more support than domestic violence. Female sexual abuse is more acknowledged than male sexual abuse. Trauma and addiction are more readily addressed in veterans' programs than in the military; if identified in the latter, it can hinder careers (National Academy of Sciences, 2013; van der Kolk, McFarlane, & Weisaeth, 1996). Cultural attitudes can also promote silencing (don't talk about what's wrong), scapegoating (a person or group is "bad"), sabotage (getting better is disloyal), and oppression (historical legacies of trauma). Yet culture can be a positive force, too—binding communities through shared language and traditions (Chu, 1992; Imhof et al., 1983; Najavits et al., 1995; Pearlman & Saakvitne, 1995) that help buffer against trauma and addiction.

Thus, part of clients' truth telling is coming to terms with how these larger forces help explain what happened to them. It moves beyond processing individual events into conversations about circles of influence. Often these have been carried forward through generations without exploration. Becoming more aware lets clients choose, as much as possible, the influences they want to carry forward or let go of.

Today's topic has five handouts. Handout 1 encourages clients to notice ways that societal influences may have created challenges and also at times may have protected them. Handouts 2 and 3 offer an exercise using the concept of a tree; clients identify their roots (past influences), leaves (current characteristics), and how they want to grow in the future. Handout 4 can be used alone or in conjunction with the other handouts. It provides an array of positive and negative influences that shaped them (specific people and events, institutions, environment, cultural heritage, and media). Finally, Handout 5 addresses large-scale societal dynamics such as social movements, societal stress, and historical legacies.

Your Emotional Reactions

As part of today's topic, clients may complain about past providers or treatments. Genuinely hearing their concerns is crucial. There's sometimes an instinctive response to defend one's profession—it must be the client's fault or a misunderstanding. The client may appear entitled or ungrateful for the help they received. Although the reality of any particular case may never be known, there are enough documented instances of malpractice, small and large, that open-minded, thoughtful listening is needed. For a long time, child abuse victims were not believed by the mental health establishment. Medications have been illegally forced on clients in institutional settings. Some counselors sexually or financially exploit clients. Clients have been subjected to humiliating exercises in addiction programs. Such practices were not always intentionally destructive, but nonetheless had serious impact. See the section "Suggestions" on page 219 for how to respond to client complaints about treatment.

Acknowledgments

The session quotation is from Beers (1907, p. 87). The use of a tree exercise (Handouts 2 and 3) has been common in narrative therapy (e.g., Denborough, 2014).

SESSION FORMAT

1. *Check-in* (per Chapter 3).
2. *Quotation.* Link the quotation to the session topic—for example, *"Today we'll talk about influences on your life—such as family and culture. The quote suggests that mental illness may have roots in these larger forces."* (*Note:* If someone comments that the quotation uses sexist language, explain that in the 19th century this is how people spoke.)
3. *Handouts* (relate the topic to clients' lives):
    Handout 1: **The Larger Context**
    Handout 2: **The Tree (Part I)**—Your *Past and Present*
    Handout 3: **The Tree (Part II)**—Your *Future*
    Handout 4: **Identify Your Influences**
    Handout 5: **Society: Helpful and Harmful**
4. *Check-out* (per Chapter 3).

SESSION CONTENT

Goals

- ☐ Explore the idea that trauma and addiction are personal but also societal.
- ☐ Identify positive and negative influences on clients' trauma and addiction.
- ☐ Try an exercise using the concept of a tree to help clients explore *past* influences, who they are in the *present*, and influences they want for their *future*.
- ☐ Discuss how society helps and harms recovery.

Ways to Relate the Material to Clients' Lives

Note: Handout 4 can be used alone but also serves to support Handouts 1, 2, and 3. It helps clients brainstorm influences that have impacted them.

★ *Encourage clients to recognize societal influences on their trauma and addiction (Handout 1).* An engaging way is to start by reading the question at the top of the handout and see how they answer it, before continuing with the handout: "For a moment and without thinking hard, what would you say if someone asked, 'Why did you become addicted?' and 'Why did trauma happen to you?'" Have them notice how much their answers do or don't reflect larger societal forces outside themselves.

★ *Do the tree exercise (Handouts 2 and 3).* This provides an active, visual way for clients to convey important influences that shaped who they are today (Handout 2). It also offers a growth plan to choose the influences they want to keep going forward (Handout 3). You can do Handouts 2 and 3 in different sessions if desired or they can be done together. See the online example at *www.creating-change.org/tree*. You can also imaginatively play with ideas relevant to the tree. For example, some tree roots are deeper than others (some influences are deeper than others). And certain conditions are needed to grow new leaves (sunlight, water)—so too in recovery, some conditions promote growth (support, guidance).

★ *Help clients identify a broad array of influences (Handout 4).* As stated above, Handout 4 can be used alone but also in conjunction with Handouts 1, 2, and 3. Often it's easier for clients to recognize influences when they see a list like this, rather than having to come up with them on their own.

Influences: Family, Community, Culture

★ *Discuss larger patterns of society (Handout 5).* This handout is educational and has a lot of information. You can help clients relate to it by asking questions such as "Are any on the list relevant to you?" and "Is there an example you want to share?"

★ *Address both positive and negative influences.* Positive societal influences are just as important as negative ones, but ensure the timing is right to address this so that it won't invalidate clients' pain. You can help clients notice whether perhaps someone intervened to help when trauma or addiction was occurring. Or some institution or treatment may have launched clients into recovery. They wouldn't be here today if some things hadn't also gone right.

★ *Discussion*
- "Growing up, what was your environment like in terms of trauma and addiction?"
- "Who most contributed to the *development* of your trauma/addiction?"
- "Who most contributed to your *recovery* from trauma/addiction?"
- "Do any media play a strong role in your trauma, addiction, or recovery? For example, music you listen to or videos you watch?"
- "Does your cultural heritage have an impact on your trauma or addiction (culture of drinking, historical oppression, etc.)?"
- "Did any organization impact your trauma or addiction (religious group, military, AA, prison, school, treatment system)?"
- "What feelings come up as you explore these influences?"

Suggestions

✦ *Understand that some clients are disconnected from their family or cultural history.* They may know their relatives only going back one generation if they are refugees or estranged from their family. This disconnection can create a sense of brokenness with the past, a lack of identity. It can be healing for clients to try family history searches to uncover their history and/or to engage in *cultural recovery* (connecting with others to keep alive their heritage and traditions; Marsh, Cote-Meek, Toulouse, Najavits, & Young, 2015).

✦ *Understand that other clients are overly tied to their family or cultural history.* The opposite of the previous issue are clients who feel doomed to relive the family "script" of multiple generations of trauma and addiction. They can benefit from recognizing that they have options now that prior generations may not have had, such as treatment, less stigma for seeking help, and access to online communities for education and support.

✦ *Don't critique clients' culture even if they do.* Today's topic can evoke clients' shame, pride, disappointment, love, anger, and other feelings about their culture. It's important for the counselor not to criticize any culture but rather to understand it from clients' point of view. For more guidance on cultural aspects, search online using the term *cultural competence*.

✦ *Help clients balance societal and personal responsibility if they go too far to either side.* Occasionally, some clients become so attached to blaming larger forces around them that it deflects from taking any personal responsibility. Other clients go too far in the other direction, blaming themselves solely for events they couldn't control, such as childhood abuse. Help clients recognize whatever mix of responsibility fits their unique story.

✦ *If a client complains about a current or past treater, navigate carefully.* It's important to respond compassionately and never dismiss a complaint without understanding more. However, some clients may unconsciously pit team members against each other, perhaps from a psychological need to re-create difficult family dynamics. Start by validating the client's *feelings*, for example, "I hear that you didn't receive the kind of help you were looking for"; "I see how hurtful that felt to you." If the complaint is significant, such as a professional boundary violation (physical, sexual, financial) or discrimination based on gender, race/ethnicity, or sexual orientation, set up a time to evaluate the situation or refer the client to whoever handles such concerns in your organization. These need further consultation and wouldn't be part of today's topic.

✦ *Highlight public apologies by governments, companies, and organizations.* Some have recognized their failures around trauma and addiction, including pharmaceutical companies that perpetuated the opioid epidemic; sports organizations that now have systems in place to prevent sexual abuse of athletes; and church leaders' apologies for harm to various groups. Public memorials such as the Vietnam Veterans Memorial in Washington, D.C., are also highly meaningful to clients.

Tough Cases

* "This makes me want to isolate; people are so horrible to each other."
* "Isn't this just avoiding responsibility for my own actions?"
* "I'm a bad influence—my kids are messed up because of me."
* "This feels too 'woke' to me."
* "Talking about this feels like I'm betraying my culture."
* "So what do I do about all this now?"

Influences: Family, Community, Culture

Quotation

"So-called madmen are too often man-made."

~ CLIFFORD BEERS, 19th-century American mental patient and mental health reformer

HANDOUT 1

The Larger Context

For a moment and without thinking hard, what would you say if someone asked, "Why did you become addicted?" and "Why did trauma happen to you?"

Most people immediately respond with how it relates to them personally: "I don't have willpower," "I was in the wrong place at the wrong time."

But it helps to consider the larger context beyond you as an individual. It's never just *you* but also culture, institutions, peers, families, and systems. All of these contribute to trauma and addiction—yet can also help heal them.

★ *Circle your answers in the table below and add comments if desired. Optional: See Handout 4, Identify Your Influences, for help in answering.*

I. Societal *Challenges*				Comments
Have **family members** (now or past generations) had: ✘ trauma? ✘ addiction?	Yes Yes	No No	Not sure Not sure	
Do you belong to a **culture** with a major history of: ✘ trauma (genocide, racism, etc.)? ✘ addiction (drinking, gambling, etc.)?	Yes Yes	No No	Not sure Not sure	
Did any **organization** (religion, military, prison, school, job, sports team, health care, etc.) play a role in your: ✘ trauma? ✘ addiction?	Yes Yes	No No	Not sure Not sure	
Did **others** ignore, cover up, minimize, or intensify your: ✘ trauma? ✘ addiction?	Yes Yes	No No	Not sure Not sure	
Any additional societal challenges relevant to your: ✘ trauma? ✘ addiction?	Yes Yes	No No	Not sure Not sure	

(cont.)

From *Creating Change* by Lisa M. Najavits. Copyright © 2024 Lisa M. Najavits. Published by The Guilford Press. Permission to photocopy this material is granted to purchasers of this book for use with your own clients or patients; see copyright page for details.

HANDOUT 1 *(p. 2 of 2)* Influences: Family, Community, Culture

II. **Societal** *Protections*				Comments
Have **family members** (now or past generations) had *successful recovery* from: ✦ trauma? ✦ addiction?	Yes Yes	No No	Not sure Not sure	
Do you belong to a **culture** that *promotes healing* from: ✦ trauma? ✦ addiction?	Yes Yes	No No	Not sure Not sure	
Did any **organization** (self-help group, religious, military, school, job, sports team, health care) play a role in *healing* your: ✦ trauma? ✦ addiction?	Yes Yes	No No	Not sure Not sure	
Did **others** *support* you during or after your: ✦ trauma? ✦ addiction?	Yes Yes	No No	Not sure Not sure	
Any additional societal protections relevant to your: ✦ trauma? ✦ addiction?	Yes Yes	No No	Not sure Not sure	

SCORING

- How many "yes" responses did you circle in Part I (challenges): _____? In Part II (protections) _____? (a maximum of 10 in each)
- How many yes responses in total across both? _____ The higher your total number, the more society has played a role in your story.

✧ **Reflections**

- Did you list more *challenges* or *protections* (which scored higher)?
- How much do you believe social factors have played a role in your addiction? your trauma? your recovery?
- Do you notice any feelings about this exercise?

HANDOUT 2　　　　　　　　　　　　　　　　　　Influences: Family, Community, Culture

The Tree (Part I)—Your *Past and Present*

This tree exercise lets you visually describe major influences that impacted you.

Optional: See Handout 4, Identify Your Influences, for help in answering.

CREATE YOUR TREE

Instructions

★ The **leaves** are your characteristics in the *present*.
★ The **roots** are *past* influences that shaped you.

Do as many leaves and roots as you want. For each leaf and root, draw a line from it and write a short description. See the next page for examples. Also see a full tree example at www.creating-change.org/tree.

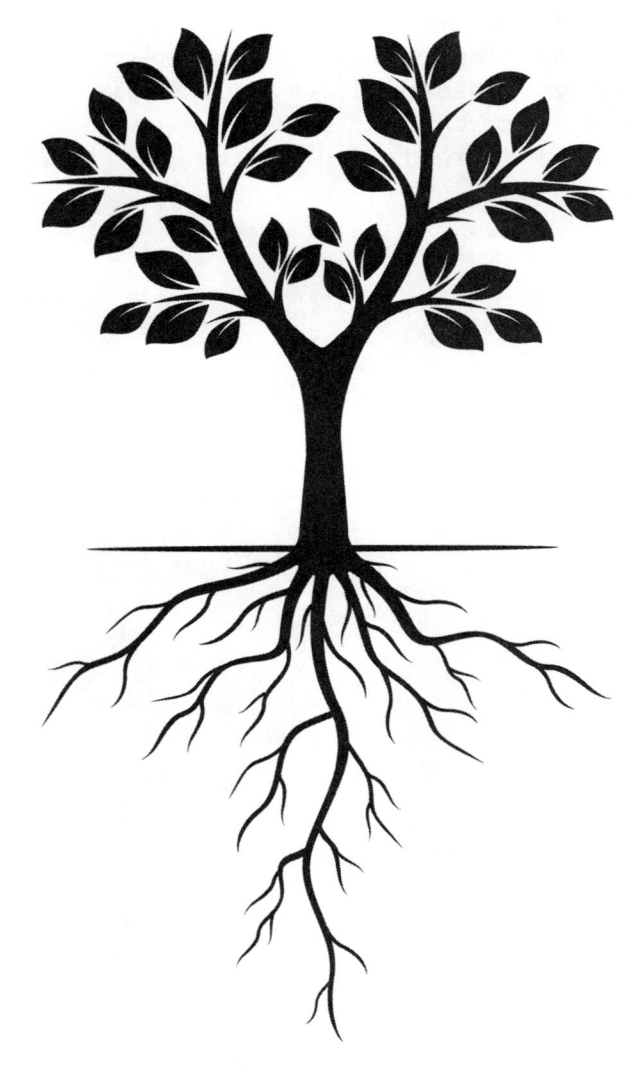

(cont.)

From *Creating Change* by Lisa M. Najavits. Copyright © 2024 Lisa M. Najavits. Published by The Guilford Press. Permission to photocopy this material, or to download and print additional copies (*www.guilford.com/najavits3-materials*), is granted to purchasers of this book for use with your own clients or patients; see copyright page for details.

HANDOUT 2 *(p. 2 of 2)*   Influences: Family, Community, Culture

Examples of Leaves (You in the Present)

The leaves are who you are in the present, including what you like about yourself (you at your *best*) and what you dislike (you at your *worst*). It's a one-word characteristic with a brief example:

- *Caring* ("My nursing work is all about helping others")
- *Workaholic* ("I never give myself a break")
- *Athletic* ("I exercise every day")
- *Sober* (6 months' abstinence)
- *"Difficult"* ("People tell me I create drama")

Examples of Roots (Past Influences)

The roots are your most important influences, both positive and negative. See Handout 4, Identify Your Influences, for ideas. It's a short phrase with a brief description:

- *Childhood diabetes*: "Made me feel weak compared to other kids."
- *Grew up in a mountain town*: "The outdoors helped me feel spiritual."
- *Rap music*: "Glorifies drug use, made me think it was OK to use."
- *Yoga classes*: "Helped me respect my body after sexual assault."
- *My baseball coach*: "Molested me and ruined my trust."

HANDOUT 3   Influences: Family, Community, Culture

The Tree (Part II)—Your *Future*

A tree's roots continue to grow throughout its life.

In this part of the exercise, you can create your growth plan to identify influences you want for a better *future*.

Recovery offers awareness and choice.

Optional: See Handout 4 to help you think about the following questions.

CREATE YOUR GROWTH PLAN

Instructions

⇧ **Strengthen the healthy roots.** These are healing or joyful influences you want to retain.
⇩ **Reduce the unhealthy roots.** These are destructive influences you want to get rid of.
⤴ **Grow new roots.** These are influences you want to add to enhance your life.

In each section, list influences relevant to you. See Handout 4 for ideas.

⇧ **Strengthen the healthy roots** *(influences you want to keep)*

Example: "I want to keep attending AA because it gives me hope."

⇩ **Reduce the unhealthy roots** *(influences you want to reduce)*

Example: "I want to cut down on watching the news as it brings me down."

⤴ **Grow new roots** *(influences you want to add)*

Example: "I want to find new friends who like to exercise, who motivate me."

From *Creating Change* by Lisa M. Najavits. Copyright © 2024 Lisa M. Najavits. Published by The Guilford Press. Permission to photocopy this material, or to download and print additional copies (*www.guilford.com/najavits3-materials*), is granted to purchasers of this book for use with your own clients or patients; see copyright page for details.

HANDOUT 4 Influences: Family, Community, Culture

Identify Your Influences

This handout helps you identify influences (e.g., for Handouts 1, 2, and 3).

◇ *Positive influences* protect you, help you recover, offer important lessons, inspire you.
♦ *Negative influences* promote your addiction; perpetuate trauma; and neglect, silence, or undermine you.

But some influences aren't purely positive or negative. Sometimes people have both positive and negative influences. Or an event that seems negative at first, such as going to rehab, can become a positive turning point.

PEOPLE

◇ *Positive.* Who loved you (even when you didn't love yourself), took care of you, sparked your interest in work or hobbies, served as a role model, positively influenced your beliefs about the world (hope, gratitude)?
♦ *Negative.* Who treated you badly, made you feel worse about yourself, scared you, ignored your needs, negatively influenced your beliefs about the world (cynicism, pessimism)?

EVENTS

◇ *Positive.* What jobs, graduations, achievements, travel, or other events made you a better person?
♦ *Negative.* Did you suffer trauma, death, loss, medical or legal problems, homelessness, poverty, addiction, children taken away, incarceration, violence?

CULTURAL HERITAGE

◇ *Positive.* What in your culture are you proud of, such as warm traditions, meaningful values, knowledge?
♦ *Negative.* What in your culture damaged you, such as sexism, drinking culture, ignorance?

MEDIA

◇ *Positive.* What healthy messages did you absorb from music, ads, social media, TV, movies (e.g., seeing the good in people, a healthy lifestyle, being responsible)?
♦ *Negative.* What unhealthy messages did you absorb from music, ads, social media, TV, movies (e.g., an unhealthy body image, glorifying addiction or violence, bullying)?

(cont.)

From *Creating Change* by Lisa M. Najavits. Copyright © 2024 Lisa M. Najavits. Published by The Guilford Press. Permission to photocopy this material is granted to purchasers of this book for use with your own clients or patients; see copyright page for details.

HANDOUT 4 *(p. 2 of 2)*   Influences: Family, Community, Culture

ENVIRONMENT

◊ *Positive.* Did you have a friendly neighborhood, safe housing, access to health care and education, leisure options (e.g., outdoors, sports, and the arts)?

♦ *Negative.* Did you have a disrupted living situation (frequent moves, foster care), unsafe housing, oppression, poverty, discrimination, violence, geographic isolation?

INSTITUTIONS

◊ *Positive.* Did you have access to good education, programs, health care, religion, sports team, jobs (e.g., ethical, respectful, caring)?

♦ *Negative.* Did you get poor education, programs, health care, religion, sports team, jobs (e.g., corruption, bias, neglect, cover-ups, favoritism)?

HANDOUT 5   Influences: Family, Community, Culture

Society: Helpful and Harmful

Societies can promote recovery or impede it.

★ *Circle any examples below that are meaningful to you.*

SOCIAL MOVEMENTS

◇ *Helpful.* Grassroots movements can support recovery. AA was created by alcoholics to help each other. Mothers Against Drunk Driving reduced highway deaths. Rape crisis centers and the #MeToo movement brought attention to sexual trauma.

♦ *Harmful.* Social groups also cause trauma and addiction, such as the Ku Klux Klan's violence against minorities as well as the rise in drug use as part of the 1960s counterculture movement.

HERD MENTALITY

◇ *Helpful.* Humans cluster in groups to survive—tribes, societies, nations. The "herd" can spring into action to help survivors after trauma such as war and natural disasters. Shared cultural values also promote lower addiction rates in minority groups.

♦ *Harmful.* Social psychology research shows that most people follow a leader even when the leader is wrong. Real-life examples include mobbing and genocide.

SOCIETAL STRESS

◇ *Helpful.* Societies strengthen or weaken under stress, just as people do. The stress of World War II inspired sacrifices that led to a huge economic boom. The stress of domestic violence led 19th-century women to rally for reduced alcohol use (the *temperance movement*).

♦ *Harmful. Collective trauma* means an entire society is traumatized (e.g., slavery or war), causing problems for generations. And substance use increases during communitywide stress such as pandemics or natural disasters.

"PECKING ORDER"

◇ *Helpful.* Social classes are part of most human societies. Sometimes these are a force for good, such as upper classes donating to the less fortunate.

♦ *Harmful.* Cover-ups and denial of trauma and addiction occur in every institution (prisons, military, sports, religions, families), and it's typically the powerful who do the covering up. Also, trauma and addiction can drag people into lower social classes.

(cont.)

From *Creating Change* by Lisa M. Najavits. Copyright © 2024 Lisa M. Najavits. Published by The Guilford Press. Permission to photocopy this material is granted to purchasers of this book for use with your own clients or patients; see copyright page for details.

HANDOUT 5 *(p. 2 of 2)*   Influences: Family, Community, Culture

MEDIA

◊ *Helpful.* Media and technology have an important role in addiction and trauma recovery—connecting people to self-help, sharing recovery stories, reducing stigma.

♦ *Harmful.* The internet, social media, music, and movies glorify substances, gambling, spending, and other addictive behavior, and media itself is addictive for some people. Media can also be traumatizing (online bullying, sex trafficking).

KNOWLEDGE

◊ *Helpful.* *Cultural recovery movements* strive to reduce alcoholism by reconnecting with knowledge of indigenous traditions. The development of *trauma-informed care* has brought greater compassion to trauma survivors.

♦ *Harmful.* Ignorance of trauma and addiction can be profoundly damaging. Cocaine was viewed as safe for a long time. Hate groups deny trauma, especially of marginalized people. Nineteenth-century psychiatry viewed child sexual abuse as just fantasy.

HISTORICAL LEGACIES

◊ *Helpful.* Awareness of your ancestors' survival can strengthen resilience. Participating in cultural traditions builds community.

♦ *Harmful.* Trauma and addiction are often *intergenerational* (repeated across family generations). Some cultures have a long history of punishing trauma and addiction: Rape victims may be shunned or jailed; addiction is punished by death in some places.

INTO THE FUTURE

Societies can change and grow just as individuals can.

As part of your recovery, consider helping others (e.g., volunteering at a shelter or AA). Individual healing helps society and vice versa.

Influences: Family, Community, Culture

Ideas for a Commitment

Commit to one action that will move your life forward!
It can be anything you feel will help you, or you can try one of the ideas below.
Keeping your commitment is a way of respecting, honoring, and caring for yourself.

✦ Option 1. How would others describe how you've influenced them? Write about that and/or ask some of them.

✦ Option 2. What is one thing you can you do this week to *increase a positive influence* or *decrease a negative one*? See examples in Handout 4.

✦ Option 3. *The wish-list imagination exercise.* If you had the power to change the world, what would you do to make trauma and addiction disappear? How would children be raised? What would schools teach? What would leaders do differently? What help would be available?

✦ Option 4. Do you enjoy a challenge? Find out what the phrase "*the thin veneer of civilization*" means. Search online or ask others.

Knowing and Not Knowing

SUMMARY

In trauma and addiction, there's often a powerful pull to *not* see certain realities. It's called *knowing and not knowing* because clients shift between awareness and lack of awareness. Today's topic helps them learn ways to face difficult truths.

ORIENTATION

"The . . . wish to hold back, control, and deny what happened by not speaking of it, the fantasy that if the words are not said, it may not be real."

"When he hits the other girls, he hits them with a closed fist—but he hits me with an open hand. That's how I know he loves me."

More than many other problems, in both trauma and addiction there's a prominence of *knowing and not knowing*, or varying levels of awareness. *Not knowing* can take many forms, most of which aren't fully conscious—for example, denial, splitting, the "pink cloud," avoidance, and the false self. It's part of the illnesses to block out the full brunt of reality, and part of counseling to bring it to light, gently but persistently. As van der Kolk et al. observed, "Unlike other forms of psychological disorders, the core issue in trauma is reality" (1996, p. 6). The same can be said of addiction.

It can be deeply painful to face truths such as "I'm an alcoholic" or "My parents didn't want me." It's sometimes called the *point of despair* when clients face essential truths they've been pushing away, even if unconsciously (Brown & Yalom, 1995). Ultimately, they'll feel better as it's emotionally exhausting to keep ignoring what needs to be accepted. Yet facing difficult truths requires courage and support.

All of the ways of not knowing can be understood as different versions of the mind shutting down as self-protection when people are overwhelmed by extreme experiences. This self-protection appears to be based on a complex blend of biology, cognition, culture, and personality. Clients respond differently in the degree and form that not knowing takes. There are, however, common themes. For example, in both trauma and addiction there's often a belief in greater control than they really have. They believe that this time they can have a drink without losing control, ignoring all the evidence from their past. They believe that if only they had worn a different outfit that day, the sexual assault would not have occurred.

Today's topic has two handouts. Handout 1 guides clients to try to recognize their ways of *not knowing*, and Handout 2 explores ways to increase *knowing*. This topic overlaps to some degree with the Creating Change topic "Respect Your Defenses." But the latter is broader in addressing behavior and relational styles (e.g., isolation, overendurance, "looking for love in all the wrong places").

Today's topic focuses solely on cognition—the client's inner experience of their own mind, which itself is a large task.

Counselors' validating role is central. One client said, "Keep encouraging people to talk . . . It takes a long time to believe. The more I talk about it . . . the more I can integrate it. Constant reassurance is very important—anything that keeps me from feeling that I was one isolated terrible little girl" (Herman, 1992, p. 179). Yet the counselor doesn't need to, indeed should not, judge the accuracy of clients' experiences. In the 1980s and 1990s, there was major controversy over whether counselors were creating false memories by asking clients biased questions. We now understand that counselors can provide strong emotional support while offering a neutral stance on factual accuracy. Validate emotional, rather than historical, truth—feelings rather than facts.

The term *knowing and not knowing* originated with Freud in relation to his cigar addiction: He smoked to the very end, dying of lung cancer, unable to give up his addiction despite knowing what he needed to do (Adeyemo, 2004). For counselors it's usually more challenging to respond to clients' not knowing about addiction than about trauma; the latter generally evokes more empathy. As Amodeo insightfully observed:

> Many counselors believe: " . . . that alcoholics and drug addicts are *unwilling* rather than *unable* to see or hear the truth. Therapists often respond to clients in denial as if the clients were engaged in purposeful efforts to deceive the counselors, rather than involved in unconscious and automatic maneuvers to protect themselves against a powerful external threat to their identity and self-esteem." (quoted in Brown & Yalom, 1995, p. 96)

Old-school addiction methods reinforced this position, using harsh confrontation and humiliating methods, sometimes called "attack therapy," to tear down defenses so that the person would be open to new, more recovery-oriented ideas (Miller & Rollnick, 1991). Interestingly, research shows that those who began with a positive self-image benefited from this approach, but those who began with a negative self-image were harmed by it (Annis & Chan, 1983). Clearly, traumatized individuals are not the right population for this type of intervention, and in general these methods are generally no longer used. Gentle, direct feedback works much better. In one famous study, the more counselors used harsh confrontation with problem drinkers, the more they drank (Miller, Benefield, & Tonigan, 1993).

Your Emotional Reactions

Notice truths you've had difficulty facing in your own life. Remember what it felt like to recognize that you failed at something; deceived yourself or others, even if unintentionally; or pretended things were better than they were. Owning such disappointments is an ongoing task for everyone seeking emotional growth. Counselors who notice their similarity to clients can provide the most useful guidance to them. Such awareness provides a deep well of empathy to draw on. It also serves as a buffer when clients appear noncompliant. Even the most experienced counselors find it challenging to respond when clients dismiss valid feedback or appear stuck in beliefs that defy reality. Counselors who understand that such blocks are based in self-protection may be better able to sustain a positive stance.

Acknowledgments

The second quotation in the "Orientation" section on page 231 is from Rachel Lloyd quoting a client (Richards, 2003). The session quotation is from Rilke (1929/1986, pp. 34–35). In Handout 1, the second quotation at the top of the page is from Harris, Fallot, and Berley (2005, p. 1294).

SESSION FORMAT

1. *Check-in* (per Chapter 3).
2. *Quotation.* Link the quotation to the session topic—for example, *"Today we'll talk about gently facing realities that are hard to face. The quotation beautifully expresses that you need to be patient with yourself as you do this."*
3. *Handouts* (relate the topic to clients' lives):
   Handout 1: **The Many Ways of *Not Knowing***
   Handout 2: **The Many Ways of *Knowing***
4. *Check-out* (per Chapter 3).

SESSION CONTENT

Goals

- ☐ Discuss *knowing* versus *not knowing* (difficulty accepting painful truths).
- ☐ Explore meaningful examples of not knowing in relation to trauma and addiction.
- ☐ Identify the positive impact of facing difficult truths.
- ☐ Highlight ways to increase awareness.

Ways to Relate the Material to Clients' Lives

★ *Ask clients to identify their typical ways of not knowing (Handout 1).* They can circle those that apply to them, and you can explain any that they don't understand. It also helps to allow time for quiet reflection to let them get in touch with what emerges.

★ *Do a real-life example using Handout 2.* Ask clients to choose any of the methods in Handout 2 to try now. Apply the methods to specific, important examples in their life; otherwise, this handout can become too abstract.

★ *Explore feelings.* Encourage clients to observe feelings as they go through the handouts, both positive (relief, self-compassion) and negative (shame, self-hatred). Moving from not knowing to knowing sometimes evokes strong feelings.

★ *Reinforce positive messages.* It's common for clients to "beat themselves up" when facing difficult truths. Reinforce positive messages that even if difficult, something good will come of it. For example, "You're doing a great job looking at what happened," "This can really help your recovery."

★ *Ensure that clients don't misinterpret not knowing to mean stupid or ignorant.* "Not knowing" in other contexts, such as school or work, is perceived negatively. Here, however, the idea is that it's a psychological process that arises for good reason and serves to protect the client. It's not about book learning, but rather how trauma and addiction impact the mind.

★ *Go beyond "denial" and "avoidance."* In the addiction field, *denial* is heavily emphasized (addiction has been called the "disease of denial"). In the trauma field, *avoidance* is a major target of treatment. Handout 1 includes these concepts but also many others. Guide clients to notice the wide variety of ways that not knowing occurs—and how all of them represent a wish for things to be different than they really are. This can also reshape the conversation from what can feel like blaming ("denial," "avoidance") to understanding the deep yearning beneath such defenses.

★ *Discussion*
- "Can you see how not knowing may have protected you?"
- "When you were growing up, how did your family deal with difficult truths?"
- "What truths might you need to face about trauma/addiction?"

- "What truths might you need to face about your past?"
- "Have you received feedback recently that's really hard for you to hear?"
- "Looking back, what's helped you face difficult truths?"

Suggestions

✦ *Understand that clients may mistrust their perceptions.* They may have been invalidated so much—lied to, disbelieved, gaslighted—that it's hard for them to rely on their own experience. Encourage them to get feedback from you and other trusted people to reality-test their perceptions (e.g., "Was it my fault that my father drank and hurt my mother?").

✦ *Recognize truth in relation to meanings, not just facts.* For example, a client may have damaged her children during her drug addiction. Coming to terms with this involves facts (what damage occurred?) but also meanings the client holds (e.g., did she intend to cause harm or not? did she try to make amends later when sober?). Allow clients to explore difficult truths in their full complexity.

✦ *Encourage clients to notice larger influences (family, peers, culture).* Sometimes these influences provide context that alleviates excessive self-blame. Growing up in a family with addiction, for example, a client may have been taught not to acknowledge what was going on and thus denied the reality of it. Or in some cultures, emotional pain is expressed in physical rather than emotional terms, which makes it hard for the client to find language for their pain.

✦ *Respect pacing.* Encourage awareness but respect clients' self-protective instincts. They may need to move slowly on facing some truths. Watch for openings in which they're willing to address something difficult.

✦ *Redirect clients if they become stuck on chasing "The Truth."* Although rare, some clients may interpret today's topic as being a call to uncover everything that happened to them and feel frustrated with gaps in knowledge about their past. Emphasize that the goal is to come to terms with something that may be hard to face—it's not about digging for information or memories they don't have. The topic "Memory" addresses this in more detail.

Tough Cases

* "Are you saying I'm lying?"
* "I often don't know who's right, me or other people."
* "I dissociate—is it my fault that I do that?"
* "If I knew what I was in denial about I wouldn't be in denial."
* "My partner tells me I'm blind to the truth; it makes me furious."
* "I'm fine."
* "Reading this makes me feel bad about myself."

Quotation

"Have patience with everything unresolved in your heart and to try to love the questions themselves. . . . Perhaps then, someday far in the future, you will gradually, without even noticing it, live your way into the answer."

~ Rainer Maria Rilke, 19th-century German poet

HANDOUT 1

The Many Ways of *Not Knowing*

"I would say, 'I need wine for that recipe,' and really believed that's why I was buying it."

"I've spent so much time lying to myself that sometimes I don't know if I could recognize the truth if I ran straight into it."

Recovery requires greater and greater awareness of *truth*. There are many terms for this awakening process:

    seeing clearly   facing illusions   owning it   acceptance   lifting the veil

In trauma and addiction, it's common not to see fully at first. You may have struggled just to survive and your mind could only accept a certain amount of reality.

It's been called *knowing and not knowing* because deep inside you have the knowledge but you're not able to connect to it at times. The phrase originated with Freud in relation to his own struggle with addiction.

It can feel too hard to admit "I'm an alcoholic" or "My parents didn't want me," for example.

Knowing and *not knowing* happens to everyone, but with addiction and trauma they're even stronger.

How about you?

1. Do you have difficulty holding on to your own truth?	Yes	Somewhat	No
2. Do you act in ways you don't want to but can't help it?	Yes	Somewhat	No
3. Do you spend too much time lost in fantasy?	Yes	Somewhat	No
4. If a difficult topic comes up, do you say, "I don't want to talk about it"?	Yes	Somewhat	No
5. Does feedback go "in one ear and out the other"?	Yes	Somewhat	No

(cont.)

From *Creating Change* by Lisa M. Najavits. Copyright © 2024 Lisa M. Najavits. Published by The Guilford Press. Permission to photocopy this material is granted to purchasers of this book for use with your own clients or patients; see copyright page for details.

HANDOUT 1 *(p. 2 of 3)*   Knowing and Not Knowing

★ *Circle any below you see in yourself. Put a question mark next to any you don't understand.*

- **Head but not heart.** You know something intellectually, but it doesn't change your behavior ("I know I shouldn't binge on junk food").
- **Blocking.** It's too hard to face something so it's blocked out, avoided ("I can't think about the rape").
- **Fantasy.** You spend too much time in an imaginary mental world that's an escape from the real world ("I spend a lot of time daydreaming").
- **Illusions.** You're caught in false beliefs that keep you stuck ("I can quit anytime," "I can't change").
- **No words.** You have difficulty describing your feelings and experiences.
- **The pink cloud.** You're overconfident, thinking it's easier than it is ("I'm fine, just out of rehab; I've got this").
- **Memory but no feelings.** You can say what happened but without emotion.
- **Justifying.** You come up with reasons but can't see your part ("She drove me to drink").
- **Hard to admit.** You have difficulty holding on to your truth ("I don't want to admit to myself that I dislike parenting").
- **Flipping.** You believe one thing at times, then the opposite at other times ("It happened/it didn't happen"; "It's my fault/it's not my fault"; "I'm great"/"I'm horrible").
- **Magical thinking.** You have superstitions ("If I had worn a different shirt that day, he wouldn't have assaulted me"; "Tuesdays are the best day to win at gambling").
- **Denial.** You're unaware. Others see it, but you don't. ("I don't have a substance problem").
- **Inner conflict.** You struggle with opposing perspectives ("I know I should enjoy sex, but I can't let myself").
- **Idealizing.** You see things as better than they are ("We were a happy family, never had problems").
- **Devaluing.** You see things as worse than they are ("I'm lower than dirt").
- **Distracting.** You react to stress by diverting your attention ("I keep scrolling social media rather than writing the report I need to do").
- **Splitting.** You ignore or reject a side of yourself, but it emerges anyway ("I'm never angry—until I blow up in rage at some small thing").
- **Assuming it's normal.** Trauma or addiction seem normal because you were surrounded by it ("It's common to grow up hearing gunshots").
- **Physical instead of emotional.** You experience emotional pain as physical (body aches, nausea, heart racing).
- **False self.** You tell yourself you're OK when you're not ("I just need some ice on my eye after he hit me").
- **Ambivalence.** It's hard to commit to a plan ("Part of me is on board with rehab, but the other part feels like there's no hope").
- **Any others?** _____

(cont.)

HANDOUT 1 *(p. 3 of 3)*   Knowing and Not Knowing

❖ **Any current example you can identify—something you may be not fully owning?**

It usually starts with "Maybe . . . "

Examples:

"Maybe I need to stop spending so much."

"Maybe I have some responsibility for the marriage failing."

"Maybe the abuse wasn't my fault."

"Maybe I couldn't have saved my friend even if I went back into the fire."

_____

_____

_____

_____

HANDOUT 2   Knowing and Not Knowing

The Many Ways of *Knowing*

Any truth can be accepted and will yield some sort of gift. In the words of people who've done it . . .

❏ "It was like letting go, surrendering to the truth." ❏ "I cried for the first time in years." ❏ "I'm proud of facing what no one in my family had the courage to face." ❏ "I was really angry with myself at first for damage I caused, but that softened into grieving." ❏ "I stopped breaking out in hives." ❏ "I learned how to stay anchored to the present." ❏ "I went back and forth for a while but came to understand what happened as a child." ❏ "I gained clarity—I knew what I needed to do next."

★ Below are ways to build awareness. Circle any that may help. Try experimenting as different strategies work better for some issues than others.

Recognize that your mind was protecting you
It shut down as an automatic survival strategy so you wouldn't be overwhelmed. Honor and respect that it helped you survive.

Try it on for size
You can explore without committing to an answer. *What if* it's true that you're addicted to marijuana? *What if* it's true that your parents didn't want you?

Become a detective
Search online for how others have handled whatever you're trying to face (e.g., "how to deal with ambivalence"). Learn all you can—from self-help books, professionals, peers.

Talk
It can be challenging to be alone with your own mind. Share with trusted others or in counseling to lift the burden, reality-test, and gain self-acceptance. Talk to multiple people, if possible, to gain perspective.

Create testimony
Write down or record important insights. This testimony gives you something to hang on to if you doubt yourself later. You can also ask others, such as your counselor, to record key messages.

Tally the evidence
If enough adds up, it can overcome doubts. How many times have you had problems because of drugs? How many friends have said your partner is abusive?

View it from a distance
If you were watching yourself as a character in a movie, what would you say and feel toward yourself? Gaining distance helps you figure out what's really going on.

Source your higher power
Have a conversation with your higher power or spiritual adviser; this can deepen insight and connect you with your truth.

(cont.)

From *Creating Change* by Lisa M. Najavits. Copyright © 2024 Lisa M. Najavits. Published by The Guilford Press. Permission to photocopy this material is granted to purchasers of this book for use with your own clients or patients; see copyright page for details.

HANDOUT 2 *(p. 2 of 2)*   Knowing and Not Knowing

- ***Notice how lack of awareness creates harm.***
  You may drive drunk, rationalizing that it's OK. You may enter an abusive relationship because you view abuse as normal.

- ***Stay aware of your body.***
  Your body offers clues. Do you feel tense when a certain topic comes up? Do you feel jittery when you're hiding something? What information does that offer?

- ***Use grounding.***
  It keeps you in the present and creates a calm feeling. Use it when you tend to lose access to yourself (e.g., for splitting, dissociating).

- ***Watch for patterns.***
  What triggers you? What thoughts and wishes keep popping up? Do certain types of people annoy you? Such patterns can reveal underlying truths.

- ***Tap intuition.***
  Notice hunches and gut feelings. Your intuition is intelligent and goes beyond logic and reason. You can also try artwork or music.

- ***Follow the trail of feelings.***
  Stay aware of vulnerable feelings in particular, such as shame, fear, and sadness. Your feelings can reveal new insights.

KEEP IN MIND

Most people want to be truthful. The ways of *not knowing* in Handout 1 are usually automatic rather than willful.

Any truth can be faced. It may bring up raw feelings like anger and shame, or make you feel weak. But it's like pulling off a bandage—it may hurt at first but gets better.

Your truth is personal and can change over time. Some truths are facts. Other truths are perceptions—how you view what happened, the meaning it holds. And as you grow in recovery, you may arrive at new truths.

Pacing. Allow yourself a manageable pace.

It's healing to face difficult truths. It improves mental and physical health, sometimes dramatically, according to research.

Knowing and Not Knowing

Ideas for a Commitment

Commit to one action that will move your life forward!
It can be anything you feel will help you, or you can try one of the ideas below.
Keeping your commitment is a way of respecting, honoring, and caring for yourself.

✦ Option 1. "The truth is my best friend." Write about this idea.

✦ Option 2. Ask a trustworthy person what you're *not* seeing. Commit ahead of time to listening without debating. You may agree or not, but the task is to fully hear that person's perspective.

✦ Option 3. Write about how your family responded to difficult truths: Were they discussed or ignored? Was there support or blame?

✦ Option 4. Sit in a calm, quiet place and choose a method from Handout 2. Explore it using any method that works for you (writing, drawing, speaking to someone else, etc.).

Your Personal Truth

SUMMARY

Clients are guided to identify their personal truth—the meanings they derive—from their experience of trauma and addiction. *Truth* is understood as an evolving perspective rather than a static set of facts. Two exercises help them explore their truth: (1) discussing a photo or other reminder from the past; and (2) "opening the door" to revisit an event from a new perspective.

ORIENTATION

Clients experienced trauma and addiction in real time from *within*, from their own perspective. They saw what they saw and felt what they felt. Part of healing now is shifting perspective to see it from the *outside*—to see the events with enough distance, enough objectivity, to bring in alternative meanings.

There are many questions one can ask to bring forth new meanings: "What do you understand now that you didn't back then?" "How could you have known if your family never taught you?" "Is it really true that you could have prevented it?" The idea is to help clients notice the conclusions they drew about themselves and the world in light of trauma and addiction. Some meanings go to the heart of human experience: why bad things happen, whether life is worth living, how someone can hurt a child, why some people get addicted but not others, whether there's a God, why there's war, who can be trusted, why evil occurs. Clients will come to their own answers, but the counselor can offer a compassionate presence to support their search.

It's important to note that today's topic doesn't try to turn negatives into positives nor to arrive at any particular conclusion. Rather, it's shifting perspective to see the past from a new vantage point. The concept of truth is a postmodern one: It's not a static set of facts, but more of a lens or filter that evolves over time. It's more like a painting than a news article.

The work relates to the concept of narratives in psychotherapy. As Johnstone and Boyle have written

> The narrative metaphor has influenced therapists from different traditions, but what they have in common is the idea that it is beneficial to develop 'rich' stories about one's life which offer opportunities for change.... When people seek professional help, their lives have often become single storied, limiting, limited and superficial rather than richly textured and multiply storied.... The aim is to help people see that they have options of which they were previously unaware. (2018, p. 120, Appendix 9)

Three handouts help clients explore their truth. The first offers general education on the topic. The second allows them to share a photo or other concrete object from their past that holds meaning for them. The third guides them to look at a scene from their past as if through a doorway, seeing it in a new way.

Your Emotional Reactions

A powerful way to explore the myriad meanings in trauma and addiction is to watch movies or read narratives of people in recovery. To locate up-to-date lists, search online for "books [videos] about trauma" and "books [videos] about addiction." However, if you're in recovery yourself, note that some have painful details, so self-care is key to prevent triggering.

Acknowledgments

The session quotation is commonly attributed to Frank Lloyd Wright. The quotation at the top of Handout 1 is from Herman (1992, p. 178).

PREPARING FOR THE SESSION

For the exercise in Handout 2 (exploring a photo or other reminder), consider whether it will occur in today's session or if you want clients to bring an item to the next session. See the section "Ways to Relate the Material to Clients' Lives" for options.

SESSION FORMAT

1. *Check-in* (per Chapter 3).
2. *Quotation.* Link the quotation to the session topic—for example, *"Today we'll talk about different ways to view your past. As the quote says, it's not just the facts of what happened but also the meaning it holds for you."*
3. *Handouts* (relate the topic to clients' lives):
    Handout 1: **Your Personal Truth**
    Handout 2: **Explore a Photo or Other Reminder of Your Past**
    Handout 3: **Open the Door to a New Perspective**
4. *Check-out* (per Chapter 3).

SESSION CONTENT

Goals

☐ Emphasize the concept of personal truth.
☐ Try an exercise in which clients discuss a photo or other reminder of their past.
☐ Conduct the "open the door" exercise (see a past event from a new perspective).
☐ Explore meanings clients hold about their trauma and addiction.

Ways to Relate the Material to Clients' Lives

★ *Discuss the concept of personal truth (Handout 1).* Handout 1 is an entry into the two exercises that follow (Handouts 2 and 3) so it can be done briefly, highlighting key points. Help clients understand that the meanings they hold about their trauma and addiction are fluid and evolve over time as they sustain recovery. They may discover all sorts of things—difficult truths, new growth, self-compassion, increased awareness of harm they did, and so on. Whatever they discover can help move them forward.

★ *Plan how you'll do the exercise on exploring a photo or other reminder (Handout 2).* The best way, if possible, is to cover just the first part of the handout in today's session ("choose a photo or other reminder to discuss"). Clients would then bring their photo or reminder to the next session and you'd go through the rest of the handout at that point. Alternatively, if you want to do the full exercise in today's session, they could pull up a photo or other reminder on their mobile phone (or even just describe one they remember, if they can't access it on their phone).

★ *Help clients take different points of view via the exercise on opening a door (Handout 3).* Encourage them to imagine a scene from different perspectives such as that of a sympathetic observer. They don't have to fully believe it at first; they can just try various ways until they arrive at what feels true. The key is that they're *observing* their younger self (and whoever else is in the scene). It's also helpful to emphasize visual aspects such as zooming in and out of the scene or watching it at a distance or from up above.

★ *Play with metaphors about opening and closing the door (Handout 3).* For example, the door may feel stuck or difficult to open. It may feel scary to push it open to see what's there. Maybe others closed the door by silencing you.

★ *Discussion*
- "What would your current self say to your younger self?"
- "Has your view of your trauma/addiction changed over time?"
- "How would you want to be able to view your trauma/addiction?"
- "Who most influenced your view of trauma/addiction?"
- "Does your culture impact the way you see your experiences?"
- "How does it feel like to 'open the door' to your past?"

Suggestions

✦ *Validate that clients may have difficulty holding on to their truth.* They may wax and wane in their understanding of what happened. It may feel real at one point and unreal at another. They may avoid parts of it, and then later be able to see it. It can be reassuring to understand that this is part of the process.

✦ *Help clients hold themselves accountable.* In addiction, for example, they may have harmed or neglected others or abandoned important responsibilities. As they go through the handouts, give them the emotional space to explore mistakes without judgment. It can be healing to acknowledge that they failed others as long as it's accurate and proportional to what they did. Some clients go too far in self-blame, while others don't admit mistakes at all.

✦ *Emphasize choice.* In Handout 2, clients choose the photo/reminder and the questions they want to answer about it. In Handout 3, clients choose to walk through the door. The exercises are voluntary, but the idea is that they have the power now, in contrast to the past where they felt powerless in the face of trauma and addiction.

✦ *Discuss how perceptions may be influenced by culture, personality, and history.* Such factors can impact the meaning clients draw from their experiences. For example, a girl growing up in a home where males are more valued than females may devalue herself without being conscious of it. Even in the same family, siblings may have very different perceptions of what occurred. There is no one truth.

✦ *Observe feelings.* A focus on meanings can sometimes become too analytic or intellectual. Watch for feelings and check in with clients; for example, "What are you feeling right now?", "Does that photo bring up feelings?"

✦ ***Explore both positive and negative meanings.*** Clients' truth may include wonderful aspects, such as people who were there for them and achievements they're proud of. It's just as important to recognize beautiful moments as to recognize painful ones. So, too, a client may have both positive and negative views of an abuser (people are complex). Allow clients their truth, although if they appear to be missing some key elements, ask questions to clarify as needed. For example, "You say your family was very happy, but you've also mentioned that no one ever talked about conflicts or problems. I'm wondering if it was more of a mixed picture?"

Tough Cases

* "Photos of my past just make me sad; why should I do this?"
* "The meaning I draw from my experiences? People suck."
* "I have no memory of most of my childhood."
* "My truth? God doesn't love me or this stuff wouldn't have happened."
* "When I look back on the worst days of my addiction, I feel lower than dirt."

Quotation

"The truth is more important than the facts."

~ Frank Lloyd Wright, 20th-century American architect

HANDOUT 1

Your Personal Truth

"Survivors of atrocity of every age and every culture come to a point . . . where all questions are reduced to . . . 'Why?' . . . [and] . . . 'Why me?'"
~Judith Lewis Herman, *Trauma and Recovery*

As your recovery expands, so does clarity about your past.

It can take a while to understand what you lived through. Your perception may shift as you let in different sides of the story.

Early in recovery from trauma, you may believe, "It's my fault" or "I'm damaged goods." In addiction you may believe, "I don't really have a problem" or "I can't picture a life without using."

With recovery, your story affirms a compassionate view of yourself, while taking personal responsibility when that's relevant.

- ❑ "I learned that I could get through tough times without using."
- ❑ "I came to understand, deep down, that the abuse wasn't my fault."
- ❑ "I found that I could love even though so little love was given to me."

Research shows that as people recover from trauma and addiction, their dreams and nightmares change (feeling more powerful, fighting back); their language changes (e.g., from *victim* to *survivor*); and their sense of purpose in life grows.

But some truths may be difficult to face:

- ■ "I realized I was addicted to anger."
- ■ "I discovered that sexual abuse goes back three generations in my family."
- ■ "I had to admit that it was up to me to get better; no one could do it for me."

GETTING TO YOUR TRUTH

It can be challenging to figure out what you really believe, especially if you were silenced in the past or told what to think. Addiction, too, can distance you from yourself.

The next two handouts offer exercises to explore your view of your past. You can integrate old and new ways of understanding.

It's more than the facts of what happened—it's about the meanings you give to them, the conclusions you draw. There's no one way and no right set of conclusions. Your truth is personal. It's a process of discovery.

From *Creating Change* by Lisa M. Najavits. Copyright © 2024 Lisa M. Najavits. Published by The Guilford Press. Permission to photocopy this material is granted to purchasers of this book for use with your own clients or patients; see copyright page for details.

HANDOUT 2   Your Personal Truth

Explore a Photo or Other Reminder of Your Past

A photo or other object can be a powerful way to explore your past that goes beyond words alone.
The idea is to share it in the session and talk about what it means to you. It can be positive or negative—bringing up pride, joy, distress, guilt, or anything else.

1. CHOOSE A PHOTO OR OTHER OBJECT TO DISCUSS

Examples of *photos*:

- Your family or other people
- A place
- You at an important age, such as before trauma or addiction
- Anything memorable (a pet, a car, etc.)

Examples of *objects from your past*:

- A letter, email, or text
- A news article about you
- Media (a song, poem, or short video)
- A small physical object, such as jewelry or a souvenir

Please be sensitive to not triggering others if you're in group treatment (e.g., no gory accident photos). If you don't bring something, you can still participate by describing what you would have brought.

2. EXPLORE THE MEANING

You can speak aloud about any of the questions below or prepare ahead by writing out your answers and then reading them aloud in the session.

Questions about your photo or object:

- Why did you choose it?
- What do you see looking at it?
- What would others see looking at it?
- Is there a story behind it?
- How old is it?
- What does it represent: isolation? belonging? injustice? yearning? pretending? love? hate? beauty? pain? strength? weakness?
- Does it bring up feelings? body sensations?
- What do you want it to mean, going forward?

For a photo, additional questions:

- What's happening outside the frame?
- Did anything important happen before or after it was taken?
- What would you have wished was in it?
- If there are people in the photo:
  - What do you see in their eyes?
  - How do they relate to each other?
  - What advice would you give to them?

From *Creating Change* by Lisa M. Najavits. Copyright © 2024 Lisa M. Najavits. Published by The Guilford Press. Permission to photocopy this material is granted to purchasers of this book for use with your own clients or patients; see copyright page for details.

| HANDOUT 3 | Your Personal Truth |

Open the Door to a New Perspective

"People tend to remember a terrible event exactly as they always have—the way it looked to them when they were living it. But viewing it from a different angle can help free them from guilt, shame and other feelings. I had always remembered, dreamed about, even smelled the first assault in the exact same way it occurred, from the eyes of my 10-year-old self. I was always part of it and so couldn't see it differently.

"One day I was reading and came upon an assault scene and I realized I felt sorry for this woman. What would happen if I viewed my assault the same way? Instead of being on the ground inside my body, feeling what I felt then, what if I stepped back and viewed the entire episode as though I was a camera person filming it? The difference was remarkable. For the very first time I saw an adult male assaulting a little boy and instantly felt a lift of guilt and shame. It wasn't permanent and I still had work to do but it was a critical moment. Change the way you view your trauma."

~DAVID, survivor of child sexual assault

In this exercise, you can see a scene from your past in a new way.

Step 1: Choose a memory to explore

It could be a difficult trauma or addiction memory, a poignant memory that shows your resilience or any other that you want to explore.

_____

_____

Step 2: Imagine that you open a door, walk through, and see the scene in a new way

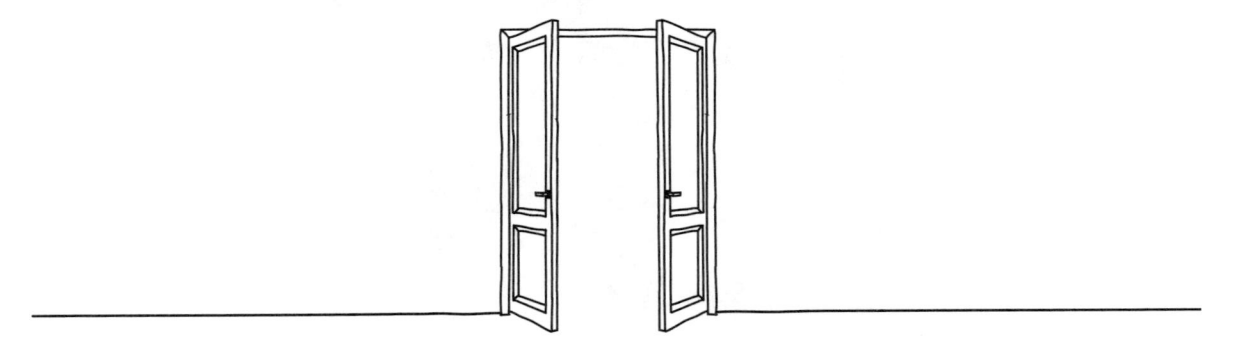

★ *Choose a perspective to view the scene:*
  ⌑ *From above* to see the big picture
  ⌑ *Zoom in* to see it closely
  ⌑ *Zoom out* to see it broadly
  ⌑ *Through your own eyes*, with compassion and honesty
  ⌑ *Through the eyes of a nurturing person* in your life
  ⌑ *Through the eyes of a kind* observer
  ⌑ As seen by *your higher power*
  ⌑ As if on a *movie screen*

  . . . or any other perspective

(cont.)

From *Creating Change* by Lisa M. Najavits. Copyright © 2024 Lisa M. Najavits. Published by The Guilford Press. Permission to photocopy this material is granted to purchasers of this book for use with your own clients or patients; see copyright page for details.

HANDOUT 3 *(p. 2 of 2)* Your Personal Truth

Step 3: Explore what the scene means to you

★ *Consider any below. You can speak, write, or draw about it.*
- What's a compassionate view of yourself in that scene?
- What do you know now that you didn't know then?
- What did you need that you didn't get?
- Do you wish you had done anything differently?
- Who were you then versus who are you now?
- How much control did you actually have?
- Were you isolated or supported during the event?
- Were you equipped to handle the situation (given your age, knowledge, maturity)?
- Did you take *too much* responsibility? ("The trauma was all my fault") or *too little* ("I'm not addicted")?
- Who was responsible for what happened? (It may be several people.)
- What do you give yourself credit for?
- What were you up against?
- What did you get, or not get, growing up that helps explain what happened?

Step 4: Come back through the door

★ *Decide what you want to do now, such as:*
- Get support from your counselor and/or group.
- Appreciate the wisdom you have gained.
- "Lock the door and throw away the key."
- Do something kind for yourself today.
- Identify how to make the future better than the past.

Ideas for a Commitment

Commit to one action that will move your life forward!
It can be anything you feel will help you, or you can try one of the ideas below.
Keeping your commitment is a way of respecting, honoring, and caring for yourself.

+ Option 1. Find a photo or object that represents *growth*, *hope*, or *health* to you. Keep it near you to remind yourself of a meaning you cherish.

+ Option 2. Are you the hero or villain of your story? Or a mix? Write about that.

+ Option 3. Expand the "open the door" exercise (Handout 3). Write, draw, or use music or art to represent how you view it.

+ Option 4. Take one of the exercises you did today and share it with someone trustworthy. Describe your perspective.

What You Want People to Understand

SUMMARY

Today's topic lets clients express what they'd want others to know about their trauma or addiction story. Two methods are described: *imaginary* conversations and *real-life* conversations. Both can be therapeutic.

ORIENTATION

Not being believed or understood is one of the most painful aspects of trauma and addiction. Clients come to doubt their reality and disconnect from what they really feel and think. An important part of recovery is learning to value their own perspective. This sometimes involves real-life conversations but also can be achieved in imaginary conversations when it's not safe to speak to a particular person or the person is deceased. Imaginary conversations also allow clients to get in touch with their own perspective before sharing it with others. If clients choose a real-life conversation, today's topic offers guidance to help it go well. For individual treatment, they can bring a safe family member or friend to a session if desired.

This approach is based on the idea that clients' view of themselves is inherently social. It's normal and human to see themselves reflected back in how others see them. Everyone absorbs messages about who they are from their family, peers, workplace, and community. In this session, clients explore, in a broad and conscious way, how they *want* others to see them, which includes how trauma and addiction impacted them. For example:

"I did the best I could, given how I grew up."
"My inner pain was always driving me."
"Everyone around me was doing it so I went along."
"I didn't know any better."
"I couldn't stop."
"I'm not a bad person."
"I'm sorry."
"I made some bad choices."

But it's not just negatives. They can express resilience; convey appreciation to people who helped them; and make amends for their own errors. They can also speak to their younger self, offering compassion for what that person lived through. Such positives can be deeply moving and release long-carried pain. As the philosopher de Botton has said, "The moment we cry in a film is not when things are sad but when they turn out to be more beautiful than we expected them to be" (n.d.).

Clients also receive guidance on whether and how to confront someone who harmed them, such as a trauma perpetrator. This is a delicate issue that requires careful thought as most of the time clients will not get the apology or validation they yearn for. Yet it can be beneficial. Seeking justice can be transformative (Herman, 2023). According to a study of female child abuse survivors, for example,

> The women that had confronted their abusers directly perceived it to have been useful despite the fact that none of the perpetrators had accepted responsibility for the abuse and that some of the women received negative reactions from other family members. Most of the survivors in the study that had found some benefit in direct confrontation referred to issues of power, responsibility for the abuse, and . . . change in relationships. (Freshwater, Ainscough, & Toon, 2003, p. 35)

However, if clients have potential for legal action against a perpetrator, ensure that they seek legal advice first so as not to undermine their own case (APA, 1998).

Today's topic has four handouts. Handout 1 raises clients' awareness of what they want others to understand about them and their past. Handout 2 offers a protocol for creating an imaginary healing conversation. Handout 3 is a protocol to prepare for a real-life conversation. Finally, Handout 4 offers important education about the pros and cons of confronting a perpetrator.

Your Emotional Reactions

It can be tempting to urge clients into real-life conversations that you believe will help them. You may want them to confront someone who has hurt them, perhaps feeling anger on their behalf that they don't feel yet. You may want them to show vulnerability and open up more. You may want them to forgive someone so they can move on. But it's essential to support clients in making their own decisions, on their own timing. There are often important reasons why they stay silent, and pushing them prematurely to confront a situation can backfire. It can also convey the message that they need to do it for you rather than for themselves. Explore whether there are aspects of your own past that compel you to want them to shift into action before they're ready for that.

Acknowledgments

Imaginary conversations have long been described, including in psychodrama (Moreno, 1964) and imagined interaction theory (Honeycutt, 2003). The session quotation is from Eliot (1860/1929, p. 79). In Handout 4, the concept of DARVO (Deny, Attack, and Reverse Victim and Offender) is from the field of interpersonal violence (Harsey, Zurbriggen, & Freyd, 2017). The quotation from Nina at the top of Handout 4 is from Cameron (2000, p. 253) and the second is from Bass and Davis (1994, p. 145). On the Commitments page, the *legacy letter* is based, in part, on the concept of a legacy will (Riemer & Stampfer, 2015), and the quotation from Enrique Peña Nieto is from a speech (Booth, 2012).

PREPARING FOR THE SESSION

Read about confronting a trauma perpetrator if you're not already knowledgeable about this challenging topic. Some resources are listed at the end of Handout 4. See also:

- *www.huffpost.com/entry/how-i-finally-confronted_b_6296342*
- *www.vox.com/first-person/2018/10/10/17953016/what-is-restorative-justice-definition-questions-circle*
- Herman (2023)

SESSION FORMAT

1. *Check-in* (per Chapter 3).
2. *Quotation.* Link the quotation to the session topic—for example, *"As the quote says, it's natural to absorb other people's views of you. In today's topic, we'll explore how to express and advocate for your own point of view."*
3. *Handouts* (relate the topic to clients' lives):
    Handout 1: **What Do You Want People to Understand?**
    Handout 2: **An Imaginary Conversation**
    Handout 3: **A Conversation in Real Life**
    Handout 4: **Deciding to Confront a Perpetrator**
4. *Check-out* (per Chapter 3).

SESSION CONTENT

Goals

- ☐ Encourage clients to express what they want others to understand about their past.
- ☐ Help them create an imaginary healing conversation with someone from their past or present.
- ☐ Plan an important real-life conversation they may want to have with a safe person.
- ☐ Discuss whether to confront a trauma perpetrator.

Ways to Relate the Material to Clients' Lives

★ *Try a role-play, empty-chair exercise, or have clients look at a photo of someone.* Handouts 2 and 3 lend themselves especially well to any of these methods. If you do a role-play, it's suggested that you (rather than a group member) play the other side as it allows you to ensure that the exercise stays therapeutic. For the empty-chair exercise, the client sits across from an empty chair and states who is "in" that chair (such as a parent, a deceased relative, the client as a young child). Then the client speaks to that "person." For the photo method, clients can pull up a photo of someone on their phone or bring a photo to the session and, while looking at it, speak to that person.

★ *Have clients write a letter to someone (but they don't have to send it).* They can take the work they've done with any of the handouts and write a letter, which they may or may not choose to send.

★ *Create a symbol that represents letting go.* For example, if they write a letter (see the point above), it can be ripped up as a symbol of letting go of that part of the past. Or after a role-play, they can write the name of the person on paper and then mark it with the word "goodbye" or put a big X across it.

★ *"Show rather than tell."* Clients can choose a creative work such as song lyrics, a poem, or art to express what they want to say to someone. If they do this, ask them to provide commentary after showing it so that the meaning is clear.

★ *Have the client bring in a safe family member or friend (individual treatment only).* This can be a powerful session if the client is interested in this option and has someone to bring in. But prepare ahead and have a structured process to keep the session helpful. Preparation can be done using Handouts 1, 2, and/or 3 (but *not* Handout 4; see below on that). It thus takes at least two sessions: one for preparation and one for the safe family member or friend (the *guest*) to attend. Choose someone who cares about the client; does not currently have a major active addiction or major mental health issue; and is not a perpetrator of physical or emotional harm.

★ The suggested session structure is as follows:
  a. *At the start, set a positive emotional tone.* Emphasize appreciation for the guest and convey the intention of supporting the client's recovery (i.e., it's not an emotional attack on the guest).
  b. *Identify that this isn't family therapy* but rather just one session, focused on the client.
  c. *State the goal:* for the client to express something important and be heard (and possibly for the guest to respond if desired by the client).
  d. *Specify the content*, which is generally one issue the client wants to express based on Handout 1, 2, or 3.
  e. *Say how much time* the client can speak and, if applicable, how much time the guest has for a response.
  f. *Clarify roles:* The guest's job is to listen without interrupting, and then the client does the same if the guest is responding.
  g. *Allow time at the end* for the guest to leave the room so that you and the client can briefly discuss how the client feels about it, and to validate the client's work.

★ ***If a client wants to resolve a conflict with another client in your program, specify how that can occur.*** You may have policies or protocols based on your setting (e.g., a house meeting or scheduling a three-way conversation with you and the two clients). If it's a very serious situation, such as physical threats between clients, consult with your supervisor. If the clients are both in the same Creating Change group, it's usually best to handle it outside of group as otherwise it can detract from a balanced focus on all clients.

★ ***Discuss the option of confronting a perpetrator—but only if this is very carefully evaluated.*** Handout 4 offers guidance for assessing whether or not to confront a perpetrator. But clients shouldn't walk out of the session and act on it without careful planning. This is typically done in individual treatment over multiple sessions until the plan is strong and safe. Handout 4 can also be covered in group or individual modality as it provides a starting point for exploring the pros and cons of confrontation. Discuss, too, how healing can occur even if a perpetrator can't be confronted (the person is deceased or unsafe to speak to). See the websites at the end of Handout 4 for more.

★ *Discussion*
  - "How are imaginary conversations powerful even if you never do them in real life?"
  - "What would it feel like if others understood better why you did what you did?"
  - "What makes it difficult for you to express your perspective?"
  - "How can you heal even if a perpetrator isn't held accountable?"
  - "If you think of confronting your trauma perpetrator, what are the pros and cons?"
  - "Is there a real-life conversation that was hard for you, but you did it anyway?"

Suggestions

✦ ***Discuss when it's good to move an imaginary conversation into a real-life one.*** This will depend on the specific client and scenario but includes identifying whether a real-life conversation is safe and likely to produce any gain. It's also good to manage expectations and potential disappointment. If the client has already attempted a conversation with the person before, evaluate what will be different this time. Some clients keep going back to a "dry well," hoping this time they will find water—"Maybe if I just say it differently, louder, longer . . . they will respond better."

Also in group modality, be careful not to let the group push a client into an unwise conversation (e.g., "You tell him! Don't hold back!"). The client may be easily influenced and it's important to arrive at a thoughtful decision.

✦ *Encourage clients to be compassionate yet realistic about their younger selves.* As they explore how they want others to see and understand them, this will unearth a lot about how they see themselves. The challenge is to be honest with themselves: neither beating themselves up ("It's all my fault") nor being totally defensive ("I've never done anything wrong"). They may have had amazing strength in difficult times yet bad judgment and poor decisions at other times. Also, their role may have been very different in trauma versus addiction. Whatever comes up, help them empathize with who they were in the past—why they did what they did, what they didn't know then that they know now.

✦ *Remind clients that conversations don't have to be dark or painful.* Sometimes positive material is incredibly poignant, such as expressing thanks to someone who stood up to their abuser. They can also hold mixed feelings, for example, appreciation and disappointment; and recognition of how someone both helped and harmed them.

✦ *Validate the importance of imaginary conversations.* Clients may assume that real-life conversations are the most valuable but imaginary ones, per Handout 2, are equally valuable and sometimes more so. They help clients get in touch with what they really need or feel. They can also release deep pain they've been holding onto.

✦ *Help clients identify who's best to share with.* In Handout 3, they may want to share their experiences with a safe family member or friend but become distressed if the person can't or won't listen. Help them understand that there are different types of relationships and some good people may just not have the emotional capacity to listen.

✦ *Educate about forgiveness.* Today's topic can bring up clients' inner conflicts about forgiveness. Help them understand that forgiving *themselves* is crucial, even if it occurs slowly over time. But forgiving others is *not* necessary for healing, despite what some people may have told them. Indeed, it can be retraumatizing to be pushed into forgiveness they don't feel. In the trauma field, it's well established that forgiving a perpetrator is optional. In the addiction field, however, it's more common to hear that forgiving others is necessary. However, that idea arose before the addiction field focused on trauma. Validate that clients don't have to decide now about forgiving others and that it's a personal choice.

✦ *For clients who are active in AA, address the 12-step concept of "making amends."* Today's topic has some convergence with that (see AA steps 8 and 9). However, it differs in not being just about harm the client did *to others* but also harm others did *to the client*. As noted in Chapter 1, AA was developed in 1935, an era in which trauma was not generally addressed. This historical context can be helpful for clients who are active in AA or other 12-step groups.

✦ *Recognize that many clients have idealized fantasies of what it'll be like to confront a perpetrator.* They may believe they'll finally feel relief or get the apology they always wanted. Yet often these don't occur. Clients may be ignored or there may be backlash. Rather than an apology, there may be anger. Rather than relief, there may be regret. Thus, if they choose to tell, they should be realistic about possible outcomes, not assuming the best-case scenario. They may still want to tell, with the idea that it's better to express their truth wherever that leads. But if there's any concern for their safety, such as confronting someone who has been violent, they should hold off until they've carefully discussed it with others to determine if it's really in their best interest. And if they're early in recovery or still actively addicted, they should wait until they are further along. It should be done from as strong a position as possible.

✦ *Refer clients for legal advice as needed.* Handout 4 is about confronting a perpetrator for its potential *therapeutic* impact. But if clients still have the option to bring legal charges against that person, have them obtain legal help first, prior to any confrontation. Lawyers typically advise not to confront the perpetrator directly as that's the purpose of the legal case. If clients already have an active case, they should follow the lawyer's instructions. Seek supervision as needed.

Tough Cases

* "It's best to forgive and forget."
* "I want to tell my mother to go to hell."
* "My family tells me I'm just looking for attention when I say how I feel."
* "I've done some really bad things to people."
* "I don't care what anyone thinks of me."
* "If I tell my family about my uncle's abuse, they'll disown me."
* "Thinking about confronting my brother triggers me to cut."

What You Want People to Understand

Quotation

"We are all apt to believe what the world believes about us."

~ GEORGE ELIOT, 19th-century British writer

HANDOUT 1

What Do You Want People to Understand?

If you have problem behaviors, they may be born out of pain rather than willful intent. Yet the world may seem unforgiving. Many people don't understand trauma and addiction.

Explore one or more of the following. You can keep it private or share it.

What do you want others to understand about . . .

❖ **How you tried to say "Help!"** What was your behavior expressing? Hurting yourself physically, starting fights, or doing poorly at school or work are distress signals that may not be seen for what they are. *Were there ways you tried to say "Help!"?*

_____

_____

❖ **What you did to survive.** If you survived a dangerous environment, you may have become dangerous. With no help for trauma, you may have turned to substances. *Did you do things you didn't want to do, just to get by?*

_____

_____

❖ **Who you are now versus then.** Maybe you've become a better parent, gone back to school, or taken responsibility for your mistakes. The "sober you" may be very different than the "addicted you." *How have you changed for the better?*

_____

_____

(cont.)

From *Creating Change* by Lisa M. Najavits. Copyright © 2024 Lisa M. Najavits. Published by The Guilford Press. Permission to photocopy this material is granted to purchasers of this book for use with your own clients or patients; see copyright page for details.

HANDOUT 1 *(p. 2 of 2)*   What You Want People to Understand

- ❖ **What you did and didn't get.** You may have been taken care of physically but not emotionally. You may have had love from one parent, but not another. *Were any of your core needs not met (e.g., love, safety, education, food, clothing, health care)?*

  _____
  _____

- ❖ **What was good about you.** Did you have a good heart? Did you try to make things better? *What was good about you that others may not have seen?*

  _____
  _____

- ❖ **How you tried to repair harm you caused.** You may have lied, neglected others' needs, been violent. *If you caused harm, how did you try to repair it?*

  _____
  _____

- ❖ **What you most regret.** Did you do things you're ashamed of? Did you fail yourself or others? *Are there regrets that weigh on you?*

  _____
  _____

- ❖ **Insight you gained.** How have you grown emotionally, intellectually, spiritually? For example, "I learned . . . to make better choices," "I learned . . . that the trauma wasn't my fault." *Are there insights you want others to understand?*

  _____
  _____

- ❖ **Other:** _____

  _____
  _____

HANDOUT 2 — What You Want People to Understand

An Imaginary Conversation

Try an *imaginary conversation* with someone, either aloud or silently. What would you say? What would you want the person to say back?

You can focus on a painful aspect of your life or a positive one, such as gratitude and love. You can address addiction, trauma, or anything else.

STEP 1

★ See examples below. Then list here, in a short phrase or sentence, an imaginary conversation you'd like to try: _____

_____

Between *you and someone in your past*

Examples ¤ You tell your deceased father how much you loved him. ¤ You apologize to a person you stole from. ¤ You confront someone who hurt you.

Between *you and yourself in the past*

Examples ¤ You forgive your 17-year-old self for mistakes. ¤ You comfort your 9-year-old self about the abuse.

Between *you and someone in the present*

Examples ¤ You reveal your gambling problem to your partner. ¤ You tell your mother how you feel when she criticizes you. ¤ You tell a friend what you're proud of overcoming.

Between *different sides of yourself*

Examples ¤ You tell the side of you that feels hopeless why you should keep going. ¤ You kindly welcome all sides of yourself, such as the young side, the angry side, the wise side.

Between *you and your higher power*

Examples ¤ You express gratitude for recovery. ¤ You ask for guidance on being a better parent.

STEP 2

★ *Now try it.*

+ Choose a method: in writing, aloud, or just in your mind.
+ Imagine the person sitting across from you, if that helps.
+ Focus on *your* perspective, what *you* want to say.
+ Notice feelings and insights that arise.

From *Creating Change* by Lisa M. Najavits. Copyright © 2024 Lisa M. Najavits. Published by The Guilford Press. Permission to photocopy this material is granted to purchasers of this book for use with your own clients or patients; see copyright page for details.

HANDOUT 3 *What You Want People to Understand*

A Conversation in Real Life

Is there an important *real-life conversation* you'd like to have?

This handout focuses on a conversation *with a safe person* in your life. (Handout 4 is about *confronting a harmful person*, such as a trauma perpetrator.)

Who?

➢ *Who do you want to speak with?* _____
_____

Choose a safe person—someone who won't lash out or harm you and has been generally supportive. If you aren't sure, ask a counselor or other trusted person for guidance.

What?

➢ *What **one issue** will you talk about?* _____
_____

Choose a meaningful topic but just one to keep it manageable. See Handouts 1 and 2 for examples.

Why?

➢ *What would you like to get out of the conversation?* _____
_____

Examples: to feel heard or accepted/to get feedback/to release something you've been holding on to/ to resolve a conflict/to obtain information/to apologize or ask for an apology

How?

➢ *How will you communicate?* _____
_____

Usually, a direct conversation is best. But you could choose email, a letter, or even a song, poem, or drawing to express yourself.

BEFORE, DURING, AND AFTER

Plan it out!

Before the Conversation

- Write notes or an outline of what you want to say.
- Identify how you'd like the conversation to go (e.g., "I want to stay calm . . . I want her to acknowledge how hard I've tried").

(cont.)

HANDOUT 3 *(p. 2 of 2)*   What You Want People to Understand

- If you've had the same conversation with this person before, what will be different this time?
- List concerns about what might not go well.
- Practice, possibly role-playing with a counselor.
- Decide if you want anyone else present.
- Identify a safe location if you're meeting in person.
- Be sober (not under the influence of any alcohol or drug).
- Plan what to do for support afterward, such as calling a friend and self-care. Include ways to prevent addictive behavior.
- *Remember:* It's a success as long as you do your part well, no matter how the other person responds.

During the Conversation

- At the start, say what you'd like from the other person ("To listen without giving me advice," "To accept my apology," "To give me feedback," etc.).
- Stay flexible as it will rarely go exactly as you imagine.
- Handle yourself well, no matter what (no yelling, sarcasm, put-downs).
- Notice your feelings and body reactions.
- Ask for a pause or end it if it's not going well.
- Anything else? _____

After the Conversation

- What worked? What didn't?
- What did you learn?
- What can you give yourself credit for?
- Is there someone you want to share it with?
- How does it help your recovery from trauma or addiction?

Praise yourself for taking a brave step, no matter how it went.

HANDOUT 4 — What You Want People to Understand

Deciding to Confront a Perpetrator

"I've been carrying this burden too long. It's your responsibility. I'm giving it back to you."

~NINA, trauma survivor

"There is no right course of action in disclosures or confrontations. There is no right time to tell, no right way to tell, and no right decision whether to tell."

~BASS AND DAVIS, *The Courage to Heal*

Confronting a trauma perpetrator means telling your truth about how the person harmed you. It can be a courageous, healing step in your recovery, but it can also backfire. Consider it carefully before deciding.

The good that can come of it

- It can be empowering to stand up to someone who hurt you.
- You can grow from it regardless of the perpetrator's response.
- It can release painful feelings, such as shame and guilt.
- It can help hold the person accountable.

Disappointments and problems

- Most survivors *don't* get an apology.
- The perpetrator may blame, gaslight, or marginalize you.
- People may side with the perpetrator rather than you.
- Most perpetrators are incapable of understanding your point of view.

To help you decide

★ *Circle any points relevant to you:*

- Recognize that you can heal from trauma and addiction whether or not you confront the perpetrator.
- Never feel pressured, even by well-intentioned people; it's always your choice.
- Consider other options, too. Perhaps you can distance yourself from the perpetrator or take legal action, depending on the situation.
- Don't rush into it. It typically takes months or years to become ready and clear on what you want to do.
- Don't do it early in addiction or trauma recovery.
- Don't do it with children present.
- Follow your lawyer's guidance if you have current legal action against the perpetrator.
- Think about what you want to gain. Remember that you'll rarely get understanding or genuine validation from the perpetrator.
- Make a plan so that it will be healing for you. Include what you'll do before, during, and after and who you'll turn to for support.
- Don't confront if you or the perpetrator are intoxicated.
- Don't confront if the perpetrator is violent.

(cont.)

From *Creating Change* by Lisa M. Najavits. Copyright © 2024 Lisa M. Najavits. Published by The Guilford Press. Permission to photocopy this material is granted to purchasers of this book for use with your own clients or patients; see copyright page for details.

HANDOUT 4 *(p. 2 of 2)*   What You Want People to Understand

- ◊ Choose the way that works best for you (letter, email, phone, or in person).
- ◊ Do a *symbolic confrontation* if it's not safe or possible to confront the person directly. You could burn a photo of the perpetrator with a supportive person present, for example.
- ◊ Learn about DARVO: Many perpetrators will <u>d</u>eny, <u>a</u>ttack, <u>r</u>everse <u>v</u>ictim and <u>o</u>ffender (they'll distort the situation and view themselves as the victim of your accusations).
- ◊ Anticipate what it'll be like if you have to keep seeing the person at family gatherings or your workplace.
- ◊ Be aware that others may support the perpetrator rather than you.
- ◊ Choose a safe, public location if you do it in person. Consider having someone come with you.
- ◊ State your boundaries, such as whether you want any further contact or not.
- ◊ Know that you never have to forgive the perpetrator to heal from trauma.
- ◊ Get input from several trustworthy people such as your counselor, sponsor, friends.
- ◊ Don't verbally or physically attack the person.
- ◊ Understand that you don't need an apology. Expecting one gives the perpetrator the power to disappoint you again.
- ◊ Choose what's right for you.

Next steps

1. Talk it over with as many trusted people as possible.

2. If you decide to confront, make a plan that keeps you safe.

3. Learn more. For further guidance, see:

    www.whatiscodependency.com/confronting-abuser-abuse-abusive-relationships

    www.havoca.org/first-step/approaching-your-abuser

    www.naasca.org/2011-Articles/062211-ForgivenessAndReconciliation.htm

Ideas for a Commitment

Commit to one action that will move your life forward!
It can be anything you feel will help you, or you can try one of the ideas below.
Keeping your commitment is a way of respecting, honoring, and caring for yourself.

- Option 1. Choose a trustworthy person and share what you wrote in the handouts today.

- Option 2. Start a *legacy journal* for family or friends to share your values and insights about what you've learned and perhaps pass along to future generations. It can be on paper or electronic, and can include media such as photos, drawings, songs, objects, and videos. You can share:

  - What you overcame
  - What you're proud of
  - Personal stories
  - What you learned
  - Important life events
  - Values you want to carry forward
  - What you appreciate about various family members

- Option 3. Write about an apology you wanted but never received.

  If you'd like to read an in-depth example, the book *The Apology* (2019) by the playwright V (formerly Eve Ensler) explores the apology she would have wanted from her abusive father.

- Option 4. Find a song, quote, drawing, or poem that expresses some important part of your experience. Choose someone safe to share it with and explain what it means to you.

- Option 5. Do you have a major regret over something in your past that you did or didn't do? Write about the quotation below, focusing on compassion for who you were then. *Note:* "Crime" does not have to be an actual crime; it can be any important regret.

  "Behind every crime is a story of sadness." (Enrique Peña Nieto, former president of Mexico)

Listen to Your Body

SUMMARY

Trauma and addiction are experienced directly in the body and also have ongoing negative impact on the body (e.g., increased health problems, greater reactivity to stress, and lower self-care). Today's topic helps clients learn how the body holds and expresses pain from the past. It also guides them to improve their relationship with their body to promote recovery.

ORIENTATION

"I feel sick to my stomach when I think about what he did to me. It gets me to see I'm not over it yet."

"I experienced physical problems for years but didn't associate it with trauma until much later. Almost every chronic medical issue I suffered was the result of PTSD or substance abuse. I had 15 years of allergies and hives, and discovered during treatment that the hives went away."

Trauma and addiction impact the body (Felitti et al., 1998; Ouimette & Read, 2014; van der Kolk, 2014). They are associated with:

- Physical health problems throughout the lifespan
- Premature death
- Lower self-care
- Greater reactivity to stress
- Decreased immune functioning
- Physical expression of emotional pain (*somatization*)
- Self-harm such as cutting, burning, and suicide
- Body addictions (binge eating disorder, compulsive sex, pornography, plastic surgery, etc.)
- Reduced medication compliance
- Brain changes
- Worse relationships with health care providers
- Impaired sexuality and unsafe sex
- Increased emergency room visits

Trauma and addiction also have strong genetic components (biological heritage within the family) and common neurobiology pathways such as the stress response (Najavits, Hyman, Ruglass, Hien, & Read, 2017; Ouimette & Read, 2014).

Helping clients gain greater understanding of the body strengthens recovery. Some clients are *oversensitive* to body sensations (overwhelmed, easily triggered); others are *undersensitive* to them (not noticing pain or injury). In today's topic, we address clients' personal patterns: What's their relationship with their body, and how is it affected by trauma and addiction (Handout 1)? They're

Listen to Your Body

encouraged to explore messages they internalized about their body growing up (Handout 2). There's an exercise to help them put into words what their body is experiencing when they focus on a positive versus a negative memory (Handout 3). And finally, there's education about the physical aspects of trauma and addiction (Handout 4).

Recognize, too, that the health care field has a known history of insensitivity and sometimes bias toward people with trauma and/or addiction. One woman said, "I told a brief version of my abuse story to one of my medical doctors, and he began to interpret all of my physical problems as emotional—like I was a hysterical woman, a whiner, a complainer. It seemed like he didn't believe me. I had to stop seeing him."

In short, the body is part of the painful experience of trauma and addiction but can also be central to their healing. The body can become ally rather than enemy.

Your Emotional Reactions

Most everyone has some sort of body issue, such as weight problems, dissatisfaction with parts of the body, or difficulty staying with healthy habits. Try the exercises in today's topic for yourself as a preview of what it's like for clients. Often deep themes emerge such as *nurturance versus deprivation*, *love versus hate*, and *control versus lack of control*. Throughout Creating Change, parallel process is helpful (observing how your own life experiences may be similar to clients'). Attitudes toward the body are a central human issue regardless of trauma or addiction.

Acknowledgments

Parts of this topic were adapted from *Finding Your Best Self*, the chapter "Body and Biology" (Naavits, 2019). The session quotation is from Moreno (1964, p. 80). Some body sensations listed in Handout 3 were drawn from the McGill Pain Questionnaire (Melzack, 1975) and the website *http:// larisanoonan.com/sensations-list*. "Surfing" a symptom is adapted from the phrase "urge surfing" in Marlatt and Gordon (1985). The phrase "the body keeps the score" is from van der Kolk (2014). The quotations at the top of Handout 4 are from Marks (2015, p. 180) and Knapp (1996, p. 83).

SESSION FORMAT

1. *Check-in* (per Chapter 3).
2. *Quotation.* Link the quotation to the session topic—for example, *"The quote is saying that we sometimes express physically what we may not be aware of emotionally. Today we'll talk about the body in relation to trauma and addiction."*
3. *Handouts* (relate the topic to clients' lives):
    Handout 1: **Your Relationship with Your Body**
    Handout 2: **Messages about Your Body**
    Handout 3: **Putting It into Words**
    Handout 4: **Trauma, Addiction, and the Body**
4. *Check-out* (per Chapter 3).

SESSION CONTENT

Goals

☐ Explore past messages clients received about their body.
☐ Discuss the physical impact of trauma and addiction.

☐ Help clients evaluate their relationship with their body in the past and present.
☐ Try an exercise on body sensations, memories, and feelings.

Ways to Relate the Material to Clients' Lives

★ *Create a small ritual to help clients let go of a message from the past (Handout 1).* Some clients like a memorable exercise such as this to help them process a painful aspect of their past. This one can be done in individual or group treatment. Ask clients to tear out from Handout 1 a negative message they want to release and a positive message they want to embrace. Put two small boxes in the middle of the room or table. One negative messages box is marked, "Leave It in the Past" or "Let Go of It." The positive messages box says, "This Is Who You Are Now" or "Embrace It." Start with the negative message box, having clients say a short personal statement as they approach the box, rip up the negative message, and drop it in the box. For example, "No one has the right to violate my physical boundaries." After clients throw away their negative message, now they do the positive message box the same way, but instead of ripping up the slip of paper, they say a positive personal statement and kiss or gently hold the message before dropping it into that box. If you're using telehealth, clients can write out the messages on paper and show themselves ripping up the negative one and holding on to the positive one.

★ *Expand on the concept of relationship with one's body (Handout 2). Relationship* is a rich concept. Ask clients what type of relationship they've had with their body in the past and what type they want to have going forward (nurturing? loving? harsh? abusive?). You can also explore their relationship with food, alcohol, self-harm, and so on. After clients fill out the reflection questions at the end of Handout 2, discuss those, too.

★ *Show clients how to search online to learn more about the mind–body connection in trauma and addiction (Handout 3).* Clients may want to understand more after the experiential exercise in Handout 3. A good starting place is the list of search terms in the fourth Commitment option on the last page of this topic. Also, offer a user-friendly description of trauma and the brain (e.g., United States Special Operations Command, 2017). For addiction, a powerful teaching tool are websites that show brain scans before and after addiction recovery (e.g., Addiction Policy Forum, 2020); this offers hope as brains do improve with abstinence. You can also find reputable short videos online by searching "TED Talks."

★ *Use an engaging question/answer format for Handout 4.* This handout has a lot of information. Make it interesting by asking thought-provoking questions such as "Why are people with trauma and addiction less likely to follow doctors' orders?" "Why do trauma and addiction lead to worse physical health?" "How do trauma and addiction impact sexuality?" "What is stress?" Clients can search for the answers in the handout or just discuss.

★ *Discussion*
- "What does it mean that the body 'remembers'?"
- "Growing up, what did you learn about how to treat your body?"
- "How has trauma affected your body?"
- "How has addiction affected your body?"
- "What does *mind–body connection* mean?"
- "Do you sometimes ignore your body and its needs?"
- "How can you improve your relationship with your body?"

Suggestions

✦ *Focus on positive, not just negative, aspects of the body.* Help clients notice what they appreciate about their body; and pleasure they get from healthy physical activity (e.g., sports, watching a sunrise, nontraumatic sexuality).

✦ ***Stay nonjudgmental unless there's a safety issue.*** Talking about the body and sexuality is highly vulnerable. These topics go to the deepest roots of identity and can evoke embarrassment, shame, and self-hatred. Stay respectful and nonjudgmental, including about sexual practices that may be unusual or unfamiliar to you, such as fetishes, as long as the client and others are not being harmed and the client does not view it as a problem.

✦ ***Convey optimism.*** Highlight how the body and brain can improve with continued recovery work, good medical care, and taking good care of the body.

✦ ***Provide medical referrals as needed.*** Clients may identify physical needs that require medical attention. Provide referrals and encourage follow-up.

✦ ***Maintain physical boundaries.*** Clients with trauma and addiction may express a wish for touch by the counselor. Unless it's a brief touch that's public and appropriate, such as a hug when graduating from the treatment program or shaking your hand at the final session, refrain from physical contact. Crossing physical boundaries can be perceived as a threat or seduction, even if that's not what you intend. If in doubt, ask a colleague.

✦ ***If desired, add a session on the biology of trauma and addiction.*** Some counselors like to educate clients on the structure of the brain and how it's affected by trauma and addiction as well as genetic versus social factors. Handout 4 briefly mentions some aspects, but this could also be expanded to an additional session after today's topic. Examples of brief, helpful online articles written for the public include Buschman (2019) and the National Institute on Drug Abuse (2019).

✦ ***Use grounding if needed.*** Body themes can bring up strong emotions, which is generally therapeutic to help clients integrate physical and emotional sides rather than these remaining split off from each other. But occasionally, a client may become triggered or dissociated. Use grounding as needed to bring down the intensity. Grounding is described in detail in *Seeking Safety* (Najavits, 2002c).

Tough Cases

* "I've been scared of sex ever since the rape. How do I change that?"
* "Are you saying my health problems are all in my head?"
* "How do I know if I'm addicted to porn?"
* "I'm overweight, but it has nothing to do with trauma or addiction."
* "I have chronic pain from a combat injury; what good is talking about it?"
* "Wearing a COVID mask is a trauma trigger for me."
* "I hate my body."

Listen to Your Body

Quotation

"The body remembers what the mind forgets."

~ Jacob L. Moreno, 19th-century Romanian psychiatrist and social scientist

HANDOUT 1

Your Relationship with Your Body

What story does your body tell? What role have trauma and addiction played in that?
★ *In each row, fill in three ratings: one for* now, *one for* at best in your past, *and one for* at worst in your past. *For ratings, use the scale provided in each section. There are no right or wrong answers.*

	Now	At **best** in your past	At **worst** in your past
For this section, use these ratings: **0** = not at all; **1** = somewhat; **2** = moderately; **3** = a great deal.			
1. Are you physically healthy?			
2. Do you take good care of your body (nourishing food; healthy level of exercise; enough sleep; sunscreen, etc.)?			
3. Do you like your body?			
4. Do you feel about positive about sex?			
5. Do you have healthy ways to cope with stress?			
6. Do you get needed medical care (doctors and dentists) *and* follow their medical advice?			
7. Do you feel safe in your body?			
8. Do you feel good about the way you look (body image)?			
9. Do you feel comfortable with touch by someone you like?			
10. Are you aware of your body, noticing its sensations and changes?			
11. Do you manage triggers safely (e.g., addiction and trauma triggers)?			

(cont.)

From *Creating Change* by Lisa M. Najavits. Copyright © 2024 Lisa M. Najavits. Published by The Guilford Press. Permission to photocopy this material is granted to purchasers of this book for use with your own clients or patients; see copyright page for details.

HANDOUT 1 *(p. 2 of 2)* Listen to Your Body

	Now	At **best** *in your past*	At **worst** *in your past*
For this section, use these ratings (they are different from the previous section): *3 = not at all; 2 = somewhat; 1 = moderately; 0 = a great deal*			
1. Is anyone, including you, harming your body (domestic violence, self-harm such as cutting, etc.)?			
2. Do you have any body-focused addiction or disorder (food, exercise, sex, pornography, tanning, substances, surgery, hair pulling, skin picking, etc.)?			
3. Do you overindulge your body (too much sugar, junk food, being a "couch potato")?			
4. Do you hate parts of your body?			
5. Do you mentally "leave" your body (*dissociate*)?			
6. Do you engage in dangerous physical activity (e.g., unsafe sex, reckless or drunk driving, high-risk sports)?			
7. Do you have ongoing stress?			
8. Do you ignore body pain or injury that you should attend to?			
9. Do you physically harm other people?			
10. Do you have *body memories* (physical sensations that remind you of trauma)?			
Now, add up the numbers in each column	Total of this column: ____	Total of this column: ____	Total of this column: ____

Higher numbers indicate a more positive relationship with your body. The highest possible score in any column is 63.

◆ Reflections

Write or think about one or more questions below.

- Does this exercise bring up emotions? body sensations?
- What do you appreciate about your body?
- How did trauma/addiction impact your relationship with your body?
- How can you improve your relationship with your body?
- If your body could speak, what would it say?
- Has your attitude toward your body changed over time? Notice words and actions: what you tell yourself about your body and how you treat it.

HANDOUT 2   Listen to Your Body

Messages about Your Body

What messages did you learn about your body from your family, peers, community, and culture? You live what you learned even if the messages weren't said aloud.

★ *Circle any* unhealthy *and* healthy *messages you absorbed.*

Unhealthy messages	versus	Healthy messages
Numb your pain with drinking, drugs, food.		Find solutions that truly work.
Live for today.		You get only one body—protect it.
Heavy drinking and drugging are normal.		Healthy people don't use heavily.
Deny your pain.		Pain is a signal to listen to.
Your only worth is your body.		You have a heart, mind, and spirit.
You're ugly.		Love yourself the way you are.
Doctors can't be trusted.		Find the best medical care you can.
Sexual feelings are bad.		Sexual feelings are normal.
Your looks are all that matters.		Who you are as a person matters.
Others can do what they want to your body.		You can set boundaries.
You're "wimpy," "slutty" (or other put-downs).		Your body deserves respect.
It's OK to eat junk and not exercise.		Your body is a gift; take care of it.
It's your fault if you become ill.		There are medical reasons for illness.
Your needs don't matter.		You have needs like everyone else.

Any others?

_____   _____

_____   _____

_____   _____

★ *Now go through the messages and put a star next to those you want to live by going forward.*

No matter what you grew up with, you can choose new messages now.

From *Creating Change* by Lisa M. Najavits. Copyright © 2024 Lisa M. Najavits. Published by The Guilford Press. Permission to photocopy this material is granted to purchasers of this book for use with your own clients or patients; see copyright page for details.

HANDOUT 3 — Listen to Your Body

Putting It into Words

It's healthy to stay aware of your body and be able to express what you're experiencing. This is called *being in your body*.

This exercise has two parts to help you put into words what your body is "saying."

PART I: AWARENESS

1. **Bring to mind a *positive* memory.**

    For example: graduation   being in love   playing with a pet   a warm bath   eating ice cream   scoring a winning goal   cuddling   something new (baby, car, job, apartment)

    ❖ **Really get in touch with that *positive* memory (close your eyes if you want). Notice *what* you feel in your body and *where* you feel it.** Circle any of these words that you notice.

    What you feel in your body

    Typical **positive** body sensations: calm   warm   light   open   excited   awake   tender   buzzing   sensitive   bubbly   electric   floating   spacious   deep   cool   expansive   releasing   alert   glowing   sweet   airy   yearning   strong   erotic   tingly   fluttery   breathy   smooth   bursting   clean   aroused   punchy   entranced   full   flushed   bittersweet   euphoric   flowing

    Others? _____

    Where you feel it in your body

    stomach   gut   heart   head   mouth   nose   ears   arms   legs   feet   soles   ankles   fingers   toes   back   neck   head   shoulders   face   thighs   chest   buttocks   genitals   skin   muscles   inside   outside   joints   knees   skin   brain   blood

    Others? _____

2. **Bring to mind a *negative* memory.**

    Start with an easier memory; later you can try a more difficult one.

    For example: craving   flashback   rejection   a fight   friend's death   job loss   break-up   trauma   loneliness   betrayal

    ❖ **Really get in touch with that difficult memory (close your eyes if you want). Notice *what* you feel in your body and *where* you feel it.** Circle any of these words that you notice.

(cont.)

From *Creating Change* by Lisa M. Najavits. Copyright © 2024 Lisa M. Najavits. Published by The Guilford Press. Permission to photocopy this material is granted to purchasers of this book for use with your own clients or patients; see copyright page for details.

HANDOUT 3 *(p. 2 of 2)* — Listen to Your Body

What you feel in your body

Typical **negative** body sensations: dizzy nauseous tired tense empty sick weak low numb pounding queasy frozen heavy winded shrinking dull knotted clenched throbbing sore gnawing burning dirty spacey sour pressure cramping aching closed wobbly itchy smothered sharp wet trapped hungry thirsty hunched light-headed hyper

Others? _____

Where you feel it in your body

stomach gut heart head mouth nose ears arms legs feet soles ankles fingers toes back neck head shoulders face thighs chest buttocks genitals skin muscles inside outside joints knees skin brain blood

Others? _____

◇ **Reflections**

- Which was easier to notice in your body—the joyful memory or the painful one?
- If you weren't able to do all or part of the exercise, what got in the way?
- If you found it difficult, practice further. Being *in your body* is an important recovery skill.

PART II: FLEXIBILITY

Now see if you can shift between emotions and body sensations.

1. **Start with a feeling** (get in touch with anger, fear, happiness, or any other feeling); then notice where you feel it in your body, *using the language of the body*.

    For example, "Anger: I feel my face flushing, my blood rising, my stomach tightening. . . ."

2. **Start with a body sensation**, then notice what feelings go with it, *using the language of feelings*.

    For example, "I'm nauseous" might be "I'm *anxious* about some bad news I got today. . . ."

Keep training yourself to connect feelings and body sensations. You'll gain greater understanding of how you store memories. You'll also develop more control over them rather than being surprised or overwhelmed.

| HANDOUT 4 | Listen to Your Body |

Trauma, Addiction, and the Body

"I'm still afraid of being hungry. . . . I never leave my house without some food."
~AVA LANDY, child Holocaust survivor

"Meg was scared of her own body, and she was scared of men's bodies . . . and alcohol took all of that away, just washed it away like the sea against sand."
~CAROLYN KNAPP, *Drinking: A Love Story*

Trauma and addiction are experienced in the *body*, as well as the heart, mind, and spirit.

BODY CHALLENGES

✶ **There are four basic responses to trauma or threat: *fight, flight, freeze, appease.*** *Fight* is attacking back; *flight* is escape; *freeze* is the body shutting down; *appease* is actively negotiating or submitting as a way to prevent greater harm. These are hardwired biological responses in both humans and animals. In trauma, your body typically decides for you—it responds instantly, before you have time to think. In some situations, such as repeated or expected trauma, you may have learned to choose your response. Either way, some people feel guilt or shame at how their body reacted, even though the body does what's natural and most protective in the moment.

➤ How did your body respond during trauma (*fight, flight, freeze, appease*, or a combination of them)?

➤ How do you feel about how your body responded?

✶ **Both trauma and addiction show up in the body** until they're dealt with emotionally. Trauma can create *body memories*, such as feeling you can't breathe or genital pain. They're like flashbacks but are physical sensations instead of visual images. Triggers can be physical too (heart racing, etc.); your body keeps reacting even when you don't want it to. And trauma and addiction are both associated with increased medical problems. It's said that "the body keeps the score" and "the body remembers."

➤ How has *trauma* shown up physically for you?

➤ How has *addiction* shown up physically for you?

✶ **Physical solutions can become addictive.** You may develop body addictions such as pornography, sports, tattooing, sex, self-harm, sun-tanning. You may overindulge your body because you're trying to comfort yourself with physical pleasure, such as eating too much. You may become too focused on your body or physical appearance. If you have physical problems (injury, illness, disability, aging, poor sleep), you may turn to substances, which then become addictive.

➤ Have you responded to *painful feelings* with addictive behavior?

➤ Have you responded to *body problems* with addictive behavior?

(cont.)

From *Creating Change* by Lisa M. Najavits. Copyright © 2024 Lisa M. Najavits. Published by The Guilford Press. Permission to photocopy this material is granted to purchasers of this book for use with your own clients or patients; see copyright page for details.

HANDOUT 4 *(p. 2 of 3)*   Listen to Your Body

✼ **You may *under*- or *overreact* physically.** *Underreacting* means your body responds too little. You may be so used to danger that you don't have the physical alerts (pit in the stomach, heart pounding) that happen for others in dangerous situations. You may also underreact to physical problems, not noticing a toothache, broken bone, hunger, or thirst. In addiction, your body may develop *tolerance* (it needs more and more to feel high). *Overreacting* is the opposite: Your body goes on high alert when there's no actual danger. You have intense triggering and hypersensitivity to physical pain. And what calms others may upset you, such as massage, sleep, sex, or closing your eyes.

> ➢ Does your body *underreact* at times?
> ➢ Does your body *overreact* at times?

✼ **Addiction and trauma increase stress.** Stress means your body is on guard due to perceived danger: muscles tighten, blood pressure rises, senses sharpen. In the short term, it helps you survive, but long term it wears down your body, leading to physical and emotional problems. Some people have been stressed for so long they forget what calm feels like. Stress is the top cause of addiction relapse and is part of the very term *posttraumatic **stress** disorder*.

> ➢ Have you had high stress over a long period of time?
> ➢ How has stress affected your recovery from trauma and addiction?

✼ **Addiction and trauma run in families.** It's estimated that half of vulnerability to addiction comes from family genes. And up to 20% of vulnerability to PTSD comes from genes. Family biology thus plays a role in both. But there are many other factors, too: social influences, peers, culture, media, and access to help and support.

> ➢ Does your mother's side have addiction or trauma?
> ➢ Does your father's side have addiction or trauma?

NEW DIRECTIONS—HEALING VIA THE BODY

Your body can also become a major resource in recovery.

⌑ **Build a better relationship with your body.** Most people have challenges in how they relate to their body, even if they don't have trauma or addiction. Struggles with weight, exercise, and aging are common. But with addiction or trauma, the challenges go deeper. If you were physically or sexually abused, you may hate your body. You may have a distorted perception of how your body looks to others, thinking you appear "damaged" or "dirty." In addiction, you may be distressed by physical reminders such as needle marks or how your body deteriorated while using. Building a healthy relationship with your body is parallel to building one with a person: Acceptance, attention, respect, and boundaries are crucial. Strive to build that relationship now, no matter what happened in the past.

> ➢ How can you improve your relationship with your body?

⌑ **Heal sexuality.** Trauma and addiction can impair sexuality: fear of sex, guilt about sexual fantasies, sexual reenactments that reflect sexual trauma, sex addiction, unsafe sex, inability to enjoy sex without substances, and so on. Sexuality runs deep. Find resources to expand your sexual recovery,

(cont.)

HANDOUT 4 *(p. 3 of 3)*   Listen to Your Body

including counseling with a sex therapist who understands trauma and addiction, self-help books, and gender-specific groups. You can become more comfortable with touch, accept your fantasies (as long as they are not hurting you or others), and stop destructive sexuality (such as unsafe sex, sex-for-drug exchanges).

> Do any aspects of your sexuality need healing or recovery?

◻ **Awaken positive physical experiences.** Build a sense of your body as a source of joy and play, not just problems. There are two main methods.

1. *Increase your physical* activity to create *energy*: dance, cycling, basketball, playing with a child or pet.
2. *Decrease your physical activity* to create *rest*: relaxing, lying down, drifting to sleep.

If there are positive physical activities you used to do such as ballet or jogging, reawaken your "muscle memory" by trying them now. Even watching some videos of these can evoke a physical connection to them.

> How can you increase positive experiences of your body?

◻ **Consider body-based help for trauma or addiction.** These include yoga, equine or dog therapy, movement therapy, acupuncture, somatic experiencing therapy, drumming/singing/dance or any other therapy that focuses on the body as a primary source of healing.

> Would a body-based method appeal to you?

◻ *Surf* **a symptom.** Like riding a wave in the ocean, you can manage addiction and trauma symptoms (urges, cravings, flashbacks) by staying focused on body sensations. You describe what your body is experiencing for 5 to 10 minutes (sometimes a bit longer), and you'll find the symptom goes down. "My chest is heavy, my stomach is fluttery, my shoulders are tense. . . ."

> Have you tried *surfing* a symptom? How did it go?

◻ **Try** *grounding* **when you're upset.** Grounding also shifts your attention away from distressing feelings but uses a wider range of methods and is more physically active than the *surfing* described above. Grounding includes running your hands under cool water, jumping, listening for sounds, clasping your hands, rolling your head, smelling essential oils or spices. The idea is to use all of your senses to get away from emotional distress.

> Have you tried *grounding*? Which methods work best for you?

Ideas for a Commitment

Commit to one action that will move your life forward!
It can be anything you feel will help you, or you can try one of the ideas below.
Keeping your commitment is a way of respecting, honoring, and caring for yourself.

- Option 1. Do you remember what it feels like for your body to be fully calm and peaceful? What can you do in the week ahead to get back to that feeling?

- Option 2. Your body is your companion as you go through life. It's silent but has a lot to "say." Write about any of the following:

    - What would it say to you? What would you say to it?
    - What do you appreciate about it? What problems do you have with it?
    - How has it let you down? How has it been there for you?

- Option 3. "The body remembers." Explore what this means to you in writing or any other method (art, collage, audio recording, etc.).

- Option 4. Search online using any of these terms, and then list five key points you learn:

    - *Stress* and the body
    - *Trauma/addiction* and the brain
    - *Body image* and trauma/addiction
    - *Brain scans and recovery* from trauma/addiction
    - *Neurobiology* of trauma/addiction
    - *Genetics* of trauma/addiction
    - *Sexuality* and trauma/addiction
    - *Health problems* in trauma/addiction
    - *Mind-body connections* in trauma/addiction
    - *Behavioral addictions*, including body addictions such as exercise, sex, and plastic surgery

- Option 5. *Surf a symptom.* Read the description in Handout 4 and after you try it, write about how it went.

Memory

SUMMARY

Today's topic explores how memory in trauma and addiction differs from regular memory. Clients identify their strengths and challenges in responding to difficult memories and learn healthy approaches to memory issues.

ORIENTATION

"I remember the exact moment when I decided to forget—I was six and I said, 'My grandfather is a good person who wouldn't hurt me. I must be making this up. I decided it was me, not him, that was the problem.'"

~Male child sexual abuse survivor

Memories are the building blocks of the past. But clients with trauma and addiction often have major challenges with memory.

"I want to remember but can't."
"I'm triggered by memories."
"I keep chasing the memory of that first meth high."
"I can talk about memories but have no feeling."
"I question whether my memories are real."
"I'll do absolutely anything to avoid my memories."
"I dig for memories, then cut myself."
"I have trouble remembering things since becoming an alcoholic."

Today's topic helps clients put their memory struggles into words and offers guidance to address them. In trauma, some clients are overwhelmed with *too much memory*—flooded and unable to escape, as in flashbacks and nightmares. They fear getting in touch with memories that will stir up new pain. Others are frustrated with *too little memory*, unable to remember important parts of the past. Or memory is expressed in body sensations or behavior rather than experienced directly.

Addiction too, especially substance addiction, is associated with memory issues (Goodman & Packard, 2016). Neuroscience research shows that substances "rewire" the brain—intense first memories of intoxication create powerful, obsessional craving for it. There are also blackouts and glorifying of substance use (suppression of bad memories). And both substance use and abstinence can evoke trauma memories that complicate recovery.

Yet during recovery, trauma and addiction have a fundamental difference with regard to memory. In trauma, the goal is to reduce a painful memory, like defusing a bomb—making it inert, removing its energy. Trauma memories aren't forgotten, but with recovery they no longer hold the intense power they had before. In contrast, in addiction recovery it helps to keep difficult memories present—the damages and losses addiction caused—as a reminder not to return to using. In alcohol addiction, it's said that one is always "just one drink" away from disaster. This session focuses primarily on education: helping clients become aware of their response to memories and how to improve it. It's less about exploring specific memories, which occurs more in other sessions. Handout 1 describes how trauma and addiction impact memory. Handout 2 helps clients observe how they respond to memories, including strengths (e.g., "I'm patient with myself when I have memory gaps") and challenges (e.g., "I glorify addiction memories"). Finally, Handout 3 suggests how to handle too much or too little memory. If clients learn how memory works and can respond in healthy ways, this can go a long way toward coming to terms with their past.

Your Emotional Reactions

You may feel caught in a bind if you try to confirm the accuracy of clients' memories, especially when the facts may not be clear (as in early child abuse). Clients understandably want you to believe them as so often their reality was negated or ignored. The most helpful approach is to validate clients' *emotional truth* rather than trying to discern the *historical truth*. Validating emotional truth means allying with the feelings and meanings the client holds (e.g., "What you're describing sounds awful; I understand how you'd be devastated by that"). Historical truth is verifying the facts, which is typically done in legal settings such as court evaluations. In short, you don't have to be "judge and jury" but instead can empathize with clients' emotional reality.

Acknowledgments

The session quotation from Rumi is per Rad (2010, p. 21). The quotations in Handout 1 are from Pitman quoted in Henig (2004); Landy in Marks (2015, p. 192); and Knapp (1996, p. 85). In Handout 1, *memory phobia* is a term from Janet (van der Kolk & van der Hart, 1990); and Janet's concept of memory being frozen and wordless is from Herman (1992, p. 37). In Handout 3, the concept of memory substitution is adapted from lab research by Hotta and Kawaguchi (2009) and others.

SESSION FORMAT

1. *Check-in* (per Chapter 3).
2. *Quotation.* Link the quotation to the session topic—for example, *"We'll be talking today about how to take a loving approach toward difficult memories as a way to try to heal them."*
3. *Handouts* (relate the topic to clients' lives):
    Handout 1: **Memory Issues in Trauma and Addiction**
    Handout 2: **How Do You Cope with Difficult Memories?**
    Handout 3: **Too Much or Too Little Memory: What You Can Do**
4. *Check-out* (per Chapter 3).

SESSION CONTENT

Goals

☐ Explore how trauma and addiction impact memory.
☐ Help clients notice how they respond to difficult memories.
☐ Offer strategies for managing *too much* and *too little* memory.

Ways to Relate the Material to Clients' Lives

★ ***Discuss how regular memory is different from trauma/addiction memories (Handout 1).*** Regular memory is easily put into words and makes sense. Handout 1, in contrast, has many examples of trauma and addiction memory issues. You can ask clients to circle any they notice in themselves. To help them understand regular memory, you could illustrate with a simple question such as "What did you have for lunch today?" or "What was the weather yesterday?" and have them notice how this type of memory is different.

★ ***Complete the Strengths and Challenges Questionnaire (Handout 2).*** This helps keep the session focused rather than overly abstract. Note that the score is not the main point, but rather helping clients observe how they respond to memories. Emphasize a compassionate approach and healthy ways of responding (e.g., not using substances).

★ ***Do a question/answer "game" on how to manage memories (Handout 3).*** For example:
- Is it good to use hypnosis to access memories? *{no}*
- What's the best way to shift away from an overwhelming memory? *{grounding}*
- Can you recover even if you have big memory gaps? *{yes}*
- What are examples of doubts about memories? *{"Did it really happen?," "Maybe it wasn't so bad."}*
- "What's mentionable is manageable"—what does this mean? *{It's helpful to put memories into words.}*
- Is it helpful or unhelpful to link emotions and memories? *{helpful}*
- Is it good to dig for trauma memories? *{no}*
- "Slower is faster": What does this mean? *{You'll make more progress in the long run if you take things slowly.}*

★ ***Have clients try new approaches for a difficult memory (Handout 3).*** For example, a client says he has an intrusive memory of a fire that killed his friend. Help him identify strategies from Handout 3 to try, rehearsing them in the session if possible.

★ ***Identify when it's good to keep painful memories alive.*** In addiction, for example, the memory of "hitting bottom" is a good reminder to stay sober. In trauma, a perpetrator of domestic violence may apologize and promise to change but never does; it's key to remember the violent actions rather than falling for the "pretty words."

★ ***Discussion***
- "Do any feelings arise as you look through the handouts?"
- "Do you think it's true that *memories can no longer harm you?*"
- "When you were growing up, how did your family deal with difficult memories?"
- "Do you tend to have too much or too little memory?"
- "How do you wish you could respond to difficult memories?"
- "What are your strengths in dealing with memories?"

Suggestions

✦ ***Emphasize hope.*** Clients typically struggle for years with difficult memories. Validate that while also helping them feel hopeful about the future. For example: "Memories can no longer harm you," and "Respect your mind for having protected you."

✦ ***Address both trauma and addiction memories.*** It's natural to focus on trauma memories but equally important to address addiction memories (e.g., overdose, getting arrested for drunk driving). Also, some memories relate to both trauma and addiction, such as being assaulted while intoxicated.

✦ ***Understand the concept of recovered memory.*** This refers to memories that come back after having been forgotten. A client may suddenly remember long-buried child abuse events, for example. This is a complex topic and it's worth reading about recovered memory if it's unfamiliar to you. Some key points are: (1) Most child abuse victims remember all or part of what happened. (2) Hypnosis or substances are not recommended for exploring memories as they can produce false memories. (3) Recovered memories can be accurate; they shouldn't be assumed to be false. (4) Don't ask leading questions such as, "You were sexually abused as a child, right?" Rather, ask neutral open-ended neutral questions such as "Did you ever experience child sexual abuse?" (APA, 1998).

✦ *Although rare, dissociative identity disorder is associated with major memory gaps.* This diagnosis used to be called *multiple personality disorder*. It arises from extreme, repeated, and typically early trauma. In addition to memory gaps, clients with this disorder have an identity that's fragmented into different *alters* (personalities) who may be different ages and genders and may not be aware of each other. You can still do Creating Change and today's topic with such clients, but they also typically need specialized treatment. Seek consultation as needed.

Tough Cases

* "I don't want to remember."
* "Maybe I made it all up."
* "I'm afraid bad memories will come up if I stop drinking."
* "I have body memories; what can I do about that?"
* "I feel awful about stuff I did when I blacked out."
* "I'm going to try hypnosis so I can remember more."

Quotation

"Through love all pain will turn to medicine."

~Jalaluddin Rumi, 13th-century Persian poet

HANDOUT 1

Memory Issues in Trauma and Addiction

Regular memories can be put into words and follow a logical sequence. But trauma and addiction memories are different.

TRAUMA

"Frequently when they remembered Vietnam, every detail came back to them—the way it smelled, the temperature, who they were with, what they heard."

~Psychiatrist who treats Vietnam veterans

"So much of my childhood between the ages of four and nine is blank. . . . It's almost as if my life was smashed into little pieces."

~Ava Landy, child Holocaust survivor

Trauma Memories May Be . . .

+ *Fragmented.* Your story may be in pieces, out of order. It may seem like a slide show of images.
+ *Re-enacted.* Trauma can show up in behavior. You may be drawn to partners who are similar to past abusers. Children may express trauma in play, such as having dolls hurt each other.
+ *Physical (body memories).* Trauma may get expressed as headaches, nausea, or other body sensations. In extreme cases, some people go blind or mute after trauma but regain their sight or voice when they come to terms with it.
+ *Intrusive.* Disturbing memories pop up, unwanted. You can't get rid of them.
+ *Lost.* You may forget events or whole blocks of time. Memory loss (*amnesia*) is more common if your trauma was very young or severe. The mind shuts down as self-protection.
+ *Recovered.* Trauma memories can emerge months or years later—awakened by counseling, abstinence from substances, or a sudden reminder such as a movie scene. These delayed memories can shift over time just as all memories can.
+ *Flashed back.* Flashbacks are intense vivid reexperiences of a trauma memory. It feels like it's happening again, in images, feelings, or senses.
+ *Feared.* You may be scared to go to sleep, afraid of trauma showing up in nightmares. You may have *memory phobia*—intense fear of your own memories.
+ *Secret.* You may have stayed silent about trauma memories to survive, or from shame or guilt.

(cont.)

From *Creating Change* by Lisa M. Najavits. Copyright © 2024 Lisa M. Najavits. Published by The Guilford Press. Permission to photocopy this material is granted to purchasers of this book for use with your own clients or patients; see copyright page for details.

HANDOUT 1 *(p. 2 of 2)* — Memory

- + *Doubted.* You may have difficulty believing yourself about what happened, especially if people around you negated your memories.
- + *Sensory.* All senses—smell, sight, sound, touch, hearing—can hold trauma memory. Sand or the smell of fuel can evoke distressing memories for soldiers, for example.
- + *Frozen.* Trauma memory is frozen, wordless, and intensely emotional, according to Janet in the 19th century, one of the first psychiatrists to describe it.

◇ **How about you?** Do you have problems with *trauma memories*?   Not at all / Somewhat / A lot

ADDICTION

"Drinking continued to work, diluting the discomfort, making things bearable. . . . At my senior prom I got blackout drunk . . . and ended up making out in a car. . . . I have no memory, no conscious memory, of what that felt like, and I suppose that was precisely the point."
~Carolyn Knapp, *Drinking: A Love Story*

Addiction Can Impact Memory . . .

This topic has been studied mostly in relation to substance use disorder but can also apply to other addictions.

- *Blackouts.* With high doses of alcohol, you may have conversations, sex, or commit a crime yet have no memory of it later even if you try.
- *Glorified memory.* You may remember only good times or see them as better than they really were. Forgetting the negative aspects perpetuates addiction, makes it seem OK.
- *"Rewiring" the brain.* Intoxication releases powerful brain chemicals. These can stamp your memory so strongly that you become obsessed with getting that feeling again.
- *Reduced memory.* Intoxication can impair memory, and long-term heavy substance use leads to difficulty learning because you can't remember things well.
- *Traumatic addiction memories.* You may have deeply disturbing memories that involve both trauma and addiction, such as seeing a friend die from an overdose or being robbed while buying drugs.
- *Coping with memory.* Addiction often develops as a way to escape from trauma memories.
- *Both substance use and substance abstinence can awaken trauma memories.* Trauma memories may surface when you're in an altered state (intoxicated) and also months into sobriety, when your brain is no longer clouded by using.

◇ **How about you?** Do you have problems with *addiction and memory*?   Not at all / Somewhat / A lot

HEALING

In recovery, trauma memory can be converted to regular memory: put into words, organized into a clear sequence, without triggering strong emotions.

So too with addiction, as you recover your brain and memory improve as well.

HANDOUT 2   Memory

How Do You Cope with Difficult Memories?

This handout helps you look at your strengths and challenges in relation to trauma and/or addiction memories.

★ *Circle an answer for each item.*

PART I: YOUR STRENGTHS

Note: If an item is not applicable, score it as a 2 in this section and list "n/a" next to the item.

	Yes	Somewhat	No
1. I can put my trauma/addiction memories into words.	2	1	0
2. I'm patient with myself when I have memory gaps.	2	1	0
3. I stay safe when triggered by memories.	2	1	0
4. I let painful memories surface and know I can get through them.	2	1	0
5. I use grounding to shift away from bad memories when needed.	2	1	0
6. I'm able to share my trauma/addiction memories with safe people.	2	1	0
7. I understand memories can't harm me.	2	1	0
8. My trauma/addiction memories don't bother me a lot.	2	1	0
9. Other strengths in dealing with memories? List here:	2	1	0

Score Part I *(add your circled numbers from these questions):* _____

(cont.)

From *Creating Change* by Lisa M. Najavits. Copyright © 2024 Lisa M. Najavits. Published by The Guilford Press. Permission to photocopy this material is granted to purchasers of this book for use with your own clients or patients; see copyright page for details.

HANDOUT 2 *(p. 2 of 2)* Memory

PART II: YOUR CHALLENGES

Note: If an item is not applicable, score it as a 0 in this section and list "n/a" next to the item.

	Yes	Somewhat	No
1. I'm often triggered by memories.	0	1	2
2. When I talk about memories, I'm numb.	0	1	2
3. I often doubt my memories.	0	1	2
4. Memories show up in my body or behavior rather than words.	0	1	2
5. I keep digging for memories, like picking at a scab.	0	1	2
6. I'm bothered by memory gaps.	0	1	2
7. I use addictive behavior in response to trauma memories (e.g., alcohol, drugs, food).	0	1	2
8. I glorify addiction memories (remembering the positive, not the negative).	0	1	2
9. Other memory challenges? List here:	0	1	2

Score Part II *(add your circled numbers from these questions):* _____

Total *(add up your scores from Parts I and II):* _____. The maximum score is 36. The higher your score, the greater your ability to cope with trauma/addiction memories.

✧ Reflection

Did you notice any feelings or insights while doing this handout?

HANDOUT 3   Memory

Too Much or Too Little Memory: What You Can Do

Memories can feel like *too much* or *too little*.

- *Too much* means feeling overwhelmed or triggered (e.g., flashbacks or drug dreams).
- *Too little* means wanting to remember more (e.g., memory gaps or blackouts).

★ *Circle any of the following that may help you.*

IF YOU HAVE *TOO MUCH* MEMORY (TRIGGERED)

- **Know** that memories may be difficult, but they can no longer actually harm you.
- **Try memory substitution.** If you reconnect a painful trigger with a new, positive memory, it can weaken the trigger. If the sound of a barking dog triggers you, for example, whenever you hear it, replace it with a positive sound, such as a bird chirping or a favorite song lyric.
- **Use grounding.** It's one of the best ways to shift away from anything too intense. Learn it, practice it, and use it anytime, anywhere.
- **Remember "slower is faster"**: Give yourself time to work through memories. Stay balanced with soothing activities and people. Take breaks.
- **Rewrite the *meaning* of a memory.** You can't change the facts of what happened, but you can change the meaning it holds. You can soften the impact. For example, can you forgive yourself for your trauma or addiction? Can you find a sense of mission by helping others in recovery?
- **Grieve the memories.** They don't disappear, but you can heal to where they no longer have emotional power over you.
- **Notice choices**. Work on memories when the timing is good. If it isn't, such as while driving, try to delay them.

IF YOU HAVE *TOO LITTLE* MEMORY (CAN'T REMEMBER)

- **Respect your mind for having protected you** from too much memory.
- **Know that you can recover even without complete memories.** Many people do. Memories are just one part of recovery.
- **Stay open to what arises,** but don't become consumed with digging for memories.
- **Be specific.** Look at calendars. Ask people who may know. Talk to a counselor or friend, which can bring up more. Let your mind drift loosely—it may take an indirect path toward memories.
- **Don't seek altered states to access memories,** such as substance use, hypnosis, or guided imagery. What you remember in normal states of mind is more accurate.
- **Tolerate uncertainty.** Some memories can be verified, others can't. That's OK.
- **Let your story develop.** It may shift as missing pieces emerge.
- **Work on addiction recovery.** The clearer your mind, the more likely memories are to surface.

(cont.)

From *Creating Change* by Lisa M. Najavits. Copyright © 2024 Lisa M. Najavits. Published by The Guilford Press. Permission to photocopy this material is granted to purchasers of this book for use with your own clients or patients; see copyright page for details.

HANDOUT 3 *(p. 2 of 2)* — Memory

MORE STRATEGIES

- **Honor your memories even if you don't like them.** What comes up can lead to something good in the long term—relief, clarity, and greater peace with your past.
- **Let go of protecting others.** Does owning your memories feel like a betrayal of others? Stay focused on your own truth for now.
- **Know that doubts are common.** "Did it really happen?" "Maybe it wasn't so bad." With time and experience, you'll arrive at your truth.
- **Follow the trail.** Let your mind and heart go where they need to. Rather than directing, it's discovery.
- **Notice emotions.** Linking memory and emotion promotes healing. What feelings emerge with your memories? How do you respond to them?
- **Seek support** from safe people. This is especially important if others have doubted or negated your experiences in the past.
- **Remember: "What is mentionable is manageable."** The more you express memories in words, the less likely they are to be expressed via other channels (your behavior, your body).
- **Keep memories alive that help your recovery.** The memory of "hitting bottom" in addiction can remind you to stay sober, for example.
- **If you have a current legal case related to trauma, get advice about memories that come up in counseling.** The concept of *recovered memory* may impact your case.
- **Stay hopeful.** Memories take time to work on, but you can make progress.

Memory

Ideas for a Commitment

Commit to one action that will move your life forward!
It can be anything you feel will help you, or you can try one of the ideas below.
Keeping your commitment is a way of respecting, honoring, and caring for yourself.

✦ Option 1. A friend says to you, "I'm afraid of my memories." What advice would you give?

✦ Option 2. Identify a *strength* in Handout 2. How can you increase it in the week ahead?

or

       Identify a *challenge* in Handout 2. How can you decrease it in the week ahead?

✦ Option 3. Write or draw using as many of these words as you choose:

    memory hope pain forgetting anger addiction trauma numb doubts honor pace overwhelmed sad recovery inner self body feel connect disconnect body

✦ Option 4. Identify a memory you want to work on in Creating Change.

Power Dynamics

SUMMARY

Power is at the core of both trauma and addiction. In trauma, people are powerless to prevent a damaging event; in addiction, people are powerless over their own behavior. Today's topic helps clients explore how they navigated difficult power dynamics in the past and how they can increase their sense of personal power now.

ORIENTATION

Most everyone wants to feel powerful; it's a healthy instinct that relates to survival. In contrast, trauma and addiction create a state of powerlessness that takes a lot of work to come back from. *Empowerment* is thus a central goal of treatment.

Today's topic focuses primarily on power dynamics in relationships (while also drawing parallels to dynamics within the self). Some clients stay stuck in a one-down position, continually acquiescing to others even when they no longer need to. Others go to the opposite extreme, dominating via power struggles and fights they feel they have to win to feel good about themselves. Some clients are afraid of wielding power, such as not wanting to have children so they won't mistreat them the way they were mistreated. Still others so deeply internalize powerlessness that it becomes a sort of identity in which suffering is overvalued. Clients' responses to power in relationships reflect a mix of their trauma and addiction history, their personality, and family and cultural messages.

Healthy use of power is often unfamiliar: mutuality, open expression, and balancing needs. Today's topic helps clients become more attuned to how they navigated power dynamics in the past under adverse conditions and how they may have overlearned responses that no longer serve them.

There are three handouts. Handout 1 explores the concept of power in relation to trauma and addiction. Handout 2 guides clients to recognize how they've navigated power, drawing on specific scenarios in their life. Handout 3 helps them identify unsafe people who may be exerting too much power over them.

One of the most compelling ways clients can experience healthy power dynamics is through positive treatment relationships. One counselor describes it beautifully:

"My work is in some sense to repair through the relationship—by clients seeing that the relationship with me and group members is different. Their feelings do count, they get to decide (have power), they will not be abused or discounted, we will listen and care. There is time for them. They start to understand that the now may initially feel the same but is not the same as then. We talk about the past and what it was like so they see the relationship between then and now. They can build trust and understand how the messages they received ('You don't count; your value is in meeting others' needs; you are never enough') affect them now. We discuss that feelings are not facts. Because you feel powerless does not mean you are."

Your Emotional Reactions

How do you experience the power dynamics in sessions? Does it feel like a healthy balance of your facilitation and clients' participation? Do they seem intimidated or at ease? Do they speak up if they disagree? Are you able to bring up sensitive topics? Do sessions feel like a smooth back-and-forth or sometimes seem like a power struggle? If the latter occurs, are you able to guide the relationship back? It's almost inevitable that challenging dynamics will arise, especially if clients' trauma and addiction are severe or chronic. Clients will bring into the room power issues from the past, even if not consciously. As an authority figure, you're likely to become the focus of their projections: They may fear you, want to compete with you, or want your approval. Indeed, from some theoretical perspectives, it's essential for them to bring such dynamics into sessions so as to work them through now.

Acknowledgments

The session quotation is per *Encyclopedia Britannica* (2020). In Handout 1, the concept of animal hierarchies is from Franz, McLean, Tung, Altmann, and Alberts (2015). On the Commitments page, the quotation in the third commitment is from the *AA Big Book* (2001, p. 30).

SESSION FORMAT

1. *Check-in* (per Chapter 3).
2. *Quotation.* Link the quotation to the session topic—for example, *"The quote expresses how important it is to be aware of the power each of us has. Today we'll explore trauma, addiction, and power dynamics."*
3. *Handouts* (relate the topic to clients' lives):
    Handout 1: **Power, Trauma, and Addiction**
    Handout 2: **Remember a Time**
    Handout 3: **Safe versus Unsafe People**
4. *Check-out* (per Chapter 3).

SESSION CONTENT

Goals

☐ Discuss how power dynamics relate to trauma and addiction.
☐ Explore how clients navigated power in the past.
☐ Teach healthy ways to build personal power.
☐ Identify unsafe people who may be exerting too much power over the client.

Ways to Relate the Material to Clients' Lives

★ *Help clients notice their habitual responses to power (Handout 1).* If someone puts them down, for example, do they tend to confront? Give in? Agree? Avoid? Stay silent? Shut down? Fight back? Assert themselves? Given a history of trauma and addiction, it's common to respond with patterns based on the past. Moreover, it's typically not just one type of response but switching between extremes, such as being overly quiet and then blowing up.

★ *Process situations from the past (Handout 2).* This handout has many options, but the goal is depth rather than trying to cover a lot of them. Guide clients to address a question with enough detail to access their feelings and beliefs about it.

★ *Emphasize strengths not just problems.* Both Handouts 1 and 2 help clients identify strengths in relation to power dynamics, not just weaknesses. For example, in Handout 1 they can identify personal power in various domains such as *social power* (e.g., ability to make friends) and *physical power* (e.g., athletic). In Handout 2, they can identify times they navigated power well versus poorly. Focusing on strengths provides a balanced perspective on the past: They had some power at times, even amid the powerlessness of trauma and addiction.

★ *Identify current unsafe relationships (Handout 3).* All relationships have ups and downs and disappointments. But Handout 3 identifies major or persistent harm that clients may be experiencing, perhaps due to a legacy of past powerlessness. If a current relationship appears unsafe, help clients evaluate it, and offer strong support for next steps. Concrete options may include leaving the relationship; domestic violence counseling; attending Co-Dependents Anonymous or Al-Anon; or, depending on the level of harm, formally reporting the situation or helping the client obtain legal help. Be sure to emphasize that clients aren't at fault for others' abusiveness. In one study of domestic violence survivors, for example, half reported that counselors blamed them for being abused, saying they were "codependent" or that they "chose" the abusive partner (Leedom, Andersen, Glynn, & Barone, 2019). Also, if clients are *themselves* harming others in any major way, seek immediate supervision on how to handle this, which may include further evaluation and mandated reporting.

★ *Encourage clients to explore opposite responses.* If they generally take a "tough guy" approach, what would it be like to show vulnerability? If they tend to appease, can they try being assertive?

★ *Discussion*
  - "Do you tend to express your power too strongly? Or the opposite, too little?"
  - "How are your relationships affected by your style of power?"
  - "What did your culture teach about how to relate to powerful people?"
  - "How did you respond during trauma (fight, flight, freeze, appease)? How do you feel about how you responded?"
  - "Do you want to change your approach to power dynamics?"
  - "Can you think of someone who navigates power well? What does that person do and not do?"
  - "Is there anyone who currently has too much power over you?"

Suggestions

✦ *Emphasize flexibility.* The goal is not to have one power style but rather to shift based on the situation. Inflexible approaches (always dominating or always hanging back) indicate an overlearned response from the past. It's doing something too much or too persistently, even when it's not useful (e.g., always fighting so as not to appear weak).

✦ *Explore cultural assumptions that disempower clients.* Clients may be devalued based on characteristics they can't control such as their age or ethnicity, or the type of trauma or addiction they experienced. Validate the reality of stigma and emphasize ways to build personal power. Some methods are provided at the end of Handout 1.

✦ *Clarify the meaning of powerlessness in the 12 steps versus trauma work.* In AA and other 12-step groups, admitting powerlessness is the first step of recovery; it means the person has the courage to face the reality of addiction. In trauma work, however, admitting powerlessness is not typically emphasized, although it's sometimes helpful for clients who inappropriately blame themselves, such as "It was my fault that I didn't stop him."

◆ *Address unhealthy power patterns sensitively.* Some that are listed in the handouts (e.g., primary victim identity, overvaluing suffering) can make clients defensive. Reinforce that these aren't character flaws but rather understandable adaptations to painful environments of trauma and addiction.

Tough Cases

- "I blame myself every day for not having fought back."
- "My kids seem scared of me when I yell at them."
- "I turned down a promotion at work because I don't want power over others."
- "I sometimes wonder if I'm in an abusive marriage."
- "In my culture, speaking up is disrespectful if you're female."
- "I don't like you having the power to report me to my parole officer."

Power Dynamics

Quotation

"The most common way people give up their power is by thinking they don't have any."

~ ALICE WALKER, 20th-century American writer

HANDOUT 1

Power, Trauma, and Addiction

Power dynamics refers to how people relate to each other when a person or group has more power than another. A teacher has power over students; a boss has power over employees, for example.

Power dynamics:

- Exist in animals, too (power hierarchies, "pecking order").
- Are unwritten rules you learn from family, peers, work, and culture.
- Are a normal part of life, invisible but always present.
- Are necessary for society to function: Some people lead at times, some follow.

HEALTHY VERSUS UNHEALTHY

But power dynamics can be healthy or unhealthy.

Healthy power dynamics	versus	*Unhealthy* power dynamics
Serve a positive purpose for all		Serve just the person in power
Open communication		Top-down communication
More flexible		More rigid
Equal opportunity to acquire power		Unequal opportunity

TRAUMA AND ADDICTION: A LOSS OF POWER

Both trauma and addiction involve a loss of power.

* Trauma means you didn't have the power to stop an external situation (e.g., assault, fire).
* Addiction means you didn't have the power to stop your own behavior (e.g., substance use, gaming).

(cont.)

From *Creating Change* by Lisa M. Najavits. Copyright © 2024 Lisa M. Najavits. Published by The Guilford Press. Permission to photocopy this material is granted to purchasers of this book for use with your own clients or patients; see copyright page for details.

HANDOUT 1 *(p. 2 of 4)*   Power Dynamics

HOW YOU HANDLE POWER

It's useful to notice how you handle power and powerlessness in relationships. Some patterns may have roots in trauma or addiction. In relating to others do you tend to . . .

- ◇ Confront or avoid?
- ◇ Lead or follow?
- ◇ Assert yourself or stay quiet?
- ◇ Make your own way or conform?
- ◇ Trust or distrust?
- ◇ Cling to power or let go of power?
- ◇ Dominate or submit?

➢ Do your typical patterns have a connection to trauma? addiction?
➢ Do your patterns vary based on the type of relationship?

PERSONAL POWER THAT HELPED YOU SURVIVE

★ *Now take stock of your personal power—what helped you survive? Circle any that have been true for you.*

Social power

    connections   makes friends easily   empathy   charisma

Intellectual power

    smart   practical   interested in learning

Physical power

    strong   tall   athletic   attractive   healthy

Emotional power

    resilient   creative   spiritual   independent   disciplined

Resource power

    money   good education   safe neighborhood   access to medical care
    positive culture   family support

Others? _____

➢ How have your personal powers helped you survive trauma? addiction?
➢ What's one way you've been more powerful than others? One way you've been less powerful?

(cont.)

HANDOUT 1 *(p. 3 of 4)*   Power Dynamics

DISEMPOWERING MESSAGES

Various negative messages about power arise in trauma and addiction, which can reduce your personal power.

Silencing

- Keep quiet.
- Keep up appearances.
- I speak, you listen.

Negating You

- You're wrong.
- You're just an addict.
- You don't matter because _____.

Threats

- Go along or you'll be hurt more.
- I'll harm someone you care about.
- Revenge is sweet.

Gaslighting

- No one will believe you.
- It's not really happening.
- You're crazy.

Rules

- Be loyal no matter what.
- Only the strong survive.
- "Kill or be killed."
- Men are in charge.
- Whoever has the money makes the rules.

These messages can be so strong that you *internalize your lack of power*. You may come to believe that:

- Your primary identity in life is *victim*.
- Powerlessness is all you're entitled to.
- The more you suffer, the more noble you are.
- You can only get power via indirect methods (by hinting or "acting out").
- You'll misuse power if you get it (fear of power).

(cont.)

HANDOUT 1 *(p. 4 of 4)* — Power Dynamics

POWER DYNAMICS DURING TRAUMA AND ADDICTION

Trauma

There are four main power dynamics when trauma is happening:

- *Fight* (attack back) • *Flight* (escape) • *Freeze* (shut down) • *Appease* (submit/negotiate)

Everyone relies on automatic instincts so it's not helpful to judge how you responded during the event. There's never a *right* response; each has its benefits and risks. For example, fighting back can help, or the opposite, can lead to worse trauma, depending on the situation.

But it's useful to understand that *you may be continuing those dynamics now*, especially if you had early or repeated trauma. If you had to appease a perpetrator, you may be appeasing people in the present even when you don't need to.

Addiction

Power dynamics in addiction often serve to maintain the addiction:

- Social pressure (e.g., to drink)
- Enabling (people make excuses for your addiction)
- Disputes (e.g., addiction-related family conflicts)

The first part of recovery is thus to face the truth—to "admit we were *powerless*" over the addiction, in the words of AA.

EMPOWERMENT—HOW TO REBUILD YOUR POWER

Rebuilding your personal power is essential after trauma and addiction. This means both power within yourself (your behavior) and with others (feeling respected). Check off ✓ those that you're already actively working on and an arrow → for those you want to work on.

- ☐ Create daily habits that reinforce your control over your own behavior.
- ☐ Notice power dynamics around you (in meetings, groups, etc.). Watch who speaks versus who listens; who's valued; who dominates; how people treat each other.
- ☐ Spend time with people who treat you with respect.
- ☐ Reinforce positive personal messages such as "I can learn and grow."
- ☐ Become aware of cultural messages about trauma/addiction, females versus males, and so on.
- ☐ "Find your voice"—express your point of view; yet also allow space for others.
- ☐ Explore how you navigated power in the past (see Handout 2).
- ☐ Limit contact with unsafe people when possible (see Handout 3).
- ☐ Pull back if you're overdominating; aim for balance among everyone present.

| HANDOUT 2 | Power Dynamics |

Remember a Time

Look back on your strengths and weaknesses in navigating power dynamics.

★ *Answer as many of the following as you want. Explore trauma or addiction examples, or others.*

STRENGTHS

Remember a time that you . . .

>**. . . stood up for yourself although it was hard.**
>For example, *"I voiced my concern about a doctor who dismissed my symptoms."*
>
>**. . . used your power strategically.**
>For example, *"I was being bullied at work and was able to get some people to stand up for me."*
>
>**. . . said "no" to a bad influence.**
>For example, *"My partner kept pressuring me to sell drugs, but I refused."*
>
>**. . . used your power to protect someone vulnerable.**
>For example, *"I protected my brother from abuse by telling a teacher."*
>
>**. . . asserted your power in some important way.**
>For example, *"I confronted my abuser in court."*
>
>**. . . set a boundary compassionately.**
>For example, *"I told my alcoholic sister I couldn't lend her more money."*
>
>**Other *strengths* in navigating power?** _____

CHALLENGES

Remember a time that you . . .

>**. . . weren't aware of power dynamics going on.**
>For example, *"My ex was gaslighting me and I kept thinking I was the problem."*
>
>**. . . had power but thought you didn't.**
>For example, *"My coach made offensive statements, and I stayed quiet."*
>
>**. . . didn't have power but thought you did.**
>For example, *"I thought I could control my cocaine habit but couldn't."*
>
>**. . . overasserted your power (rage, intimidation, etc.).**
>For example, *"I sent threats to people online when I didn't agree with their politics."*

(cont.)

From *Creating Change* by Lisa M. Najavits. Copyright © 2024 Lisa M. Najavits. Published by The Guilford Press. Permission to photocopy this material is granted to purchasers of this book for use with your own clients or patients; see copyright page for details.

HANDOUT 2 *(p. 2 of 2)* — Power Dynamics

. . . perpetuated an unhealthy power struggle.
For example, *"I kept trying to make my partner jealous because he didn't love me enough."*

. . . had no power, through no fault of your own.
For example, *"My uncle abused me and got away with it."*

Other *challenges* in navigating power? _____

◆ **Reflections**

- Did any feelings or body sensations come up during this exercise?
- What were the unwritten rules of who had power in your family?
- How did trauma/addiction impact your sense of personal power?
- What can help you feel more empowered in the future?

HANDOUT 3 — Power Dynamics

Safe versus Unsafe People

As you explore power dynamics, you become better at seeing who's safe versus unsafe. The more that people have the following unsafe traits, the more likely they are to have too much power over you.

- Constantly finding fault with you
- Punishing you with silence or withdrawal
- Abusive, angry
- Lying, deceiving, having gaps in their story
- Gaslighting (telling you there's no problem when there is)
- Blaming everyone but themselves
- Repeatedly getting you to cover them financially
- Extremely self-centered
- Unable to learn from experience
- Communicating that rules and morality don't apply to them
- Criminal acts
- Faking an identity, living a double life (e.g., two wives)
- Casting people aside when no longer useful to them
- Manipulating, acting, faking emotions
- Lacking empathy or care for others
- Taking pleasure in others' suffering

Trauma and addiction can make you vulnerable to unsafe people

If you had a tough past, you may be less skilled at setting boundaries and getting out of unsafe relationships. You may so yearn for love that you dive in too quickly, rather than slowly building trust. You may give up too much of your personal power. However, some unsafe relationships, such as intimate partner violence, are not possible to leave without expert support and guidance.

What to do

✡ *Get others to weigh in; you may be in too deep to see clearly.* Ask as many trusted people as possible. Be totally honest with them about what's going on. Be open to their feedback even if it's difficult.

✡ *Keep watching behavior, not just words.* Every relationship has ups and downs. It can take time for people to change. But if you see no concrete progress, consider your options.

✡ *Remember that "love is never enough."* It's common to believe that your love will heal the person. But no matter how loving you are, if the person is not making active efforts to change, no amount of love will be enough.

✡ *Protect yourself.* If needed, get away from the person and protect your assets. If you can't get away, minimize contact, set firm boundaries, and seek support.

✡ *Try support groups* such as Al-Anon and Co-Dependents Anonymous. These are free and available online as well as in person.

✡ *If you believe you may be harming others, get help.* If the list of unsafe traits reflects how you act toward others (family, friends, partners), it is crucial to get help to prevent further harm.

◆ **Reflections**

- Are you currently in any relationship that may be unsafe?
- Do you tend to stay too long in unsafe relationships?
- Do you have enough safe people in your life?
- Are you concerned that you may be harming others?

From *Creating Change* by Lisa M. Najavits. Copyright © 2024 Lisa M. Najavits. Published by The Guilford Press. Permission to photocopy this material is granted to purchasers of this book for use with your own clients or patients; see copyright page for details.

Power Dynamics

Ideas for a Commitment

Commit to one action that will move your life forward!
It can be anything you feel will help you, or you can try one of the ideas below. Keeping your commitment is a way of respecting, honoring, and caring for yourself.

✦ Option 1. Write a letter to your younger self: What have you learned about empowerment?

✦ Option 2. Choose from these words to fill in the sentences below:

love   leave   abuse   avoid   admire   trust   dismiss   respect   misunderstand reject   value   enjoy   ignore   use   put down   cherish   others? _____

  a. *In the past*, I was the kind of person who others _____.

  b. *Now* I am the kind of person who others _____.

✦ Option 3. Write what this quote means to you, from the *Big Book* of Alcoholics Anonymous:

  "The idea that somehow, someday he will control and enjoy his drinking is the great obsession of every abnormal drinker. The persistence of this illusion is astonishing. Many pursue it into the gates of insanity or death."

✦ Option 4. Search online for *how to know if you're in an abusive relationship*.

✦ Option 5. What can you do this week to expand your personal power in a positive way? How can it help your recovery from trauma/addiction?

Deepen Your Story

✢

SUMMARY

This topic offers a multitude of ways to explore the past. The goal is to continue to expand clients' trauma and/or addiction narrative, based on the idea that there's no one right way, but many.

ORIENTATION

Telling the trauma and addiction narrative is not one event and doesn't end when treatment ends. For many clients, it's a lifelong path to keep "turning it over" as they address different aspects of their story with new insights.

Clinical experience as well as the literature on past-focused methods offer a wealth of methods and, at this point, there's no clear evidence that particular methods are better than others (per Chapter 2). Today's topic draws from this rich history.

Handout 1 provides general guidance as clients often feel judged, by themselves or others, that they are doing it wrong. The handout includes reassurance such as "It's about discovery; you don't have to know exactly what to say" and "Express compassion for who you were, even if you made mistakes."

Handout 2 encourages clients to try methods that appeal to them, with 30 different exercises to explore their past (e.g., "Try slow motion," "Trace a trigger," "Describe a 'flashbulb memory,'" "Write a survivor letter"). Handout 3 is an inventory to take a long view at patterns across their lives, including both positive and negative aspects of their story.

Across the exercises there's a range of intensity to allow for different settings and needs, which can help build increasing levels of awareness. Ella, a trauma survivor, said,

> "For me there were at least three different levels of telling. The first was telling the story and not feeling anything. Telling it as a third-party story. Saying 'I' but not really meaning it happened to me. At that point I still didn't really believe it happened. . . . Then there was a really painful, scared level of telling. The tone of my voice changed. . . . And it hurt. That's the place I discovered my feelings. . . . The last way I've told has to do with stepping back and seeing the bigger picture. I looked at family dynamics. . . . I saw what happened and why it happened." (Bass & Davis, 1994, p. 107)

The experience evolves over time: "Each time you tell is a different experience. Telling your therapist or your support group, telling your partner or a new lover, telling a friend, telling publicly, telling in writing, will all feel different" (Bass & Davis, 1994, p. 107).

Your Emotional Reactions

Many counselors have experienced trauma and/or addiction and have done important recovery work themselves. It may feel natural to steer clients toward methods that worked for you. But notice which ones appeal to clients without imposing strong ideas of how it ought to look. Clients differ in their degree of emotion, their willingness to speak aloud on difficult topics, and their level of motivation. So too, some prefer creative methods, going wherever their heart and mind lead, while others prefer more structure. Stay aware of what it brings up for you when clients go about the work in ways that differ from your preferred methods.

Acknowledgments

Strategies in Handout 1 are drawn from numerous sources such as "hot spot" (Grey, Holmes, & Brewin, 2001); "empty chair," "imaginary conversation," and "psychodrama" (Moreno, 1964); "speak in the present tense" and "slow motion" (Foa & Rothbaum, 1998); "focus on the body" (Shapiro, 1995); "reminders," which are equivalent to *in vivo* exposure techniques; "shift perspective" (Pennebaker & Evans, 2014); "use all senses" (Wolfe, quoted in Herman, 1992, p. 177); "observe fantasies" and "surface feelings" (the latter adapted from the concept of adaptive vs. maladapted emotion; McCullough, 2003); "stuck points" and "manufactured emotions" (Chard et al., 2009); "creative methods" (Herman, 1992); the "storybook" idea (Hanney & Kozlowska, 2002); "try mapping" (Dees, Dansereau, & Simpson, 1994); "talk about someone else" (derives from the concept of displacement in psychodynamic treatment); the examples of interoceptive exposure in "focus on the body" (Taylor, 2006); "replay it with a different ending" (derives from imagery rehearsal therapy; Krakow et al., 1993); "'sit' with feelings" (from many different therapies using terms such as affect tolerance, exposure to affect, and distress tolerance). Finally, some suggestions on conducting the topic in group modality are from Foy, Ruzek, Glynn, Riney, and Gusman (2002). More broadly, see Chapter 1 for earlier origins of past-focused treatments, including Wolpe (who developed the principles of Exposure Therapy), and Janet, Freud, and others who developed catharsis-based treatments. In Handout 2, the idea of using chapter titles to tell one's story (per item 25, "Tell it in sections") is from Ackerman (2017). Negativity bias is from various sources, including Vaish, Grossmann, and Woodward (2008).

SESSION FORMAT

1. *Check-in* (up to 3 minutes per client). See Chapter 3.
2. *Quotation* (briefly). See page 304. Link the quotation to the session. For example, *"In today's topic, we'll explore many different ways to tell your story. You can return to these again and again, as long as you need to."*
3. *Handouts* (relate the topic to clients' lives in-depth; most of the session):
   a. Ask clients to look through the handouts:
      Handout 1: **Supporting Yourself**
      Handout 2: **30 Ways to Deepen Your Story**
      Handout 3: **The Long View**
   b. Help clients relate the topic to current and specific problems in their lives. See "Session Content" (below) and Chapter 3 for suggestions.
4. *Check-out* (briefly). See Chapter 3.

SESSION CONTENT

Goals

☐ Help clients explore different ways to talk about the past.
☐ Identify clients' preferred methods.

☐ Discuss how to take a supportive approach.
☐ Emphasize *deepening*: getting to new layers of insight.

Ways to Relate the Material to Clients' Lives

★ ***Reinforce a supportive approach to the work (Handout 1).*** Many clients grew up in families that didn't speak about trauma or addiction, or they may have felt so much shame or guilt that they couldn't talk about these until now. Handout 1 provides education on overarching strategies to promote a positive experience regardless of which particular methods are used in subsequent handouts. Have clients identify points on Handout 1 that are especially relevant to them. If you're conducting group treatment, also see the topic "Tell Your Story" for ways to reinforce a supportive approach among group members.

★ ***Have clients identify which methods appeal to them (Handout 2).*** They can mark the sheet as noted (a star next to ones they want to try; a question mark next to ones they want to learn more about). If desired, you can discuss their choices briefly, such as why they chose particular ones, and which ones they tried in the past. However, don't let this become lengthy as the goal is to move into the actual exercises. It can create anxiety to *talk about* it rather than just doing it. Remember, too, that you may want to adjust the intensity based on your knowledge of the clients, so once you hear which ones appeal to clients, steer them toward those you think will work best. See also Chapters 2 and 3 for key principles that are especially relevant to today's topic, such as the need for pacing. Remember, too, that greater emotional intensity in and of itself doesn't produce greater healing.

★ ***Try one or more methods (Handout 2).*** In *individual treatment*, the client simply begins and you could spend the whole session and even multiple sessions using just one method. Or you can try various ones in turn. For *group treatment,* after hearing their preferences, it's best for you to decide on one for everyone to try (if they're willing) as conducting many different methods in the same session is typically too fragmented. But be clear that each exercise is voluntary so any client can choose just to watch rather than participate. Also note that some exercises lend themselves to clients all doing the same exercise at the same time, silently (e.g., "Create a 10-word story," "Do a mind map"), and then discussing what they wrote. Other exercises are for one person to share aloud at a time (e.g. "Do an empty-chair exercise"). For the latter type, see the protocol in the topic "Tell Your Story" for ways to share time between group members.

★ ***Help clients make use of Handout 3.*** The goal is to take stock of significant experiences across their lives and not limited just to trauma or addiction. The reflection questions at the end of the handout help them identify meanings they draw from their experiences.

★ ***If clients are familiar with Seeking Safety, you can also trace a Seeking Safety topic into the past.*** For example, using the Seeking Safety topic "Honesty," you could explore the origins of clients' issues with honesty with questions such as, "Did people lie to you a lot when you were growing up?," "What happened in the past that led you to hide what was really going on?," and so on.

★ ***Discussion***
- "Why is it important to take a supportive approach (Handout 1)?"
- "What does it mean to 'let your story evolve'?"
- "How does it feel to share about your past?"
- "Which ideas in the handouts are new to you?"

Suggestions

✦ ***Discuss the concept of "deepening."*** It means growing, expanding, strengthening. Clients have already shared some aspects of their past in Creating Change and now they're given additional methods for continuing the work. In addition to the ideas in today's handouts, you can inquire whether they have specific events or ways of exploring the past that they want to focus on.

✦ ***Emphasize optimism about healing, but also realistic time frames.*** Everyone can recover, but no method is a quick fix, especially for clients with a complex or lengthy history of trauma or addiction. Also, any method can be used multiple times to help process some important part of their history.

✦ ***Suggestions for the empty-chair method in Handout 2.*** If you use this method, it's not recommended to have the client take the perspective of a violent or abusive person (e.g., when switching roles) as the goal is not to have the client empathize with a perpetrator. Some counselors do, in fact, do that (Shaw, 2023), but if you choose to, proceed with extreme caution.

Tough Cases

* "How will this help me stay sober?"
* "I don't like any of these methods."
* "I'm afraid of getting too angry if I talk about my trauma."
* "I feel triggered just reading this."
* "How do I know I can trust you?"
* "I don't remember most of my childhood."

Quotation

"You tell your story until you don't need to tell it anymore."

~ ANONYMOUS

HANDOUT 1

Supporting Yourself

Keep these ideas in mind to help you explore your past. Mark any that are important to you.

- Choose "hot" events (ones that really matter to you).
- It's OK to have feelings and also OK not to; start with where you are.
- You found a way to survive; notice your strengths.
- Observe how trauma and addiction were linked, if you had both.
- Don't judge yourself for your feelings, your story, or how you tell it.
- Tell your truth as best as you can.
- Express compassion for who you were, even if you made mistakes.
- It's about discovery; you don't have to know exactly what to say.
- It's always your choice what to reveal or not.
- Let your story evolve; it may change over time.
- Follow where your mind goes; something good can come of it.
- Notice how feelings come in waves, rising and falling.
- Appreciate the people who helped along the way.
- Pace yourself; take breaks.
- Give your counselor feedback (e.g., "I'd like to focus on this part, not that").
- Express yourself safely (use *words* not *actions*).
- Describe details: what was said or done, sights, sounds, and so on.
- It's OK to cry, to have anger or any other feelings.
- If it gets too intense, use grounding as needed.
- Healing doesn't happen all at once; there are layers of telling.
- You can do this—it's within every human being to overcome the past.

Other ideas?

_____

_____

From *Creating Change* by Lisa M. Najavits. Copyright © 2024 Lisa M. Najavits. Published by The Guilford Press. Permission to photocopy this material is granted to purchasers of this book for use with your own clients or patients; see copyright page for details.

HANDOUT 2 — Deepen Your Story

30 Ways to Deepen Your Story

There are many ways to understand your story in a new way. Try any below that interest you. They vary in intensity so choose what's right for you.

Remember, too, that your story includes *pain* but also *resilience*, and *harm* by others but also *help* by others. Let your story reflect all sides of what happened.

★ *Put a star (★) next to any method you want to try. Put a question mark (?) next to any you want to hear more about.*

1. **Embrace gifts of clarity.** What wisdom have you gained about your trauma and addiction? It may be facts or insights. For example, "I came to accept that my mother would never change." "I learned to love myself even if others didn't." "I discovered that my father wasn't really my father." "I realized there are things I care about more than drinking."

2. **Create a 10-word story.** Choose just 10 words to tell about your past. Examples:
   - "I almost gave up, but I am glad I didn't."
   - "For a while I felt dead inside. I came alive."
   - "I was abandoned at birth. Yet I thank God every day."

3. **Fill in the blank.**

   "I remember _____."

   "I most wanted _____."

   "I wish I had said _____."

   "I'm proud of myself for _____."

   "I never told anyone that _____."

   "I am angry because _____."

   "If people really knew me _____."

4. **Write a survivor letter.** This is a letter you don't have to send. It's about what you survived and how you did it. You can write it to the world, a person, your family, or a whole category of people ("to others who have been abused" or "to the people who hurt me"). Say whatever you want to say.

5. **See it in slow motion.** Picture an event from your past as clearly as possible in slow motion. This brings out details and helps you see aspects you may not have noticed before.

6. **Notice daydreams about the past.** You may wish for revenge, an apology, love, or different choices. Explore your daydreams and fantasies about the past. What do they reveal?

7. **Make a "list of 5."** List 5 difficult events and 5 best events you went through; list 5 people who harmed you and 5 who helped you; or other lists of 5 (balancing 5 positives and 5 negatives per list). Creating short lists can bring forth important themes.

8. **Draw what you feel in your heart** when you think about your trauma/addiction.

9. **Identity inner conflicts.** Are there nagging questions, points of confusion, or other inner conflicts about some aspect of your past? List those. For example, "Part of me still feels it was my fault even though I know in my head it wasn't."

(cont.)

From *Creating Change* by Lisa M. Najavits. Copyright © 2024 Lisa M. Najavits. Published by The Guilford Press. Permission to photocopy this material is granted to purchasers of this book for use with your own clients or patients; see copyright page for details.

HANDOUT 2 *(p. 2 of 3)* 	Deepen Your Story

10. **Use all your senses.** Remember a scene using all your senses (sight, sound, smell, taste, touch). This helps you access it more fully.
11. **Notice what's missing.** What you don't say is as important as what you do say. Are there details you're too embarrassed to talk about? Memories you're afraid to look at? It's common in trauma and addiction to have secrets based in shame, guilt, and denial.
12. **Name losses.** Did you lose innocence? time? health? opportunities? people? money? self-respect? Which losses still affect you? Which have you already come to terms with?
13. **Close your eyes.** Close your eyes to make it more vivid. If you prefer not to close them, look at a neutral area on the wall or floor.
14. **Identify patterns** (both positive and negative). For example:
    "I was so hungry for love that I tolerated stuff I shouldn't have."
    "I always did the best I could with the options in front of me."
    "I've given up too easily (on sobriety, relationships, etc.)."
    "My family always supported me no matter how badly I relapsed."
    "Growing up it was 'say nothing,' so now it's hard for me to open up."
15. **Notice it in your body.** As you access difficult memories, notice what you feel in your body. Heaviness? tingling? nausea? And when you want to shift away from the past, what helps your body feel calm?
16. **Welcome all sides of yourself.** Everyone has different sides at different times: the loving side, the angry side, the weak side, the playful side. In trauma and addiction, it's common to have sides of the self that are split off. For example, you may have anger that erupts suddenly, surprising even you. Is there a side of yourself you need to explore?
17. **Relate to someone else's story.** Watch a movie or read online about someone else's trauma or addiction recovery. Sometimes it's easier to feel for others than yourself.
18. **Say it as if it's happening now** (e.g., "I open the door and . . . ").
19. **Do an empty-chair exercise.** This classic counseling exercise helps you express your perspective. Place a chair across from you and identify who or what is in the chair that you want to speak to. It can be a person (anyone, alive or dead); you at a younger age; or an abstraction (your addiction, your trauma, your "inner critic," your "fearful self"). Speak aloud as your counselor listens. You can also switch roles and sit in the other seat so you speak to "yourself" from that other perspective. Afterward, talk about what came up.
20. **Notice what moves you.** An animal, a child, a movie, heroic stories, goodness, nature, music, people who overcame hardship? What you identify with can give insight into your own experience.
21. **Trace a trigger.** This means linking the trigger to your past. Someone cuts you off in traffic and you're furious rather than just annoyed. There are often deep roots to small events. It may connect to a boundary violation in trauma or feeling that no one cared about your needs. To trace a trigger, ask, "Why do I feel so strongly about it? Is it out of proportion to what's going on? Does it relate to my past? What does it remind me of?"
22. **Compare *then* versus *now*.** Take an important event in your past and notice how you viewed it then versus now (using any of the rows shown in the table). This can help identify what's changed and what still needs work.

Then	versus	Now
Harsh toward yourself		Compassionate toward yourself
Unclear		Clear
Narrow perspective		Broad perspective
Child point of view		Adult point of view

23. **Describe a "flashbulb memory."** This refers to an extremely vivid memory, as if a flashbulb were lighting the scene. You remember exactly where you were, what you were doing, what you felt.

(cont.)

HANDOUT 2 *(p. 3 of 3)*   Deepen Your Story

Many people in the U.S. remember 9/11 this way, for example. Describing a vivid memory to someone else can provide comfort so you're not alone with it. You can also try reengineering the memory by imagining how a kind person would talk you through the situation ("You're a good person, you are so strong to get through it; it's not your fault").

24. **Find the *hot spots*.** Also known as *stuck points*, these are the parts of your story that are hardest for you. An assault survivor said a hot spot for him was the moment he realized he couldn't get away. A person with meth addiction said her hot spot was guilt about stealing from her mother to pay for drugs. Talking about these can release their emotional power over you.

25. **Tell it in sections.** You could describe *before, during, after* (trauma or addiction). Or you could create chapter titles for important events and stages of your life. One person wrote the title "Awkward and Uncertain," with this description: "My teenage years were dominated by a sense of uncertainty and confusion in a family of seven." You can also include "The Future" as the last chapter: What comes next? Who do you want to become?

26. **Picture a different outcome ("what if").** Talk about how you would have wanted things to go. Although it didn't happen that way, it can bring out poignant perspectives that help you access feelings. For example, what if you had received help sooner? What if you had made different choices?

27. **Tell a larger story.** Start with a headline (a phrase); then go a bit larger (a sentence); then larger (a paragraph), like bigger and bigger circles. Be sure to include self-compassion as you enlarge the story. For example, the headline is "Terrible car accident"; then a few details ("I didn't see the stop sign, and then the truck came toward me"); then more ("After the crash, I felt so guilty. I see now that I was sleep-deprived; I had neglected myself for too long"). *Note*: This is a very brief example; yours can be longer.

28. **Be the hero of your story.** Research shows that people notice negatives far more than positives (*negativity bias*). You may have made mistakes; everyone does. But try telling your story from the point of view of what you did right—surviving against the odds, overcoming adversity, seeking help.

29. **Do a *mind map*.** Start with a key word or phrase, such as *the assault*, and then notice what pops into mind. Notice themes and connections. You can add colors and symbols (e.g., circles for feelings, squares for memories, triangles for actions, arrows for next steps). You can draw it or search online for "free mind-mapping program" and "how to mind map."

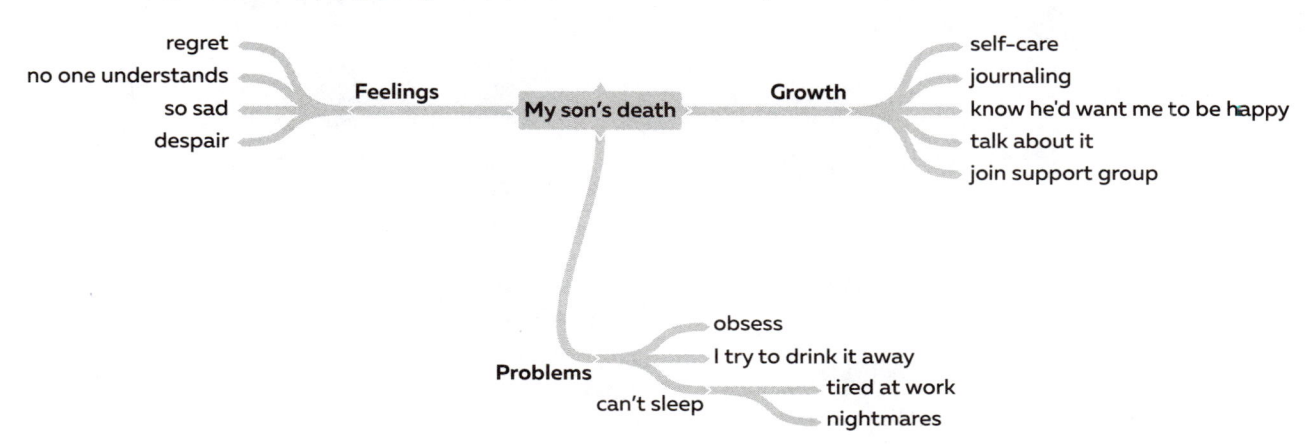

```
       regret                                                     self-care
no one understands       Feelings              Growth             journaling
       so sad         ─────────► My son's death ─────────►        know he'd want me to be happy
       despair                                                    talk about it
                                                                  join support group

                                    │
                                    ▼
                                                obsess
                                                I try to drink it away
                                Problems
                                                tired at work
                                    can't sleep
                                                nightmares
```

30. **Look back on who you hoped to become.** When you were younger, did you have an idea of what you wanted for your life? being a parent? a specific career? where you wanted to live? surrounded by certain types of people? What dreams did you accomplish? Are there any you still want?

Any other methods you'd like to try? _____

_____

HANDOUT 3   Deepen Your Story

The Long View

This exercise helps you take stock of major experiences across your life.

★ *Fill in as many in as you want (you don't have to do three for each). Then see the reflection questions at the end.*

1. ***Best/worst events in my life*** [up to three of each]

    Examples of *best events*: captain of high school football team; birth of my first child; 5 years cancer-free

    Examples of *worst events*: bullied in school; drug overdose; mental breakdown; sister's suicide

    ❖ *Best events in my life*

    1.
    2.
    3.

    ◆ *Worst events in my life*

    1.
    2.
    3.

2. ***Proud of/regret*** [up to three of each]

    Examples of *proud of*: survived my childhood; got 1-year AA chip; first one in family to graduate from college

    Examples of *regret*: lost custody of my kids due to drugs; stole from my family; wasted too much time

    ❖ *I'm most proud of*

    1.
    2.
    3.

    ◆ *I most regret*

    1.
    2.
    3.

3. ***People who helped/harmed*** [up to three of each]

    Examples of *people who helped*: aunt who adopted me; 5th-grade teacher who noticed something was wrong; best friend Callie for always being there

    Examples of *people who harmed*: my father, for all the abuse; my dealer; the doctor who didn't listen and I got sicker

    (cont.)

From *Creating Change* by Lisa M. Najavits. Copyright © 2024 Lisa M. Najavits. Published by The Guilford Press. Permission to photocopy this material is granted to purchasers of this book for use with your own clients or patients; see copyright page for details.

HANDOUT 3 *(p. 2 of 3)*   Deepen Your Story

- *The people who helped*
    1.
    2.
    3.
- *The people who harmed*
    1.
    2.
    3.

4. **Best/worst influences (including media, culture)** [up to three of each]

    Examples of *best influences:* my cultural traditions; religion; superhero movies

    Examples of *worst influences:* friend who got me into gambling; social media

    - *Best influences on me*
        1.
        2.
        3.
    - *Worst influences on me*
        1.
        2.
        3.

5. **Growth/stayed stuck** [up to three of each]

    Examples of *growth:* understood the trauma wasn't my fault; learned to take care of my body (lost 25 pounds)

    Examples of *staying stuck:* never leaving home; choosing toxic partners; continuing to use substances

    - *Ways I've grown*
        1.
        2.
        3.
    - *Ways I've stayed stuck*
        1.
        2.
        3.

6. **Needs that were/were not met** [up to three of each]

    Examples of *needs that were met:* food, shelter, basic education

    Examples of *needs that were not met:* not enough friends; not feeling loved for who I am; no help for trauma early on

(cont.)

HANDOUT 3 *(p. 3 of 3)* Deepen Your Story

* *Needs that were met*
    1.
    2.
    3.

* *Needs that were not met*
    1.
    2.
    3.

7. Best/worst aspects of trauma recovery [up to three of each]

Examples of *best aspects of trauma recovery:* less alone; fewer nightmares

Examples of *worst aspects of trauma recovery:* unable to fully talk about what happened; panic attacks; urges to drink when triggered

* *Best aspects of trauma recovery*
    1.
    2.
    3.

* *Worst aspects of trauma recovery*
    1.
    2.
    3.

8. Substances (or other addiction) gave me/cost me [up to three of each]

Examples of *substances (or other addiction) gave me:* excitement; comfort; relaxation

Examples of *substances (or other addiction) cost me:* too much money; health problems; self-esteem

* *Substances gave me*
    1.
    2.
    3.

* *Substances cost me*
    1.
    2.
    3.

✧ Reflections

- Was it easier to identify positive or negative events?
- Do you notice any patterns across time?
- What has mattered most—relationships? work? recovery? something else?
- Did this exercise bring up feelings?

Ideas for a Commitment

Commit to one action that will move your life forward!
It can be anything you feel will help you, or you can try one of the ideas below.
Keeping your commitment is a way of respecting, honoring, and caring for yourself.

- Option 1. Talk to someone who knew you when you were younger. What were you like back then? (Be sure to choose a trustworthy, safe person.)

- Option 2. Search online for a TED Talk of an inspiring story of recovery from mental illness, trauma, or addiction. List an insight you gained from it.

- Option 3. Write a dialogue between *you now* and *you in the past*. What advice would you give your younger self?

- Option 4. Create scrapbook pages titled: "Past," "Present," and "Future." What would you put on those pages?

- Option 5. Take one of the ideas in Handout 2 and write or use art (e.g., music, photos, video, drawing) to explore it.

Growth

SUMMARY

In this final topic, clients identify their progress and future goals, explore feelings about ending, and share feedback about the treatment. There's also discussion of posttraumatic (and addiction) growth—how suffering can bring forth positive new meanings and sense of purpose.

ORIENTATION

We are never finished with grief. It is part of the fabric of living.
~V. S. NAIPAUL, *The Strangeness of Grief*

By now clients have learned *how* to process pain from the past, which is essential knowledge they can draw on anytime in the future. They have, it's hoped, experienced how to explore deep feelings and emotions and seen that something good can come of it.

The concept of something good arising from suffering has been studied extensively in the trauma field, with terms such as *posttraumatic growth*, *trauma wisdom*, and *stress-related growth*. Estimates indicate that 40–70% of people who survive a trauma develop some new, positive understanding from it (Calhoun & Tedeschi, 1999). It's been categorized into three main types: closer relationships, improved perceptions of self, and changed philosophies of life (Linley & Joseph, 2002). Sometimes the growth is paradoxical, such as "I am more vulnerable, yet stronger" (Tedeschi, 2004).

The addiction field, too, emphasizes that recovery means not just stopping addictive behavior (being "dry") but also developing new values, sense of purpose, and service to others (being "sober"). Addiction recovery is often viewed as a lifelong pursuit of these goals.

Today's topic has four handouts. Handout 1 explores the idea of posttraumatic (and addiction-related) growth. Handout 2 helps clients identify changes they notice in themselves. Handout 3 encourages them to take stock of where they are in their recovery, what the treatment has meant to them, and what they hope for in the future. Handout 4 offers the option to share their perceptions of different aspects of the treatment. (Counselors can also complete the questionnaire and send it to the book author.)

Clients often hold a mix of positive and negative views on these topics. Allow space for them to express their truth. Some recover without experiencing new growth (Tedeschi, 2004), so it's not helpful to create an expectation of a right way to view the work or to force a positive interpretation. Some may continue to focus mostly on their pain ("I still wish I could turn back the clock"). Recovery will be lifelong for some clients. They can say goodbye while also understanding the end as a continuation of the work.

It's best to allow multiple sessions for this topic if time allows, especially if the treatment has been lengthy or especially meaningful.

Your Emotional Reactions

Vicarious resilience is the opposite of the more well-known concept of *vicarious traumatization* (Hernández, Gangsei, & Engstrom, 2007). The latter refers to counselors becoming emotionally damaged when working with traumatized clients. The former refers to counselors becoming emotionally *stronger* from the work. Hearing clients' stories of resilience can increase your own personal and professional resilience. In a study of counselors working with survivors of torture, Hernández et al. noticed "the inspiration and strength they drew from working with clients they sometimes described as 'heroes'" (2007, p. 230). One counselor said, "This work generates a positive change as you generally may become more resourceful, less fearful, more dynamic, more resolute, more active and eager to question yourself. . . . When you witness someone coping with something like a kidnapping, you question why you don't cope better with your own losses. In other words, you develop your potential" (p. 237). Another said, "I learned about how human beings have so many resources to face tragedy, the importance of spirituality, tolerance and the ability to survive" (p. 236). Both vicarious resilience and vicarious traumatization can coexist in the same counselor, and both are important. In today's topic, as you hear clients' views on how they've changed, notice how you've changed as well.

Acknowledgments

The quotation at the start of the "Orientation" section is from Naipaul (2019). The session quotation is from Simmons (2003, p. ix).

SESSION FORMAT

1. ***Check-in*** (per Chapter 3).
2. ***Quotation.*** Link the quotation to the session topic—for example, *"As we end today, I want to honor your having shared so much about your life—both the pain and the resilience. As the quote suggests, life is a mix."*
3. ***Handouts*** (relate the topic to clients' lives):
    Handout 1: **From Pain to Growth**
    Handout 2: **Progress**
    Handout 3: **Past, Present, Future**
    Handout 4: **Creating Change Feedback Questionnaire**
4. ***Check-out*** (per Chapter 3).

SESSION CONTENT

Goals

- ☐ Discuss posttraumatic (and addiction) growth.
- ☐ Help clients notice their progress.
- ☐ Explore how it feels to end the treatment.
- ☐ Identify clients' goals and hopes for the future.
- ☐ Elicit feedback about the treatment.

Ways to Relate the Material to Clients' Lives

★ *Help clients identify growth arising from pain (Handout 1).* This is the concept of post-traumatic (and addiction-related) growth. The handout briefly describes the concept and asks clients to notice whether they've experienced it. But it's important not to push clients to find something positive. As one client said, "Oh, here's where I'm supposed to find the silver lining to rape." Some clients may feel nothing positive has come of their adversity and that needs to be respected.

★ *Recognize clients' progress (Handout 2).* The list in the handout can help clients honor changes they've made thus far. It's written as quotes from clients so as to be emotionally powerful rather than simply a list of symptoms.

★ *Share your perception of how each client has changed (Handout 2).* It's very moving for clients to hear what you notice about them. The more specific you are, individualizing your feedback to each client, the more meaningful it is. You can also reflect on realistic ups and downs you observed and what you view as their next steps in recovery.

★ *Process the ending of the treatment (Handout 3).* Handout 3 offers discussion questions. You can let each client choose one to speak about. Or, depending on available time, clients can write out answers to several, perhaps one from each section, and then read their answers aloud. Emphasize that there are no right or wrong reactions. Some may be anxious or sad about ending; others may feel relieved. Some may be appreciative of the work; others may be disappointed at not achieving as much progress as they hoped for or may feel pessimistic about their future.

★ *Encourage honest feedback about the treatment (Handout 4).* Clients may have ideas on how to improve the delivery of Creating Change or feedback for you as a counselor. Even if you don't agree with their point of view, validate their honesty. "Thanks for sharing that" is typically enough of a response, especially if it's the final session. Clients can give you their Creating Change Feedback Questionnaire once they complete it. In addition, if you or they want to provide feedback to the author, there's an online version of the form at *www.creating-change.org*, or it can be mailed or emailed. The feedback can help improve the model, and clients like to know that their opinions have an impact.

★ *Express your feelings about ending.* This is also an opportunity for you to model how to say goodbye and how to sit with feelings of sadness and loss. For example, "I'm so impressed by what you've done here over these many months. It's bittersweet that this is our last session. I welcome you to send me updates any time."

★ *Discuss the concept of* **victim, survivor,** *and* **thriver.** This recovery framework arose in the trauma field but is also relevant to addiction. After describing each of these, ask clients which they identify with most.

Victim. A trauma *victim* is overwhelmed by the trauma. The term is often used judgmentally in the culture at large ("She's such a victim!") but is actually a natural starting point in recovery. People who never acknowledge being a victim may be in denial about what happened, rather than recognizing their vulnerability. In addiction, the term *victim* wouldn't be used, but rather being "powerless over the addiction" or "admitting an addiction problem."

Survivor. This is someone who's actively working on healing. Even while still struggling with the impact of trauma or addiction, there's a sense of hope and increased strength.

Thriver. Thrivers live with a sense of purpose, have a healthy outlook, practice self-care, maintain positive relationships, and enjoy life.

★ *Address aftercare.* Offer referrals and clarify whether clients have the option to return to treatment with you in the future. Emphasize the importance of reaching out for help as needs arise in the future.

★ *Discussion*
  • Handout 3 has the discussion questions for today's topic.

Suggestions

✦ ***Allow two or more sessions to process the ending, depending on your treatment context.*** The number of sessions will depend on your setting (whether clients are ending treatment altogether or just Creating Change), modality (individual vs. group), type of group (closed or open), length of treatment, and level of attachment that developed. Allow enough time to process the ending in a way that feels complete. One challenge in open groups is clients ending at different times. For that scenario, you could take a few minutes at the end of the session to allow the departing client to say goodbye.

✦ ***Consider offering a certificate.*** Clients value this and you can either reward *attendance* (listing how many sessions they came to) or treatment *completion* (if you had a minimum number of required sessions, typically 12 or more). Chapter 3 has an attendance certificate or you can search online for other examples.

✦ ***Encourage clients to fill out a brief assessment on trauma and/or addiction.*** You can search online for "free validated trauma symptom assessment" and "free validated addiction assessment." Choose reputable sites from universities, nonprofit agencies, or government. Help clients score the measure and learn what the scores mean.

Tough Cases

* "I don't feel any better."
* "Am I done working on the past?"
* "Posttraumatic growth sounds like BS."
* "Can I call you when I'm in trouble?"
* "I'm afraid of becoming suicidal with treatment ending."

Growth

Quotation

"Life is both more and less than we hoped for. . . .
We've known the dark woods but also the moon."

~ Philip E. Simmons, 20th-century American writer

HANDOUT 1

From Pain to Growth

Has a difficult event made you stronger or better in some way?

In the trauma field, this is called *posttraumatic growth* or *trauma wisdom*. It also applies to addiction recovery.

For example, some people find that overcoming difficulties leads to:

✦ Closer relationships
✦ An improved sense of self
✦ Greater appreciation of life
✦ Spirituality
✦ A new sense of purpose

But it's not saying you would have chosen trauma or addiction or that it was good these things happened. There's also no pressure to find something positive if you don't feel it.

Painful experience	⇨	**Growth that came from it**
My husband died.	⇨	I learned how to grieve.
I became an alcoholic.	⇨	I discovered spirituality in AA.
I was bullied online.	⇨	I reduced social media and expanded my real life.

✧ **And you?**

Has your trauma or addiction led to growth?

Painful experience		**Growth that came from it**
_____	⇨	_____
_____	⇨	_____

Add more: How did the growth come about? What about it are you most proud of?

_____
_____
_____

From *Creating Change* by Lisa M. Najavits. Copyright © 2024 Lisa M. Najavits. Published by The Guilford Press. Permission to photocopy this material is granted to purchasers of this book for use with your own clients or patients; see copyright page for details.

HANDOUT 2   Growth

Progress

> "When you've been down so long, hating yourself, you don't take for granted what it feels like to be up. There's a greater sense of appreciation. You don't forget."
> ~MELANIE, in long-term recovery from trauma and addiction

Below are quotes from people who progressed in recovery.

★ *Check off any that are true for you and add your own as well. If desired, circle ones that you haven't yet accomplished but want to in the future.*

___ 1. "I can forgive myself. I really feel it. It's not just words."
___ 2. "I take better care of my body."
___ 3. "When I get addiction cravings, I can let them pass."
___ 4. "I'm no longer afraid of my memories."
___ 5. "I learned who my real friends are."
___ 6. "I'm more responsible; my word means something now."
___ 7. "I found things I care about more than drinking."
___ 8. "I became a better parent by nurturing myself more."
___ 9. "I learned I don't have to rebel to be seen and heard.'"
___ 10. "I'm stronger than I thought I was."
___ 11. "I stopped keeping secrets."
___ 12. "I'm more than my trauma/addiction."
___ 13. "I know who I am now. I'm not a stranger to myself anymore."
___ 14. "I learned it's OK to feel what I feel."
___ 15. "Things that used to throw me, I can handle now."
___ 16. "I came to see my worst behaviors as expression of pain."
___ 17. "I can be sexual now without getting triggered."
___ 18. "I don't lie as much."
___ 19. "I figured out why things went the way they did."
___ 20. "I discovered that I want to live."
___ 21. "I learned to protect myself more."
___ 22. "I see that progress is possible, even with ups and downs."
___ 23. "I've become able to reach out for help."
___ 24. "I understand now that facing the truth is always best."
___ 25. "I can choose people who treat me well."
___ 26. "I no longer lash out at people."
___ 27. "I have a future to look forward to."
___ 28. Others? _____

From *Creating Change* by Lisa M. Najavits. Copyright © 2024 Lisa M. Najavits. Published by The Guilford Press. Permission to photocopy this material is granted to purchasers of this book for use with your own clients or patients; see copyright page for details.

HANDOUT 3 Growth

Past, Present, Future

★ *Choose one question or more and share your answers.*

About Your Recovery

- What does *recovery* mean to you?

- How solid is your addiction recovery? Your trauma recovery?

- What are you most proud of?

- What helped along the way?

- What wisdom would you offer other survivors of trauma/addiction?

About This Treatment

- How does it feel to end?

- What was most/least helpful about this treatment?

- Are there particular moments that were especially meaningful for you?

- Is there anything about the treatment you wish had been different?

- What are the top three things you learned?

About the Future

- How do you still want to change?

- What can you put in place to help achieve your goals?

- How can you hold on to what you've already gained?

- What would you like to contribute to the world?

Would you like to provide feedback about Creating Change?

Visit *www.creating-change.org* to share your suggestions, or you can complete Handout 4 (Creating Change Feedback Questionnaire).

From *Creating Change* by Lisa M. Najavits. Copyright © 2024 Lisa M. Najavits. Published by The Guilford Press. Permission to photocopy this material is granted to purchasers of this book for use with your own clients or patients; see copyright page for details.

HANDOUT 4   Growth

Creating Change Feedback Questionnaire

Your honest feedback is greatly appreciated.

Answer only the questions you choose to. At the end, you'll see instructions for sending it.

Thank you!!

How many sessions of Creating Change have you done? _____ [fill in number]

How many sessions did it take you to feel *comfortable* with this treatment? _____ [fill in number]

Please rate the questions below from 0% (not at all) to 100% (greatly):
- How helpful is Creating Change *overall*? _____%
- How helpful is Creating Change for *trauma*? _____%
- How helpful is Creating Change for *addiction*? _____%
- How *much will you use* what you learned in this treatment in the future? _____%
- How *easy to understand* is this treatment? _____%
- How *innovative* (creative, new) is this treatment? _____%
- How much would you *recommend* this treatment to someone else? _____%

How helpful are the *parts* of the book:
- The focus on the *past*? _____%
- *Integrated* treatment (addressing trauma and addiction together)? _____%
- The *quotations*? _____%
- The *session format (check-in/check-out, etc.)*? _____%
- The *handouts*? _____%
- The *commitments* (homework between sessions)? _____%

In your own words:
- What do you consider the *best/worst aspects* of this treatment model?

- What *modifications* would you like to see (e.g., topics to add or delete?)

- Did you experience any negative impact of the treatment (significant problem or harm)?

- Are there specific *types of people* you feel the program is especially helpful/unhelpful for?

- Any *other comments*?

You can hand in this questionnaire to your counselor and/or send it to Dr. Lisa Najavits, the author of *Creating Change*, in any of the following ways:

    Online form: *www.creating-change.org*
    Email: info@treatment-innovations.org
    Mail: Treatment Innovations, 28 Westbourne Rd., Newton, MA 02459

From *Creating Change* by Lisa M. Najavits. Copyright © 2024 Lisa M. Najavits. Published by The Guilford Press. Permission to photocopy this material, or to download and print additional copies (*www.guilford.com/najavits3-materials*), is granted to purchasers of this book for use with your own clients or patients; see copyright page for details.

Growth

Idea for a Commitment

✦ *Continue to grow in your recovery.* Let yourself grieve when you need to. Keep learning. Take pride in who you are and what you survived. Find others who share your vision of what life can be. Always remember that it is within you to change.

Extra Topic
Understanding Trauma and Addiction

SUMMARY

Today's topic offers education about trauma and addiction and conveys the message that *recovery is possible*. It also includes a screening tool for behavioral addictions, which is recommended for all clients as these often go undetected (e.g., food, pornography, shopping, work, gambling). If desired, you can engage the client's family or other important supports in the session as well. This topic is "extra" because some clients are already knowledgeable about trauma and addiction, but others can benefit from deepening their understanding. It can be conducted at any time based on your view of client needs.

ORIENTATION

Trauma and addiction are experienced every day in clients' lives, among the most common of experiences, yet often remain hidden and silent, steeped in shame. For a long time, these issues went unaddressed in treatment programs, in the media, and in the culture at large. It's thus healing, in and of itself, for clients to learn more about trauma and addiction. They may have these issues yet not be educated about them.

For clients with both trauma and addiction, it's also important for them to understand the linkages between them. Jade, a survivor of child sexual abuse, said, "If you get sober as you work on trauma, it will save you years of grief."

Yet even with greater attention to trauma and addiction in recent decades, there's typically attention to just one or the other. Clients with addiction enter addiction treatment, where trauma often goes unaddressed. Clients with trauma enter mental health treatment, where addiction often goes unaddressed. *Integrated treatment*—treating both at once, by the same provider—is still not the norm in many places.

In addition to educating clients, today's topic is useful for exploring clients' attitudes toward trauma and addiction. How do they talk about these? How compassionate are they? Do they see the linkages between them if they have both? How hopeful are they about recovery from each?

There are four handouts. Handout 1 teaches the basics of trauma; Handout 2 teaches the basics of addiction; Handout 3 is an educational tip sheet for people in clients' life; and Handout 4 is the Excessive Behavior Scale, which assesses for behavioral addictions that often go undetected.

When possible, it's also helpful to use today's topic to involve clients' social support network: family, friends, advocates, sponsors, or other helpers. It's said that for every person with addiction it impacts five others around them (and the same can be said for trauma). Handout 3, the tip sheet, is written for them, but you can guide clients to share the other handouts as well. This builds increased empathy for clients and encourages others to seek out their own help if they too have trauma or addiction. The goal is a widening circle of understanding of trauma and addiction.

As a reminder, however, clients don't have to have trauma or addiction to participate in Creating Change. The model can be used with anyone who wants to come to terms with the past, related to a wide range of problems, such as interpersonal conflicts, loss, depression, and self-esteem issues. Many problems have roots in the past.

Your Emotional Reactions

Trauma and addiction evoke wide-ranging and sometimes intense emotional responses, including:

- Rescue fantasies
- Disappointment when clients don't progress
- Frustration when clients lie or hide addiction
- Guilt at not being able to do enough
- Judgment about clients' decisions and actions.

Many emotional reactions that counselors experience stem from a sense of needing to do more, better, faster. The pressure comes from identification with clients' suffering and also from treatment systems that expect so much from their staff. Yet the problems and solutions are long term, a marathon rather than a sprint.

All of the usual methods can be helpful: Keep working on your own emotional growth, talk with supportive colleagues, and seek supervision when possible. Another method that's less commonly emphasized is getting on the internet with clients during the session to teach them how to search for help outside of your sessions. Outside resources create a wider safety net that can alleviate your sense of sole responsibility. The more clients engage other supports, the easier it is to sustain yourself through the ups and downs of treatment.

Acknowledgments

The session quotation is a modernized version, widely available online, of the actual Douglass quote from his 1882 speech about freed slaves: "Judge them leniently, and measure their progress, not from the heights to which they may in time attain, but from the depths from which they have come." All of the handouts are adapted from Najavits (2019). In Handout 1, the concept of trauma as physical events is from DSM-5-TR (American Psychiatric Association, 2022); trauma as emotional events is from SAMHSA (2014); see also online Appendix A, "Key Terms" (*www.guilford.com/najavits3-materials*). In Handout 2, the opening quotation is from Weiss and Schneider (2015).

PREPARING FOR THE SESSION

Several optional free brief screening tools are mentioned later in this chapter (in the bullet point "Offer clients a free screening tool for trauma, PTSD, and/or addiction" on page 324). If you plan to use any, obtain them ahead of time either electronically or in hard copy.

Extra Topic: Understanding Trauma and Addiction

SESSION FORMAT

1. *Check-in* (per Chapter 3).
2. *Quotation.* Link the quotation to the session topic—for example, *"Today we'll talk about trauma and addiction. The quote encourages compassion for your challenges (the depths you have to climb)."*
3. *Handouts* (relate the topic to clients' lives):
    Handout 1: **What Is Trauma?**
    Handout 2: **What Is Addiction?**
    Handout 3: **Tip Sheet to Support the Client**
    Handout 4: **Excessive Behavior Scale (Behavioral Addictions)**
4. *Check-out* (per Chapter 3).

SESSION CONTENT

Goals

- ☐ Provide education on trauma and addiction.
- ☐ Help clients identify whether they have trauma and/or addiction problems.
- ☐ Offer a screening tool for behavioral addictions.
- ☐ Discuss how clients' safe supports can help.
- ☐ Emphasize that recovery is possible.

Ways to Relate the Material to Clients' Lives

★ *Ask clients to circle symptoms they've experienced (Handouts 1 and 2).* Each lists different types of trauma and addiction and examples of symptoms. These can launch a meaningful conversation.

★ *Conduct a brief knowledge game in group treatment (Handouts 1 and 2).* Before showing the handouts, you could do a group game, giving a point to anyone who can "name three trauma symptoms," "say what 'PTSD' stands for," "give two examples of behavioral addictions," and so on.

★ *Encourage clients to involve their safe supports (Handout 3).* Coach clients on how to share the handout effectively. For example, they can say what they'd like others to understand (e.g., "I just want you to know that I'm working hard on my recovery and it's not easy"). You could also have clients invite in any of their trusted others for an educational support session to go over the handouts, but this would typically be done only in individual treatment. For more on that process, see the section "Consider Inviting the Client's Safe Supports (e.g., Family or Friends) to Specific Sessions" in Chapter 3. Additional guidance is in the book *Seeking Safety* (the topic "Getting Others to Support Your Recovery") and in the book *Finding Your Best Self* (the appendix "How Others Can Help—Family, Friends, Partners, Sponsors"). An excellent free resource is Al-Anon for family and friends of people with addiction. Also, refer clients to family treatment as needed.

★ *Help them fill out the Excessive Behavior Scale (Handout 4).* The instructions are straightforward, but clients may need guidance in moving through the measure. Behavioral addictions—those that don't involve substances—may be unfamiliar as they're typically not assessed in treatment programs. The scale is an efficient way to evaluate a wide range of addictions, but you may also want to provide validated measures for specific ones.

★ *Show clients how to get additional information on trauma and addiction.* Model a spirit of curiosity and persistence. Only the most motivated clients will pursue resources on their own, so taking time in the session to demonstrate the learning process is useful. Using their mobile phone or sitting at a computer together, you can show clients how to search the internet, emphasizing reputable sources. Use search terms for areas that are important to them ("trauma treatment for veterans," "gender differences in addiction," etc.). Help them identify good trauma and addiction mobile apps as well, for example, to track their symptoms.

★ *Offer clients a free screening tool for trauma, PTSD, and/or addiction.* There are many validated screens online including the following.

For **trauma**:
- Stressful Life Experiences Screening Questionnaire
- Life Events Checklist for DSM-5
- Child and Adolescent Trauma Screen (includes a PTSD screen)

For **PTSD**:
- PTSD Checklist for DSM-5
- Primary Care PTSD Screen for DSM-5

For **addiction**:
- CAGE Questionnaire
- Michigan Alcohol Screening Scale (MAST)
- Drug Abuse Screening Test
- Brief Addiction Monitor
- Binge Eating Disorder Screener–7 (seven-item version)
- Lie/Bet Screen for gambling disorder

★ *Evaluate for diagnoses, if needed.* It may be relevant to also assess clients for psychiatric diagnoses related to trauma and addiction, rather than just using the screening tools above. Many clients don't know they have such diagnoses even if they've had them for years (e.g., PTSD, substance use disorder, depression, anxiety disorders). Refer clients to a trained assessor unless you're able to conduct a diagnostic assessment yourself. A full diagnostic workup of all major psychiatric disorders is optimal, if possible, as trauma and addiction are comorbid with other conditions that should be directly treated as well.

★ *Discussion*
- "What trauma problems do you most want help with?"
- "What addiction problems do you most want help with?"
- "Have you ever talked to anyone about your trauma? your addiction? How did it go?"
- "Do you believe that recovery is possible for you?"
- "Do any feelings come up as you look at these handouts?"
- "Is there anyone you want to share the handouts with?"

Suggestions

✦ *Help clients bring compassion toward their trauma and addiction.* Offer warm, generous statements such as "You deserve a lot of credit for surviving all that you have"; see Chapter 3 for more examples. In today's list of Commitments, there's also a link to a self-compassion scale that's useful to do in the session if you have time.

✦ *Adjust the focus based on clients' level of knowledge.* It's common for clients to have greater knowledge of one area over another (trauma or addiction) based on their prior history of services. If they had primarily addiction treatment, for example, they may know much less about trauma. Provide education and assessment as needed to ensure a solid foundation in whatever areas apply to them.

✦ *Create a plan to reduce addictive behavior.* See the section "Best Practices in Addiction Treatment" in Chapter 4 for essential, practical ideas to reduce addiction, including a written plan specifying limits on the amount of use.

Extra Topic: Understanding Trauma and Addiction

✦ *If behavioral addictions are identified, provide referrals.* There are 12-step groups for many behavioral addictions, such as Overeaters Anonymous, Gamblers Anonymous, Sexaholics Anonymous, and Co-Dependents Anonymous, and there are phone and Zoom meetings for those who can't attend in person. Also, encourage clients to search online to learn more about behavioral addictions.

✦ *Offer clients a list of crisis helplines.* There is an extensive list of them in Handout 2 in the topic "Trust versus Doubt."

✦ *Consider adding some Seeking Safety topics.* Some that are especially relevant to today's topic are "PTSD: Taking Back Your Power" (more detail on trauma and how to take a compassionate approach toward it); "When Substances Control You" (more detail on addiction and how to reduce it); and, as mentioned earlier, "Getting Others to Support Your Recovery" (education on trauma and addiction for clients' family or close friends).

Tough Cases

* "I have to keep gambling to win back what I lost."
* "Have you had trauma? I can't trust you unless I know."
* "I work three jobs because I need the money. Do I have work addiction?"
* "In AA they say don't sit on the 'pity pot,' so why are you going on about trauma?"
* "People tell me I'm addicted to _____, but I know I'm not."
* "I don't have any supportive people in my life."

Extra Topic: Understanding Trauma and Addiction

Quotation

"You are not judged by the height you have risen, but from the depth you have climbed."

~ Frederick Douglass, 19th-century American escaped slave, writer, activist

HANDOUT 1

What Is Trauma?

"Starting at the moment that the bomb went off, I had a mental video and audio of that day's experiences that played 24 hours a day, along with everything else I was doing."

~Paul Heath, survivor of the Oklahoma City bombing

TRAUMA MEANS "WOUND"

Trauma comes from the Greek word for "wound." It's a serious, unwanted, harmful event that may lead to lasting pain. The wounds may be physical, emotional, or both. Most people have at least one in their lifetime and some have many.

Although the past can't be redone, you can change how you relate to it. You can heal.

TYPES OF TRAUMA

Traumas can be *physical events:*

• car accident • sexual assault • military combat • physical violence • fire hurricane or other natural disaster • major illness or injury • domestic violence • sudden death of someone close to you • industrial accident • terrorist incident • chronic physical pain

Traumas can also be *emotional events:*

• emotional abuse • bullying • growing up with mentally ill parents • neglect • abandonment • homelessness • major loss • severe social rejection • poverty • discrimination

They may happen directly to a person or be threatened or witnessed.

(cont.)

Adapted from *Finding Your Best Self, Revised Edition: Recovery from Addiction, Trauma, or Both* by Lisa M. Najavits (2019). Permission to photocopy or download this material (*www.guilford.com/najavits3-materials*), is granted to purchasers of this book for use with your own clients or patients; see copyright page for details.

HANDOUT 1 *(p. 2 of 3)*   Extra Topic: Understanding Trauma and Addiction

WHO EXPERIENCES TRAUMA?

In earlier eras, trauma was only identified in men coming back from war, with terms such as *shell shock* and *combat fatigue*.

But it's now clear that trauma occurs across all types of people. It also occurs in organizations such as sports teams and religious groups. Whole communities can be affected by trauma as well, such as during natural disasters.

TRAUMA PROBLEMS

Trauma can have direct and sometimes lasting impact, including . . .

> \+ depression + distrust + nightmares + relationship problems + anger + spaciness + flashbacks + shame, guilt + dissociation (the mind shuts down) + wanting to die + impulse to hurt yourself or others + physical health problems + fear of being attacked even when there's no threat + poor concentration + difficulty remembering parts of the trauma + physical problems that your doctor can't explain + panic + paranoia + giving up + a belief that you're no good + thoughts that you can't get out of your mind

In children, trauma problems may show up in play rather than in words.

It's Not a Personal Failure

You're not weak or crazy for having trauma problems. They've been called *a normal reaction to abnormal events*—your reactions make sense after what you've been through.

Yet people react differently to the same type of trauma. The intensity of trauma problems varies based on various factors:

- *How physically damaging the trauma was.* Being raped is more distressing than witnessing a street fight, for example.
- *How others reacted.* Some people get compassionate support after trauma; others are isolated and shamed.
- *How well you were doing before trauma.* If you were having a hard time, trauma may be harder to deal with than if you were feeling strong and happy.
- *Your family history.* A history of mental illness or addiction in your family can make you more likely to develop problems after trauma.

It's Medical

Trauma can lead to various mental health conditions:

- *Acute stress disorder* is immediate distress that lasts up to a month after a trauma.
- *Posttraumatic stress disorder* (PTSD) lasts for more than a month and sometimes for years.
- *Adjustment disorder* refers to difficulty coping with a stressful event. Adjustment disorders usually resolve quickly.
- *Dissociative identity disorder* is rare but can arise from extreme, repeated childhood trauma. The main characteristic is having fragmented identity—different "alters" (personalities).

(cont.)

HANDOUT 1 *(p. 3 of 3)* Extra Topic: Understanding Trauma and Addiction

Trauma impacts both the brain and the body. In addition to mental health conditions, trauma, especially if repeated and severe, is associated with physical health problems, too.

Learn More

Search online using terms such as "the impact of trauma," "PTSD," "mental health and trauma," "physical health and trauma." You can also find free online measures to identify trauma problems, such as the *PTSD Checklist*.

HANDOUT 2 — Extra Topic: Understanding Trauma and Addiction

What Is Addiction?

> "In those rare times lately when I sit back and take stock of myself, I can see that I'm spending hour after hour, evenings and weekends, just sitting around staring at porn. Instead of actually having 'a life,' I've lost precious hours, days, weeks, months, even years in isolation and loneliness. . . . I don't know what it is to have a real relationship because all I've ever experienced is webcam hookups and porn."
> ~Client with sex addiction (quoted in Weiss & Schneider, 2015)

People can become addicted to anything that gives pleasure or relief. Everyone wants to enjoy life, but if you can't put the brakes on a behavior that's causing problems, it's time to look at it clearly yet with compassion.

Addiction is an illness—it's not just wanting to have a good time or lack of willpower. It has biological and social causes, "nature and nurture."

ADDICTION MEANS "CAN'T STOP"

Addiction comes from Latin roots for *enslavement*, which perfectly describes what serious addiction feels like.

Addiction can be *mild*, *moderate*, or *severe*.

Addiction means that you continue a behavior even when it's causing harm:

- You drink after your doctor tells you it's causing liver disease.
- You gamble despite being in debt.
- You have affairs even if it means your partner leaves you.

People without addiction would stop. People with addiction may want to stop but can't—they feel more and more out of control. Or they think it's not a problem even though others can see it.

KEY SIGNS OF ADDICTION

Signs of addiction include:

+ You feel ashamed of it.
+ You're unable to stop.
+ You lie or hide to cover it up.
+ You can't imagine life without it.
+ Others complain, but you don't think it's a problem.
+ It takes up too much time or money.
+ You need to do it more and more.
+ It becomes too big a part of your life.
+ It gets in the way of being responsible at work, as a parent, and so on.

(cont.)

From *Creating Change* by Lisa M. Najavits. Copyright © 2024 Lisa M. Najavits. Published by The Guilford Press. Permission to photocopy this material, or to download and print additional copies (*www.guilford.com/najavits3-materials*), is granted to purchasers of this book for use with your own clients or patients; see copyright page for details.

HANDOUT 2 *(p. 2 of 2)*   Extra Topic: Understanding Trauma and Addiction

You may have a problem even if you don't fit the classic image of an addict. You may be successful in other areas of your life, may be kind and decent, and may take good care of yourself otherwise. People who look good on the outside are the least likely to be noticed as having an addiction, such as professionals and those who are well-off.

MANY TYPES OF ADDICTION

Substance Addiction

Substance addiction is common and what most people think of as "addiction." There are four basic types:

- *"Downers"* (*depressants* such as alcohol, Valium, and Seconal)
- *"Uppers"* (*stimulants* such as cocaine, Ecstasy, speed, and methamphetamine)
- *Opioids* (such as heroin and OxyContin)
- *Hallucinogens* (such as LSD, peyote, and hallucinogenic mushrooms)

And some substances are a mix, such as marijuana.

Behavioral Addictions

Other behaviors can also become addictive, such as:

• gambling • shopping or spending • sex, pornography • electronics (e.g., gaming, television, social media) • work • exercise • hobbies • self-harm such as cutting

Behavioral addictions are less studied than substance addiction but are recognized more and more. They can be just as addictive as substances and evoke similar brain changes.

A NEW PERSPECTIVE LINKING ADDICTION AND TRAUMA

It's now clear that addiction and trauma often go together.

Usually, trauma occurs first, then addiction. It makes sense—substances and other addictive behavior can be an attempt to cope with emotional pain. After trauma, people often want to feel *more* of something, such as energy or calm; or *less* of something, such as rage, hurt, or self-hatred.

RECOVERY IS POSSIBLE

Whatever type of addiction you have, it can get better. David, a man in recovery from trauma and addiction, wrote:

"Living in recovery is like gradually waking up from a long, nightmare-filled sleep. It is discovering pale days slowly fading into warm, colorful transforming experiences rich with meaning and joy."

LEARN MORE

Keep learning. Search online using terms such as "definition of addiction," "the impact of addiction," "alcohol and drug problems," "addiction and trauma," "how to identify addiction problems," and "screening measures for addiction/trauma." See also Handout 4, the Excessive Behavior Scale.

HANDOUT 3 Extra Topic: Understanding Trauma and Addiction

Tip Sheet to Support the Client

★ *You can give this sheet to anyone in your life who's supportive and safe for you (partner, family, friends, sponsor, advocate, or others). You can also share other handouts from today's session or future sessions, if you want.*

❖ **How you can support the client during Creating Change counseling**

- Provide warm support as the person goes through this treatment.
- Learn about trauma and addiction (search online and see the resources listed below).
- Obtain help you need for yourself (counseling? Al-Anon?).
- You can invite the person to tell you about the content of counseling sessions but please never insist.
- Be patient with ups and downs.
- Allow the person emotional space to feel what comes up, without judging the feelings as right or wrong.
- Please don't encourage the person to explore the past with you; it's best if this occurs only in counseling for now.
- Be supportive but remember you should never tolerate any physical danger or emotional abuse.
- **If you become concerned about the person, be sure to contact the counselor below;** the goal is safety. *Note:* You can always provide information to the counselor even if the counselor cannot share details with you (the client would have to sign off on that).

❖ **How to reach the counselor (name, phone, and/or email)**

_____

_____

❖ **Emergency plan**

- Dial or text 988 for crisis/suicide hotline (free, confidential, 24/7)
- List additional emergency plans, if applicable, here:

_____

_____

❖ **For more information**

- *Creating Change counseling*
  www.creating-change.org
- *Addiction*
  www.samhsa.gov (click on "Find Help" or "Public Messages")
  www.al-anon.org
- *Trauma*
  www.nctsn.org (for families and children)
  www.ptsd.va.gov

From *Creating Change* by Lisa M. Najavits. Copyright © 2024 Lisa M. Najavits. Published by The Guilford Press. Permission to photocopy this material, or to download and print additional copies (*www.guilford.com/najavits3-materials*), is granted to purchasers of this book for use with your own clients or patients; see copyright page for details.

HANDOUT 4 — Extra Topic: Understanding Trauma and Addiction

Excessive Behavior Scale (Behavioral Addictions)

PART I: TYPES OF EXCESSIVE BEHAVIORS

Almost any behavior can become a problem if you do it too much. This screening tool allows you to identify excessive behaviors that might be *behavioral addictions*.

Some people have a problem with too much gambling, eating, sex, shopping, work, exercise, social media, pornography, hair pulling, skin picking, tanning, or tattooing.

You may notice an excessive behavior based on any of the following signs:

- You spend too much time on it.
- You can't stop.
- The toll it takes—money problems, family or social problems (people complaining about the behavior), medical or legal problems.
- Control issues: Sometimes it makes you feel more in control, but other times like you've lost control.
- The compulsion to do it.
- Craving it.

If you identify any problem behavior here, you can ask your counselor or other mental health support for guidance. You can also find information online.

★ **Circle each behavior that *may have been excessive for you for at least 1 month in the past year*.**
Base it on what you notice about yourself or what others say about you. You don't have to be certain about it. Be honest even if you are embarrassed or unsure.

	Excessive for at least 1 month in the past year?
Gambling (lottery, sports betting, poker, keno, etc.)	Yes / Maybe / No
Alcohol or drugs (cocaine, marijuana, heroin, oxycodone, etc.) List which (if more than one, pick the worst):	Yes / Maybe / No
Working (beyond what is needed)	Yes / Maybe / No
A leisure activity (TV; a hobby such as fishing, crafting, fantasy football) List which:	Yes / Maybe / No
Exercising or doing a sport (running, baseball, etc.)	Yes / Maybe / No
Food (too much or too little, i.e., bingeing or restricting) List which:	Yes / Maybe / No

(cont.)

From *Finding Your Best Self, Revised Edition: Recovery from Addiction, Trauma, or Both* by Lisa M. Najavits. Copyright © 2019 Lisa M. Najavits. Adapted in *Creating Change* (The Guilford Press, 2024). The scale cannot be adapted without advance written permission from info@treatment-innovations.org. Permission to photocopy this material, or to download and print additional copies (www.guilford.com/najavits3-materials), is granted to purchasers of this book for use with your own clients or patients; see copyright page for details.

HANDOUT 4 *(p. 2 of 3)*   Extra Topic: Understanding Trauma and Addiction

	Excessive for at least 1 month in the past year?
Electronics (texting, email, internet, social media, computer games) List which:	Yes / Maybe / No
Body improvement (such as tattooing, plastic surgery, tanning) List which:	Yes / Maybe / No
A nervous habit (such as hair pulling, skin picking, chewing ice) List which:	Yes / Maybe / No
Sex-related activities (such as pornography, sex, sexual fetishes) List which:	Yes / Maybe / No
Too loose with money (such as shopping or overspending) List which:	Yes / Maybe / No
Too tight with money (such as acquiring or hoarding money) List which:	Yes / Maybe / No
Hurting self or others physically (cutting, burning, hitting, etc.) List whether self or others: List which type of behavior:	Yes / Maybe / No
Criminal activity (stealing, setting fires, etc.) List which:	Yes / Maybe / No
Relationships (co-dependency or "love addiction") List which:	Yes / Maybe / No
A specific emotion (anger, sadness, etc.) List which:	Yes / Maybe / No
Others? List which:	Yes / Maybe / No

(cont.)

HANDOUT 4 *(p. 3 of 3)*   Extra Topic: Understanding Trauma and Addiction

PART II: SCREENING QUESTIONS

Step 1. Take the *first* excessive behavior that you checked as "yes" or "maybe" in Part I and answer the eight questions below in relation to that behavior.

For example, if you checked "yes" or "maybe" for *gambling*, answer the eight questions in relation to it.

In the Comments box, list any details that clarify your answers.

When you think about your worst month* of that behavior in the past year . . .					Comments?
1. How much were you caught up in the behavior (doing it, thinking about it, craving it, etc.)?	Not at all (0)	Somewhat (1)	A lot (2)	A great deal (3)	
2. How ashamed are/were you about the behavior?	Not at all (0)	Somewhat (1)	A lot (2)	A great deal (3)	
3. How serious a problem was the behavior?	Not at all (0)	Somewhat (1)	A lot (2)	A great deal (3)	
4. Did you have losses from the behavior? (relationships, job, home, time, money, physical or emotional health, opportunities, etc.)	Not at all (0)	Somewhat (1)	A lot (2)	A great deal (3)	
5. How successful were you at decreasing the behavior?	Not at all (0)	Somewhat (1)	A lot (2)	A great deal (3)	
6. How much control did you have over the behavior?	Not at all (0)	Somewhat (1)	A lot (2)	A great deal (3)	
7. How much did others say you had a problem with the behavior?	Not at all (0)	Somewhat (1)	A lot (2)	A great deal (3)	
8. Any other sign that the behavior was excessive? List the sign: _____ Rate it on the scale.	Not at all (0)	Somewhat (1)	A lot (2)	A great deal (3)	

*"**Worst month**" means the month in which you were most excessive in the behavior. For example, if your behavior was gambling, it would be the month in the past year in which you spent the most time/money on gambling or suffered the most severe consequences of gambling (getting into a major fight over it, losing your job over it, etc.). Note that "worst" is not a judgment of you—it's just identifying the most severe month of the behavior, in your opinion.

Step 2. Scoring: Add up the numbers you circled (one per row). The minimum score is 0; the maximum is 24. The higher your score, the more likely you have a problem.

Step 3. Now go back to your list in Part I, take the next behavior where you checked "yes" or "maybe," and fill in the same eight questions for that behavior. Continue to do that for each behavior you said "yes" or "maybe" to in Part I.

WHAT'S NEXT?

If you identify any problem behavior, seek information and help. Talk to anyone who is helping you with recovery, such as your counselor or sponsor. Also search online using terms such as "I have a problem with _____" or "I am doing _____ too much." Be honest with yourself and others about problem behaviors so you can work on them.

Extra Topic: Understanding Trauma and Addiction

Ideas for a Commitment

Commit to one action that will move your life forward!
It can be anything you feel will help you, or you can try one of the ideas below.
Keeping your commitment is a way of respecting, honoring, and caring for yourself.

- Option 1. Fill out the *Self-Compassion Scale* (link below). How can you increase self-compassion for your trauma or addiction?

    https://self-compassion.org/test-how-self-compassionate-you-are

- Option 2. Write about today's quotation. What is the "depth you have climbed"? What is the "height" you want to rise to?

- Option 3. Fill out Handout 4. If you identify problem behaviors, seek more information (the bottom of the handout has suggestions).

- Option 4. Learn more about trauma and/or addiction. Search online, find a library book, or ask your counselor, sponsor, or other recovery support person.

Extra Topic
Recovery Strengths and Challenges

SUMMARY

Today's topic addresses client strengths and challenges that may relate to participation in Creating Change (e.g., current psychosis, domestic violence). It can be used at the start of treatment or at any point. This topic is "extra" because many clients won't need it. You may already know the client well and/or the client appears ready to start Creating Change (or the three-session try-out of the model per Chapter 3).

ORIENTATION

Clients who engage in Creating Change span a wide range of severity and settings. The model was specifically designed for this breadth per the features described in Chapter 1. It's been used successfully with highly vulnerable clients as part of both clinical implementation and research per the "Evidence Base" section in Chapter 1.

Yet sometimes it's important to evaluate clients' level of functioning. At the start of treatment, you may not know a client well or may have concerns based on what you do know. During the course of treatment, clients' symptoms may increase, and it can be useful to evaluate how they're doing. If clients are in fact struggling with major impairments, the goal is to collaborate on a plan for improvement.

Today's topic offers several methods to serve these purposes. Handout 1 evaluates clients' strengths and challenges relevant to participation in Creating Change. Strengths include "I know what grounding is and when to use it"; challenges include "I've attempted suicide or been violent in the past." This handout can be conducted as an interview or filled out by the client. It was developed based on a close read of the treatment literature that identifies characteristics impacting past-focused treatment. Handout 2 creates a plan for improvement. For example, if a client doesn't have strong coping skills, you could encourage a coping skills group while participating in Creating Change. Handout 3 is a mental health advance directive to specify client preferences during a psychiatric emergency, such as statements that calm them and people who help them feel safe.

However, none of the handouts should be used as a definitive test of clients' capacity to participate in Creating Change. There are no cutoff scores in Handout 1 because many combinations of clients and settings can succeed with the model. A very severe client who's a good fit while in a residential setting may be less suited for it as an outpatient. Factors such as close monitoring and longer length of stay all serve to support the work. Thus, use your judgment and consult with colleagues as needed to identify options in your setting. Someone who's actively psychotic would typically need medication consultation and/or basic stabilization before starting any past-focused trauma treatment, for example.

One of the best ways to evaluate clients' capacity for Creating Change is to let them experience it directly by trying any three sessions (the *three-session try-out* described in Chapter 3). Today's topic can count as one of the three or you can choose others. If a client doesn't like the model or becomes overly disturbed by the materials beyond a moderate level of reactivity, you likely wouldn't continue without further stabilization. You could later redo Handout 1 in a few weeks or months to identify the client's fit at that point.

It's also highly recommended to assess trauma and addiction symptoms over time, especially if you have concerns about a client. There are many free, brief validated measures online (for examples, see the extra topic "Understanding Trauma and Addiction"). But there are no required assessments in Creating Change because programs typically have their own assessment protocol, and choice of assessments varies based on factors such as staffing and time burden.

Today's topic is generally best conducted individually rather than in group modality as the handouts are designed to develop an individual recovery plan. But it can be done in groups as long as clients understand they don't have to share sensitive personal information with others.

Your Emotional Reactions

There's sometimes a tendency to overprotect clients, identifying more with their vulnerability than their strength, which can lead to believing they're not ready to work on the past. Creating Change allows clients to pace themselves and choose the level of intensity. It also uses a theme-based approach and is highly flexible, evoking rather than directing. We thus find that most clients have the capacity to participate, absorbing what they can and letting go of the rest. They can "find their level." It's also useful to remember that clients may interpret overprotection by the counselor in negative ways: "I'm weak," "I'll never get better," "The counselor doesn't understand me." In sum, it's usually best to have them try it out. Validate their resilience and all they've survived thus far, and shore up supports as needed.

Acknowledgments

The session quotation is often attributed to Lily Tomlin but is from an earlier unknown author per Popik (2012).

SESSION FORMAT

1. *Check-in* (per Chapter 3).
2. *Quotation.* Link the quotation to the session topic—for example, *"Today we'll talk about your recovery strengths and challenges. The quote is hopeful—it's saying that it's always possible to make things better."*
3. *Handouts* (relate the topic to clients' lives):
    Handout 1: **Strengths and Challenges Questionnaire**
    Handout 2: **Next Steps Plan**
    Handout 3: **Mental Health Advance Directive**
4. *Check-out* (per Chapter 3).

SESSION CONTENT

Goals

- ☐ Identify client strengths and challenges that may impact participation in Creating Change.
- ☐ Help clients create a *next steps plan* to strengthen their recovery.
- ☐ Encourage clients to try Creating Change for a few sessions (unless there's a significant reason not to).
- ☐ Offer a *mental health advance directive* for clients to specify preferences if a crisis arises or their symptoms worsen.

Ways to Relate the Material to Clients' Lives

★ *Help clients identify current strengths and challenges (Handout 1).* You can do it together during the session or have them fill it out prior to the session and go over it. Be sure clients' answers make sense to you as you may need to clarify inconsistencies. For example, if a client marks "yes" for strength question 5 ("I have positive coping skills") but can't name any, change the "yes" to "no." If a client marks "don't know," try to get more information.

★ *Interpret clients' answers on Handout 1.* The total score ranges from 0 to 36, with higher scores indicating greater stability and functioning. There's no defined scoring cutoff and no automatic exclusion. For example, some clients currently self-harm but it's not frequent or severe and they do fine in Creating Change. Others have low scores on the handout but do well because they're in a supportive setting such as residential, inpatient, or a halfway house. Emphasize that the goal is to identify domains that need strengthening. Also, when looking at client scores, be sure to read their written responses (the questions in italics) as those are just as important as the numbers.

★ *Create a Next Steps Plan (Handout 2).* Collaborate on a roadmap of actions that will aid clients' participation in Creating Change. Prioritize goals they want to work on. Focus on a few domains with the option to add additional ones as they progress. For complex client issues or anything beyond your scope of practice or knowledge, consult with a supervisor as needed. Clients may also need referrals to treatments outside of Creating Change. Below are examples of questions in Handout 1 and action steps in Handout 2.

a. ***Strength** examples*
- *Strength 3: "I take psychiatric medication as prescribed."* If a client lists "no" or "not sure," get more information and consult with the client's medication prescriber if needed. There are many reasons a client may not take a medication as prescribed, some of which are concerning (taking more than prescribed) and others that may require case management (side effects or lack of money to pay for the medication). Action steps could include encouraging the client to discuss side effects with the prescriber and helping the client apply for public assistance to pay for the medication.
- *Strength 4: "I have a written plan for what to do in a mental health crisis (who to contact, where to get help)."* Verify that the client can describe the plan and also has it in writing. It may include resources such as the National Suicide and Crisis Lifeline (dial 988), the National Domestic Violence Hotline (800-799-SAFE), and the local emergency room. Action steps could include creating a plan if the client doesn't have one, copying it onto the client's phone, rehearsing when to use the plan, and sharing it with safe family and friends.
- *Strength 5: "I have positive coping skills."* The client should be able to name various specific skills. The "Safety" chapter in the *Seeking Safety* book provides a list of over 80 safe coping skills for trauma and/or addiction that can be used in any treatment. It's also in the

book *Finding Your Best Self* (see the chapter "Safe Coping Skills") or there's a free version at *www.seekingsafety.org/training/materials/handouts* (Basic Handouts, pp. 5–6).

  b. ***Challenge* examples**
   - *Challenge 3: "I've attempted suicide or been violent in the past."* It's unfortunately common for clients with significant trauma or addiction to have suicidal thoughts (and, more rarely, violent thoughts). They can participate in Creating Change if they have no immediate plan or intent to act on it. If they do have an immediate plan or intent, consult with a supervisor for next steps, such as a thorough assessment and referral to additional care. For example, the Columbia-Suicide Severity Rating Scale is a free, brief validated suicide risk assessment. If clients only have a past history of suicide or violence, they can typically participate in Creating Change. The client's current context is also relevant: Is the client in residential treatment with ongoing monitoring?—that would be a positive factor. Is the client currently undergoing severe and multiple stressors with little support?—that would be a negative factor. Also see Chapter 3 for more on emergency situations.
   - *Challenge 6: "I have a current diagnosis of dissociative identity disorder ('multiple personality disorder')."* Dissociative identity disorder (DID) is rare, affecting less than 2% of the population, and is associated with severe trauma, typically in childhood. Clients with the disorder can still participate in Creating Change, but action steps include accurate assessment and referral to specialized therapy. If you don't know about DID, consult a supervisor.
   - *Challenge 7: "I have a current diagnosis of bipolar disorder or a psychotic disorder."* If the answer is "yes" and the disorder is under control, this means clients aren't experiencing severe current symptoms, in which case they can participate in Creating Change in most cases. But if the disorder is not under control, work on that first. Action steps could include getting medication and joining a support group relevant to the diagnosis.

★ **Work on a mental health advance directive (Handout 3).** Help clients identify their preferences. Trauma and addiction can lead to lack of awareness of their needs and wants, so it may require more than one discussion to complete the handout. You can also incorporate elements from Handout 1 into the advance directive such as their favorite grounding, coping skills, and safe people. After Handout 3 is complete, make a plan for clients to share it with relevant others (e.g., family, friends, sponsor, staff) and follow up to find out if they did so. When possible, include security staff, too, as they may need to calm clients during emergencies.

★ **Provide as many supports as possible.** This includes additional screening, treatment referrals, and ongoing monitoring. The specifics will depend on the clients and setting. If you use Seeking Safety, see the topic "Introduction to Treatment/Case Management" for a structured way to approach it.

★ ***Discussion***
  - "What are your most important strengths?"
  - "How do you feel about where you're at in recovery?"
  - "What kinds of support would improve your recovery?"
  - "What are your goals for the next 3 months?"
  - "Who can you share your mental health advance directive with?"

Suggestions

✦ ***Let the client try up to three sessions of Creating Change.*** This is called the "three-session try-out" as discussed in Chapter 3. It's the best way to identify if it's a good fit unless there's an important reason not to. Remember that many clients can participate in Creating Change even if they have current substance use disorder or another addiction (as long as they're not intoxicated during the session) and even if they have self-harm, homelessness, criminal justice involvement, or other major vulnerabilities.

+ *See the other extra topics.* Each takes a different approach toward improving clients' participation in Creating Change. The topic "Understanding Trauma and Addiction" offers basic education on trauma and addiction for those who need that. The topic "Relationships" helps them improve their style of relating while in treatment.

+ *Express optimism.* There's opportunity for progress no matter how long-standing or severe clients' problems are. So too, emphasize clients' strengths rather than just challenges.

+ *Try some topics from Seeking Safety.* Topics such as "Safety," "Detaching from Emotional Pain (Grounding)," and "Asking for Help" are especially useful to build stabilization. You can also encourage the client to attend Seeking Safety while in Creating Change. It uses the same style and approach but focuses on coping skills in the present, including practical tools such as a safety plan and safety contract. See *www.seekingsafety.org*; see also Chapter 3 for how to combine the two models.

+ *Learn more about mental health advance directives.* They're also called psychiatric advance directives and are viewed as a legal document in many states. Clinically, they promote client empowerment and can improve care. The end of Handout 3 lists resources to learn more about them.

+ *If Creating Change is not currently a good fit, offer reassurance.* You can say, for example:
  - "We can return to Creating Change when the timing is right."
  - "There are many ways to work on recovery."
  - "It's helpful to accept, with a generous heart, where you're at now."
  - "I want you to get the help that's best for you."
  - "You have many strengths; recovery is possible."

Keep in mind, too, that if some clients aren't ready for past-focused treatment, this can create a high- versus low-status dynamic in which clients perceive exclusion from the treatment as a personal failure. This is all the more likely in settings where clients interact, such as intensive outpatient programs and residential care. Provide a compassionate explanation that emphasizes the need to tailor care to each individual. As one client said, "It sounds like you all know what you're doing. . . . I just needed to know what you were doing, too."

Tough Cases

* "I know what I need to do but just can't do it."
* "These questions make me feel bad—nothing I do is ever enough."
* "My problem is the people around me."
* "I don't want more treatment."
* "People say I have an anger problem, but I don't."
* "I want to work on trauma, not addiction."

Extra Topic: Recovery Strengths and Challenges

Quotation

"The road to success is always under construction."

~ Anonymous

HANDOUT 1

Strengths and Challenges Questionnaire

Today's date: _____ Your name or initials: _____

Everyone has strengths and challenges in recovery. This questionnaire helps identify yours so you can build a plan to move forward.

★ *Instructions*

* You can fill this out or your counselor may do it with you.
* Answer for **the past month** unless it says otherwise.
* If you mark "yes" or "not sure," answer the question in italics as well.
* There are no right or wrong answers.
* If you don't understand a question, mark "not sure."
* For more space, use the back of the page.

PART I: STRENGTHS

		2 Yes	0 No	Not sure
Strength 1	**I attend addiction and/or mental health treatment regularly** (counselor, psychiatrist, 12-step groups, etc.). *List which treatment(s) and how often:*			
Strength 2	**I have safe people I call for support or when I need help** (family, friends, hotline, sponsor). *List who you call:*			
Strength 3	**I take psychiatric medication as prescribed.** *List how often you take it:* Or if you're not on psychiatric medication and don't need it, mark here: ☐			

(cont.)

From *Creating Change* by Lisa M. Najavits. Copyright © 2024 Lisa M. Najavits. Published by The Guilford Press. Permission to photocopy this material, or to download and print additional copies (www.guilford.com/najavits3-materials), is granted to purchasers of this book for use with your own clients or patients; see copyright page for details.

HANDOUT 1 *(p. 2 of 3)* Extra Topic: Recovery Strengths and Challenges

		2 Yes	0 No	Not sure
Strength 4	**I have a written plan for what to do in a mental health crisis** (who to contact, where to get help). *List the plan:*			
Strength 5	**I have positive coping skills.** *List some of your positive coping skills:*			
Strength 6	**I know what grounding is and when to use it.** *List how you do it and how often:*			
Strength 7	**I stay within specific limits for my addictive behavior** (e.g., substances, gambling, spending). *List the addiction(s) and specific limits, such as abstinence or other plan:* Or if no addiction, mark here: ❏			
Strength 8	**I live in a safe environment or a place that monitors my safety** (residential treatment, inpatient, halfway house, etc.). *List it:*			
Strength 9	**Any other current major strengths?** *List them:*			

Counselor: Score each "yes" = 2, each "no" = 0, each "don't know" = 0. For questions 3 and 7, if the box is checked, score each as 2 points.

List strengths score here: _____

PART II: CHALLENGES

		0 Yes	2 No	Not sure
Challenge 1	**I'm currently in a damaging relationship** (e.g., being harmed physically or emotionally). *List the relationship harm:*			
Challenge 2	**I have a current major life stressor** (e.g., legal problem; divorce; job loss or financial problem; serious medical problem such as chronic pain or cancer; homelessness or unsafe living environment). *List your current major life stressor(s):*			

(cont.)

HANDOUT 1 *(p. 3 of 3)* Extra Topic: Recovery Strengths and Challenges

		0 Yes	2 No	Not sure
Challenge 3	**I've attempted suicide or been violent in the past.** *List for suicide how many times and approximately when:* *List for violence how many times and approximately when:*			
Challenge 4	**I have access to an *illegal* or *unsecured* gun or other major weapon.** *List the weapon(s):*			
Challenge 5	**I have a behavior I can't control (or others say I do).** Examples include *physical harm to self or others* (cutting, burning, hitting, etc.); *emotional harm to others* (verbal abuse, neglect); or *any possible addiction* (alcohol, drugs, food, spending, internet, gaming, exercise, work, sex, pornography, gambling, etc.). *List the behavior(s) and a brief description of how it's a problem for you:*			
Challenge 6	**I have a current diagnosis of dissociative identity disorder ("multiple personality disorder").**			
Challenge 7	**I have a current diagnosis of bipolar disorder or a psychotic disorder.** *If "yes," list the disorder(s):* *If "yes," is it currently under control (no major symptoms)?* Yes / No			
Challenge 8	**I have a mental health disorder not already named above** (e.g., depression, panic disorder, social phobia, anorexia, personality disorder). *List the disorder(s) here:*			
Challenge 9	**Any other major current challenges?** *List your other major challenges:*			
Counselor: Score each "yes" = 0, each "no" = 2, each "don't know" = 0, except for question 7. For question 7, if it's currently under control, score it as 2 points. **List challenges score here:** _____			

Scoring:
   Grand total _____ = *strengths* score (from Part I) _____ plus *challenges* score (from Part III) _____
   The higher your score, the stronger your recovery is.

HANDOUT 2 — Extra Topic: Recovery Strengths and Challenges

Next Steps Plan

Today's date: _____ Your name or initials: _____

What next steps can strengthen your recovery? Please be specific.

EXAMPLES

Current issue	Goal	Next step	When
1. I stopped taking my psych medication due to side effects.	Talk to my doctor about options.	Call my doctor.	Within 24 hours
2. When I'm stressed, I drink a lot.	Reduce my drinking.	Try SMART Recovery; find a meeting.	This week

YOUR PLAN

Current issue	Goal	Next step	When
1.			
2.			
3.			
4.			

Anything else that can help?

_____

_____

ACCEPTANCE

If you're ready and interested in exploring the past in Creating Change, your clinician will work with you on it. If you're not ready or interested, accept this with a generous heart. What does that mean?

- There's no one right way—there's just what's right for you, right now.
- You're listening to your needs.
- Don't judge yourself as less than or weak.
- Remember that many different types of treatment are effective.
- You can focus on strengthening your recovery.
- Your counselor will guide you when the timing is right.

From *Creating Change* by Lisa M. Najavits. Copyright © 2024 Lisa M. Najavits. Published by The Guilford Press. Permission to photocopy this material, or to download and print additional copies (*www.guilford.com/najavits3-materials*), is granted to purchasers of this book for use with your own clients or patients; see copyright page for details.

HANDOUT 3   Extra Topic: Recovery Strengths and Challenges

Mental Health Advance Directive

This handout lets you specify in advance how you want people to respond if you're having a mental health crisis or your symptoms worsen. It's also called a *psychiatric advance directive*.

★ *Answer as many questions as you want. Then share this document with anyone you choose, such as treatment staff, family, and a sponsor. You can also ask for their feedback on it.*

ACTIVITIES

1. **What *helps you feel better* when you're upset?** For example, favorite activities, types of grounding, calming statements you want to hear.

2. **What *makes you feel worse* when you're upset?** What's best for you not to do (e.g., drinking, scrolling social media)? What should others not do (e.g., make loud noise, give advice)?

3. **Do you have *any material* that should be temporarily removed to protect you?** For example, a gun or other weapon, medication you may take too much of, triggering books. *If "yes," include what are they and who knows where they are other than you.*

PEOPLE

4. **Do you prefer to be *alone or around others* when you're upset?** *If you want people around, list details such as specific people or if you just want to be in a public space.*

5. **Is there *anyone we can contact* to help you?** For example, to speak with you, give you a ride, help with tasks: a partner, roommate, friend, sponsor, or hotline. *If "yes," provide the names and contact information (phone/email) and any details such as when to reach them and how they can help.*

6. **If you're in treatment, which *staff feel best to talk to* when you're upset?**

(cont.)

From *Creating Change* by Lisa M. Najavits. Copyright © 2024 Lisa M. Najavits. Published by The Guilford Press. Permission to photocopy this material is granted to purchasers of this book for use with your own clients or patients; see copyright page for details.

HANDOUT 3 *(p. 2 of 2)*   Extra Topic: Recovery Strengths and Challenges

TREATMENT

7. **Are there *any treatments to increase* when you're upset?** For example, counseling, medication, self-help groups.

8. **Are there *any treatments you don't want*?** For example, specific medications.

9. **Do you have *preferences for more intensive treatment*?** For example, name of hospital, emergency room, or program.

OTHER

10. **What else *helps keep you safe* when you're in crisis or have intense symptoms?**

NEXT

➢ **Who do you want to share this with?** List names and specify how you'll share it with them (such as email or meeting with them).

➢ **Can we put a copy of this document in your treatment chart so staff will understand your preferences?** Yes / No

Client signature: _____ Date: _____

Client name, printed: _____

LEARN MORE

Additional resources on mental health advance directives:

➢ *www.nrc-pad.org*
➢ *https://mhanational.org/creating-psychiatric-advance-directive*

Extra Topic: Recovery Strengths and Challenges

Ideas for a Commitment

Commit to one action that will move your life forward!
It can be anything you feel will help you, or you can try one of the ideas below.
Keeping your commitment is a way of respecting, honoring, and caring for yourself.

+ Option 1. What's one of your greatest personal strengths? How can you use it to improve your recovery?

+ Option 2. What's one of your greatest personal weaknesses? How can you minimize it to improve your recovery?

+ Option 3. Search online for "famous people who overcame adversity." List three key points you learn from that search.

+ Option 4. What's one action you can take *today* to strengthen your recovery?

Extra Topic
Your Relationships

SUMMARY

Clients learn how to improve their relationships to support recovery (including their relationship with you). This topic is "extra" as not all clients need it. It's typically used early on if you're concerned that a client's style of relating would interfere with treatment. Or it can be used at any point if you begin to see such difficulties.

ORIENTATION

To the extent that clients with trauma and addiction engage others to support and encourage them, they have a great asset to help them through.

But too often, due in large part to the nature of these problems, they end up with damaged relationships that are a reflection of their internal state. They may alienate people who started out wanting to help them, by breaking promises or lying about addiction. They may repeatedly get involved with people who hurt them. They may strain relationships with what seem like unending needs. They may have intense anger, sometimes lashing out. They may abandon or neglect others, perhaps repeating what was done to them. Chu describes clients who survived major child abuse: "Unfortunately, the ability to relate to and feel supported by others is a primary area of disability in many patients with a history of severe childhood abuse. . . . Instead of being able to trust in others to support them, they fully expect abandonment and betrayal. In addition, they unconsciously reenact the abusive style of their families of origin in their current relationships" (1992, p. 353). In short, when clients most need the comfort and support of strong relationships, they may be least likely to obtain them.

The counseling relationship is no exception. Counselors are subject to behavior that can imperil the treatment. Clients may miss appointments, engage in risky behavior, pull for boundary violations (wanting more time or contact than the counselor can give), and struggle with crises that stress the counselor and the system. It's a well-known truth that clients will reenact, in treatment, relationship problems that occur on the outside. The hope is that by successfully resolving these with the counselor, it will create a ripple effect to improve their outside relationships, too.

In today's topic, clients are offered a handout on how to promote positive relationships, with ideas such as *observe your impact on others*, *seek feedback*, and *try not to compare suffering*. However, this is not to imply that clients alone are responsible for all of their relationship problems. They may be involved with unsafe people who exploit or neglect them, and this will be an important aspect to explore in their ongoing work in Creating Change. But to the extent that some clients relate in sessions in ways that interfere with their own or other group members' progress, it's important to address those directly. A second handout in today's topic is the Agnew Relationship Measure that can be filled out separately by you and the client to identify the quality of your working relationship, also known as the *therapeutic alliance*.

The goal is to help clients bring out the best in themselves and others, which in turn will support their recovery.

Your Emotional Reactions

No matter how caring you are, working with clients who have trauma and addiction raises relationship challenges. Counselors need a wide range of skills including the ability to set limits, give negative feedback at times, and recognize when their own or clients' frustration is rising, particularly in its more subtle forms such as distancing, pessimism, overprotectiveness, and "never feeling angry." When there's a problem, the confusing part is to identify what each of you is contributing. If a client feels hurt by you, it may reflect the client's past relationships and have little to do with you; it may genuinely reflect something you did; or in many situations, it's a mix of these. It takes strength to look squarely at such dilemmas and, if you've made an error, to own that directly so the client can experience what a healthy resolution feels like. However, if there's an ongoing, unresolvable lack of fit between you and the client, seek consultation with a supervisor, or refer the client to someone else. See also Chapter 4, which has extensive discussion of these issues.

Acknowledgments

The session quotation is per Schirmacher (2003).

SESSION FORMAT

1. *Check-in* (per Chapter 3).
2. *Quotation.* Link the quotation to the session topic—for example, *"Today we'll talk about how to sustain positive relationships as you work on recovery. The quote beautifully conveys how one person can help another."*
3. *Handouts* (relate the topic to clients' lives):
    Handout 1: **Strengthen Your Relationships**
    Handout 2: **Agnew Relationship Measure—*Client Version***
4. *Check-out* (per Chapter 3).

SESSION CONTENT

Goals

- ☐ Explore how to promote positive relationships while in recovery.
- ☐ Identify difficulties in current relationships that may impact treatment.
- ☐ Have both you and the client fill out a measure to evaluate the strength of your relationship.
- ☐ Discuss how trauma and addiction affect relationships.

Ways to Relate the Material to Clients' Lives

★ ***Discuss ways to strengthen relationships to support recovery (Handout 1).*** As you go through the handout, ask clients for specific current examples from their life. For *expect conflicts*, you could ask whether they have any current conflicts with anyone. For *seek feedback*, you could ask who they typically get feedback from. Highlight and build on their current relationship strengths as well as identifying areas in need of improvement.

★ ***Fill out the Agnew Relationship Measure—Client Version (Handout 2).*** The client can fill out Handout 2, and you can fill out the counselor version on page 352. This free, brief validated scale assesses the quality of the counseling relationship (Cahill et al., 2012), which can launch an open discussion of how the client feels toward you and the work. Help the client understand that you invite honest feedback at any point during treatment and you can work together to resolve any issues that arise. However, the counselor scale is for your information; it's not advised to tell the client your score. For group treatment, it's best to ask members to fill it out anonymously to obtain the most honest results. You don't necessarily need to discuss the results in group but can use it as information. *Note:* Typically, client ratings are higher than counselor ratings (Lambert, 2013), but if there's a large difference or if the client ratings are very low, you may want to seek supervision.

★ ***Gauge clients' social support.*** Some clients have strong support, others are highly isolated, and some are in unhealthy relationships. This information can aid treatment planning and provide insights relevant to other Creating Change sessions (e.g., capacity for intimacy and power dynamics in relationships).

★ ***Provide referrals to help clients improve their social supports.*** Examples include social skills training, couples/family treatment, 12-step groups, SMART Recovery, and also local social connections such as *www.meetup.com* and *www.nextdoor.com* to help them expand their network. If a client has a current domestic violence concern, be sure to get expert advice on this, including contacting the National Domestic Violence Hotline (800-799-7233).

★ ***Discussion***
- "How do trauma and addiction impact your relationships?"
- "What is one thing others like about you? One thing they dislike?"
- "How lonely do you feel?"
- "What does a healthy relationship look like?"
- "How can you strengthen your relationships as you do this treatment?"
- "Do you have any concerns about our counseling relationship?"

Suggestions

✦ ***Validate that relationship issues are normal.*** Let clients know that there are likely to be bumps in any ongoing relationships and that continual adjustment is part of the process. Clients with trauma and addiction sometimes hold unrealistic views that relationships should be easy or, at the other extreme, that they're always painful. Emphasize the need to see people clearly and respond accordingly (e.g., protecting themselves from unsafe people).

✦ ***Identify relationship aspects that are specific to trauma and addiction.*** Examples of challenges include distrust, codependency, boundary problems, being used or exploited, isolation, self-blame, and difficulty leaving toxic relationships. Examples of positive relationship aspects include mutual support via 12-step groups, empathy for other trauma survivors, and positive bonding as part of treatment and recovery.

✦ ***Build hope.*** Clients often have long-standing relationship issues that feel impossible to change. They may resist noticing their role in relationship problems or the opposite, may blame themselves too much. Strive to create optimism that they can build healthy relationships as they continue in treatment.

✦ ***Reinforce positive group dynamics if you're conducting group.*** Consider having clients fill out the Group Climate Questionnaire (Johnson et al., 2006) to assess how helpful the group feels; it's free, validated, and easily found online. Also invite discussion of the importance of positive group dynamics, such as members being supportive yet honest with each other in group.

Tough Cases

* "Why don't people like me?"
* "I'm there for everyone, but no one's there for me."
* "I prefer to be alone."
* "I get attracted to people who end up hurting me."
* "I've never felt loved."
* "I'm too depressed to bother with relationships."

Extra Topic: Your Relationships

Agnew Relationship Measure—*Counselor Version*

Please fill this out about your client.

	Strongly disagree	Disagree	Slightly disagree	Neutral	Slightly agree	Agree	Strongly agree
1. I feel supportive.	1	2	3	4	5	6	7
2. My client and I agree about how to work together.	1	2	3	4	5	6	7
3. My client and I have difficulty working as a partnership.	7	6	5	4	3	2	1
4. My client has confidence in me and my techniques.	1	2	3	4	5	6	7
5. I feel confident in myself and my techniques.	1	2	3	4	5	6	7

Scoring: Total your score. The higher your score, the more positive your view of the alliance with your client.

From the five-item version of the scale by Cahill et al. (2012). Adapted with permission from the authors. Permission to photocopy this material, or to download and print additional copies (*www.guilford.com/najavits3-materials*), is granted to purchasers of this book for use with your own clients or patients; see copyright page for details.

Extra Topic: Your Relationships

Quotation

"At times our own light goes out and is rekindled by a spark from another person."

~ ALBERT SCHWEITZER, 20th-century German physician and philosopher

HANDOUT 1

Strengthen Your Relationships

Do you have challenges . . .
- ❖ *finding* positive relationships?
- ❖ *maintaining* positive relationships?
- ❖ *knowing* what a positive relationship is?

Relationships can support your recovery, helping you rise beyond what you thought possible. But they can also descend into tension and difficulty, creating more stress.

Here are ideas to strengthen your relationships.

Seek Feedback from Trustworthy People
Honest feedback can be hard to hear but promotes growth. Stay open to feedback even when it's negative, as long as it's from a trustworthy source.

❖ *Are you able to hear feedback even when it's negative?*

Build Connections beyond Trauma and Addiction
If trauma and addiction are your only bond with others, your identity can become overly tied to these. Build relationships with safe people outside of recovery: Connect on sports, hobbies, children religion, or anything else.

❖ *Do you have a balance of relationships?*

Resolve Conflicts
In any close relationship, conflicts arise. In the past, you may have had to avoid conflicts to survive toxic or dangerous people. But now you can face conflicts and find solutions.

❖ *Are you able to address conflicts in healthy ways?*

Build Trust Stepwise
You may be so hungry for connection that you open up too much too soon with people you don't know well enough. Or the opposite, you may hold back so much that you stay isolated. Aim for the middle, building trust stepwise.

(cont.)

From *Creating Change* by Lisa M. Najavits. Copyright © 2024 Lisa M. Najavits. Published by The Guilford Press. Permission to photocopy this material is granted to purchasers of this book for use with your own clients or patients; see copyright page for details.

HANDOUT 1 *(p. 2 of 2)*   Extra Topic: Your Relationships

❖ *Are you able to share, but in a paced way?*

Observe your Impact on Others

Do people warmly move toward you or subtly distance themselves? Are they often annoyed with you? Are they intimidated? Admiring? Do they confide in you? Notice the patterns even if it's not pleasant.

❖ *What patterns do you notice?*

Find a Few People Who Can Understand

Some people don't want to know about trauma or addiction or just can't "go there" because it's too much for them. It's fine to have some lighter relationships that don't delve into difficult topics. But find a few people who can understand.

❖ *Do you have a few people who understand you?*

Get Help to Leave Toxic Relationships

Carefully evaluate, with the help of your counselor or trusted others, *if*, *when*, and *how* to leave relationships that are so destructive that there's no hope for change. It can be really hard to figure out a path (and especially if there's potential for violence, you'll need a lot of guidance).

❖ *Do you have any relationship(s) that you may need to leave?*

Try Not to Compare Suffering

All people compare themselves to others. But comparisons about trauma and addiction are unhealthy if it means competing for who has it the worst. Or sometimes it's the opposite—comparing who's making more progress.

❖ *Do you compare yourself to others too much?*

Be the Instrument of Change

There's sometimes a deep wish to have others save you. And people who care about you would if they could. But they can only guide and support. Recovery is a road you pave yourself.

❖ *Are you doing all you can for your recovery?*

Keep Others on Your Side

Trauma and addiction can erode relationships (breaking promises, lashing out even at those who are trying to help, etc.). Try to preserve relationships by being responsible and respecting boundaries. If you make an error, work to repair the relationship.

❖ *Can you improve how you treat others?*

Tell Your Counselor If You Have Concerns

Fill out the scale in Handout 2. If your score is low or if you have any other concerns, let the counselor know. (Or, if there is an ethical violation such as sexual contact, seek immediate help from a supervisor.)

❖ *Are you able to discuss concerns about the counseling?*

Any other ideas for strengthening your relationships? _____

_____

HANDOUT 2   Extra Topic: Your Relationships

Agnew Relationship Measure—*Client Version*

Please fill this out about your Creating Change counselor.

Be fully honest (you don't need to try to protect the counselor).

	Strongly disagree	*Disagree*	*Slightly disagree*	*Neutral*	*Slightly agree*	*Agree*	*Strongly agree*
1. My counselor is supportive.	1	2	3	4	5	6	7
2. My counselor and I agree about how to work together.	1	2	3	4	5	6	7
3. My counselor and I have difficulty working as a partnership.	7	6	5	4	3	2	1
4. I have confidence in my counselor and the counselor's techniques.	1	2	3	4	5	6	7
5. My counselor is confident in him/herself and his/her techniques.	1	2	3	4	5	6	7

Scoring: Total your score. The higher your score, the more positive your view of your counselor.

From the five-item version of the scale by Cahill et al. (2012). Adapted with permission from the authors. Permission to photocopy this material, or to download and print additional copies (*www.guilford.com/najavits3-materials*), is granted to purchasers of this book for use with your own clients or patients; see copyright page for details.

Ideas for a Commitment

Commit to one action that will move your life forward!
It can be anything you feel will help you, or you can try one of the ideas below.
Keeping your commitment is a way of respecting, honoring, and caring for yourself.

- Option 1. Ask a trustworthy person, "What is best about me in relationships?" and "How can I improve my relationships?"

- Option 2. Create a *vision board* to express how you want to grow your relationships. Read online about vision boards (they can include writing, pictures, quotations, souvenirs, goals, etc.).

- Option 3. Write about how trauma and/or addiction impacts your relationships.

- Option 4. Answer the questions in Handout 1 in more detail.

References

Abueg, F. R., & Fairbank, J. A. (1991). Behavioral treatment of the PTSD-substance abuser: A multidimensional stage model. In P. Saigh (Ed.), *Posttraumatic stress disorder: A behavioral approach to assessment and treatment* (pp. 111–146). Pergamon Press.

Ackerman, C. E. (2017, June 18). *19 Best narrative therapy techniques and worksheets.* https://positivepsychology.com/narrative-therapy.

Addiction Policy Forum. (2020, September 2). *Addiction and the brain.* www.addictionpolicy.org/post/addiction-and-the-brain.

Adeyemo, W. L. (2004). Sigmund Freud: Smoking habit, oral cancer and euthanasia. *Nigerian Journal of Medicine, 13*(2), 189–195.

Alcoholics Anonymous World Services. (2001). *Alcoholics Anonymous Big Book* (4th ed.). Author.

Alighieri, D. (1996). *The inferno* (J. Ciardi, Trans.). Signet. (Original work published 1321)

American Psychiatric Association. (2022). *Diagnostic and statistical manual of mental disorders* (5th ed., text rev.). Author.

American Psychological Association. (1998). Final conclusions of the American Psychological Association Working Group on Investigation of Memories of Child Abuse. *Psychology, Public Policy, and Law, 4,* 933–940.

American Psychological Association. (2017). *APA Clinical Practice Guideline for the Treatment of PTSD in Adults: How long will it take for treatment to work?* www.apa.org/ptsd-guideline/patients-and-families/length-treatment.

Andreasen, N. C. (2011). What is post-traumatic stress disorder? *Dialogues in Clinical Neuroscience, 13*(3), 240–243.

Annis, H. M., & Chan, D. (1983). The differential treatment model: Empirical evidence from a personality typology of adult offenders. *Criminal Justice and Behavior, 10*(2), 159–173.

Aviv, R. (2021, July 19). The German experiment that placed foster children with pedophiles. *The New Yorker.* www.newyorker.com/magazine/2021/07/26/the-german-experiment-that-placed-foster-children-with-pedophiles.

Back, S. E., Dansky, B. S., Carroll, K. M., Foa, E. B., & Brady, K. T. (2001). Exposure therapy in the treatment of PTSD among cocaine-dependent individuals: Description of procedures. *Journal of Substance Abuse Treatment, 21,* 35–45.

Back, S. E., Foa, E. B., Killeen, T. K., Mills, K. L., Teesson, M., Dansky Cotton, B., . . . Brady, K. T. (2015). *Concurrent Treatment of PTSD and Substance Use Disorders Using Prolonged Exposure (COPE): Therapist guide.* Oxford University Press.

Back, S. E., Killeen, T., Badour, C. L., Flanagan, J. C., Allan, N. P., Ana, E. S., . . . Brady, K. T. (2019). Concurrent treatment of substance use disorders and PTSD using prolonged exposure: A randomized clinical trial in military veterans. *Addictive Behaviors, 90,* 369–377.

Back, S. E., Killeen, T., Foa, E. B., Santa Ana, E. J., Gros, D. F., & Brady, K. T. (2012). Use of an integrated therapy with prolonged exposure to treat PTSD and comorbid alcohol dependence in an Iraq veteran. *American Journal of Psychiatry, 169*(7), 688–691.

Back, S. E., Killeen, T. K., Teer, A. P., Hartwell, E. E., Federline, A., Beylotte, F., & Cox, E. (2014). Substance use disorders and PTSD: An exploratory study of treatment preferences among military veterans. *Addictive Behaviors, 39*(2), 369–373.

Bailey, K., Trevillion, K., & Gilchrist, G. (2019). What works for whom and why: A narrative systematic review of interventions for reducing post-traumatic stress disorder and problematic substance use among women with experiences of interpersonal violence. *Journal of Substance Abuse Treatment, 99*, 88–103.

Bass, E., & Davis, L. (1994). *The Courage to Heal* (3rd ed.). *Revised and Expanded: A Guide for Women Survivors of Child Sexual Abuse*. HarperCollins.

Baumeister, R. F., Bratslavsky, E., Finkenauer, C., & Vohs, K. D. (2001). Bad is stronger than good. *Review of General Psychology, 5*(4), 323–370.

Beck, A. T., Wright, F. D., Newman, C. F., & Liese, B. S. (1993). *Cognitive therapy of substance abuse*. Guilford Press.

Becker, C. B., Zayfert, C., & Anderson, E. (2004). A survey of psychologists' attitudes towards and utilization of exposure therapy for PTSD. *Behavior Research and Therapy, 42*(3), 277–292.

Beers, C. W. (1907). *A mind that found itself*. Longmans, Green and Co.

Bemak, F., & Young, M. E. (1998). Role of catharsis and group psychotherapy. *International Journal of Action Methods, 4*, 166–184.

Bjornestad, J., Svendsen, T. S., Slyngstad, T. E., Erga, A. H., McKay, J. R., Nesvåg, S., . . . Moltu, C. (2019). "A life more ordinary." Processes of 5-year recovery from substance abuse: Experiences of 30 recovered service users. *Frontiers in Psychiatry, 10*, 689.

Black, C. (2020). *It will never happen to me: Growing up with addiction as youngsters, adolescents, and adults*. Central Recovery Press.

Booth, W. (2012, December 1). Peña Nieto sworn in as Mexico's president, vows big change. *Washington Post*. www.washingtonpost.com/world/the_americas/pena-nieto-sworn-in-as-mexicos-president-vows-big-change/2012/12/01/4dcc72bc-3c00-11e2-9258-ac7c78d5c680_story.html.

Briere, J. (2019). *Treating risky and compulsive behavior in trauma survivors*. Guilford Press.

Briere, J. N., & Scott, C. (2014). *Principles of trauma therapy: A guide to symptoms, evaluation, and treatment (DSM-5 Update)*. SAGE.

Brown, S., & Lewis, V. (1995). *The alcoholic family: A developmental model of recovery*. Jossey Bass.

Brown, S., & Yalom, I. D. (Eds.). (1995). *Treating alcoholism*. Jossey-Bass.

Brown, V. B., Huba, G. J., & Melchior, L. A. (1995). Level of burden: Women with more than one co-occurring disorder. *Journal of Psychoactive Drugs, 27*, 339–346.

Burroughs, A. (2003). *Dry: A memoir*. St. Martin's Press.

Buschman, H. (2019, October 8). *Large study reveals PTSD has strong genetic component like other psychiatric disorders*. https://health.ucsd.edu/news/press-releases/2019-10-08-study-reveals-ptsd-has-strong-genetic-component.

Cacioppo, J. T., Cacioppo, S., & Gollan, J. K. (2014). The negativity bias: Conceptualization, quantification, and individual differences. *Behavioral and Brain Sciences, 37*(3), 309.

Cahill, J., Stiles, W. B., Barkham, M., Hardy, G. E., Stone, G., Agnew-Davies, R., & Unsworth, G. (2012). Two short forms of the Agnew Relationship Measure: The ARM-5 and ARM-12. *Psychotherapy Research, 22*(3), 241–255.

Calhoun, L. G., & Tedeschi, R. G. (1999). *Facilitating posttraumatic growth: A clinician's guide*. Routledge.

Cameron, C. (2000). *Resolving childhood trauma: A long-term study of abuse survivors*. SAGE.

Camus, A. (1968). *Lyrical and critical essays*. Knopf.

Carruth, B., & Burke, P. A. (2006). Psychological trauma and addiction treatment. *Journal of Chemical Dependency Treatment, 8*(2), 1–14.

Castonguay, L. G., & Hill, C. E. (Eds.). (2017). *How and why are some therapists better than others?: Understanding therapist effects*. American Psychological Association.

Catherall, D. R. (1997, Spring). Family treatment when a member has PTSD. *National Center for PTSD Clinical Quarterly, 7*, 19–21.

Center for Victims of Torture. (2021). *Professional Quality of Life: Health Worker, Version 1*. https://proqol.org/proqol-health-measure.

Chard, K. M., Resick, P. A., Monson, C. M., & Kattar, K. A. (2009). *Cognitive processing therapy: Veteran/ military version: Therapist's group manual.* Department of Veterans' Affairs. www.div12.org/wp-content/uploads/2014/11/Group-CPT-Manual.pdf.

Chemtob, C. M., Novaco, R. W., Hamada, R. S., & Gross, D. M. (1997). Cognitive-behavioral treatment for severe anger in posttraumatic stress disorder. *Journal of Consulting and Clinical Psychology, 65,* 184–189.

Chu, J. A. (1988). Ten traps for therapists in the treatment of trauma survivors. *Dissociation: Progress in the Dissociative Disorders, 1,* 24–32.

Chu, J. A. (1992). The therapeutic roller coaster: Dilemmas in the treatment of childhood abuse survivors. *Journal of Psychotherapy Practice and Research, 1,* 351–370.

Cienfuegos, A. J., & Monelli, C. (1983). The testimony of political repression as a therapeutic instrument. *American Journal of Orthopsychiatry, 53*(1), 43–51.

Clark, C., & Fearday, F. (2003). *Triad women's project: Group facilitator's manual* (Publication No. 415). University of South Florida Mental Health Law & Policy Faculty.

Cloitre, M., Courtois, C. A., Charuvastra, A., Carapezza, R., Stolbach, B. C., & Green, B. L. (2011). Treatment of complex PTSD: Results of the ISTSS expert clinician survey on best practices. *Journal of Traumatic Stress, 24*(6), 615–627.

Cloitre, M., Koenen, K. C., Cohen, L. R., & Han, H. (2002). Skills training in affective and interpersonal regulation followed by exposure: A phase-based treatment for PTSD related to childhood abuse. *Journal of Consulting and Clinical Psychology, 70,* 1067–1074.

Coffey, S. F., Dansky, B. S., & Brady, K. T. (2002). Exposure-based, trauma-focused therapy for comorbid posttraumatic stress disorder-substance use disorder. In P. Ouimette & P. J. Brown (Eds.), *Trauma and substance abuse: Causes, consequences, and treatment of comorbid disorders* (pp. 209–226). American Psychological Association Press.

Coffey, S. F., Schumacher, J. A., Nosen, E., Littlefield, A. K., Henslee, A. M., Lappen, A., & Stasiewicz, P. R. (2016). Trauma-focused exposure therapy for chronic posttraumatic stress disorder in alcohol and drug dependent patients: A randomized controlled trial. *Psychology of Addictive Behaviors, 30*(7), 778.

Cook, J. M., Dinnen, S., Thompson, R., Simiola, V., & Schnurr, P. P. (2014). Changes in implementation of two evidence-based psychotherapies for PTSD in VA residential treatment programs: A national investigation. *Journal of Traumatic Stress, 27*(2), 137–143.

Courtois, C. A. (2004). Complex trauma, complex reactions: Assessment and treatment. *Psychotherapy: Theory, Research, Practice, and Training, 41,* 412–425.

Covington, S. S. (2000). Helping women recover: A comprehensive integrated treatment model. *Alcoholism Treatment Quarterly, 18*(3), 99–111.

Covington, S. S. (2003). *Beyond trauma: A healing journey for women.* Hazelden.

Crawford, L. (2020, June 25). Novelist Lacy Crawford writes about her sexual assault while she was a student at St. Paul's School. *Vanity Fair.* www.vanityfair.com/style/2020/06/novelist-lacy-crawford-writes-about-her-sexual-assault.

Crits-Christoph, P., Siqueland, L., Blaine, J., Frank, A., Luborsky, L., Onken, L. S., . . . Moras, K. (1997). The NIDA Cocaine Collaborative Treatment Study: Rationale and methods. *Archives of General Psychiatry, 54,* 721–726.

Crocq, M.-A., & Crocq, L. (2000). From shell shock and war neurosis to posttraumatic stress disorder: A history of psychotraumatology. *Dialogues in Clinical Neuroscience, 2*(1), 47–55.

Cuijpers, P., Reijnders, M., & Huibers, M. J. H. (2019). The role of common factors in psychotherapy outcomes. *Annual Review of Clinical Psychology, 15,* 207–231.

Damasio, A. (2003). Feelings of emotion and the self. *Annals of the New York Academy of Sciences, 1001*(1), 253–261.

Das, G. (1993). Cocaine abuse in North America: A milestone in history. *Journal of Clinical Pharmacology, 33*(4), 296–310.

Davis, B. (2006). Psychodynamic psychotherapies and the treatment of co-occurring psychological trauma and addiction. *Journal of Chemical Dependency Treatment, 8*(2), 41–69.

Dayton, T. (2000). *Trauma and addiction: Ending the cycle of pain through emotional literacy.* Simon & Schuster.

de Botton, A. (n.d.). *A quote by Alain de Botton.* www.goodreads.com/quotes/330942-the-moment-we-cry-in-a-film-is-not-when.

De Jongh, A., Resick, P. A., Zoellner, L. A., Van Minnen, A., Lee, C. W., Monson, C. M., Feeny, N. (2016). Critical analysis of the current treatment guidelines for complex PTSD in adults. *Depression and Anxiety, 33*(5), 359–369.

Dees, S. M., Dansereau, D. F., & Simpson, D. D. (1994). A visual representation system for drug abuse counselors. *Journal of Substance Abuse Treatment, 11*(6), 517–523.

Denborough, D. (2014). *Retelling the stories of our lives: Everyday narrative therapy to draw inspiration and transform experience.* Norton.

DiClemente, C. C., & Crisafulli, M. A. (2022). Relapse on the road to recovery: Learning the lessons of failure on the way to successful behavior change. *Journal of Health Service Psychology, 48,* 59–68.

Donovan, B., Padin-Rivera, E., & Kowaliw, S. (2001). Transcend: Initial outcomes from a posttraumatic stress disorder/substance abuse treatment study. *Journal of Traumatic Stress, 14,* 757–772.

Douglass, F. (1882, May 30). We must not abandon the observance of Decoration Day. *Rochester Daily Union and Advertiser, 38*–52.

Ehlers, A., Clark, D. M., Hackmann, A., McManus, F., & Fennell, M. (2005). Cognitive therapy for posttraumatic stress disorder: Development and evaluation. *Behavior Research and Therapy, 43*(4), 413–431.

Eliot, G. (1929). *The mill on the floss.* Heath. (Original work published 1860)

Encyclopedia Britannica. (2020, March 25). *Alice Walker.* www.britannica.com/explore/100women/profiles/alice-walker.

Estés, C. P. (1992). *Women who run with the wolves: Myths and stories of the wild woman archetype.* Ballantine Books.

Evans, K., & Sullivan, J. M. (1995). *Treating addicted survivors of trauma.* Guilford Press.

Febos, M. (2022, November 12). Opinion: How I learned the art of seduction. *New York Times.* www.nytimes.com/2022/11/12/opinion/how-i-learned-the-art-of-seduction.html.

Felitti, V. J., Anda, R. F., Nordenberg, D., Williamson, D. F., Spitz, A. M., Edwards, V., . . . Marks, J. S. (1998). Relationship of childhood abuse and household dysfunction to many of the leading causes of death in adults. The Adverse Childhood Experiences (ACE) Study. *American Journal of Preventive Medicine, 14*(4), 245–258.

Finney, J. W., Hahn, A. C., & Moos, R. H. (1996). The effectiveness of inpatient and outpatient treatment for alcohol abuse: The need to focus on mediators and moderators of setting effects. *Addiction, 91*(12), 1773–1796.

Foa, E. B. (2000). Psychosocial treatment of posttraumatic stress disorder. *Journal of Clinical Psychiatry, 61*(Suppl. 5), 43–48; discussion 49–51.

Foa, E. B., McLean, C. P., Zang, Y., Rosenfield, D., Yadin, E., Yarvis, J. S., . . . STRONG STAR Consortium. (2018). Effect of prolonged exposure therapy delivered over 2 weeks vs 8 weeks vs present-centered therapy on PTSD symptom severity in military personnel: A randomized clinical trial. *Journal of American Medical Association, 319*(4), 354–364.

Foa, E. B., & Rothbaum, B. O. (1998). *Treating the trauma of rape: Cognitive-behavioral therapy for PTSD.* Guilford Press.

Foa, E. B., Rothbaum, B. O., Riggs, D. S., & Murdock, T. B. (1991). Treatment of posttraumatic stress disorder in rape victims: A comparison between cognitive-behavioral procedures and counseling. *Journal of Consulting & Clinical Psychology, 59*(5), 715–723.

Foa, E. B., Yusko, D. A., McLean, C. P., Suvak, M. K., Bux, D. A., Oslin, D., . . . Volpicelli, J. (2013). Concurrent naltrexone and prolonged exposure therapy for patients with comorbid alcohol dependence and PTSD: A randomized clinical trial. *Journal of the American Medical Association, 310*(5), 488–495.

Ford, J., Kasimer, N., MacDonald, M., & Savill, G. (2000). *Trauma Adaptive Recovery Group Education and Therapy (TARGET): Participant guidebook and leader manual.* University of Connecticut.

Forman-Hoffman, V., Middleton, J. C., Feltner, C., Gaynes, B. N., Weber, R. P., Bann, C., . . . Green, J. (2018). *Psychological and pharmacological treatments for adults with posttraumatic stress disorder: A systematic review update* (Report No. 18-EHC011-EF; Comparative Effectiveness Review, No. 207). Agency for Healthcare Research and Quality.

Foy, D. W. (1992). *Treating PTSD: Cognitive-behavioral strategies.* Guilford Press.

Foy, D. W., Ruzek, J. I., Glynn, S. M., Riney, S. J., & Gusman, F. D. (2002). Trauma focus group therapy for combat-related PTSD: An update. *Journal of Clinical Psychology, 58*(8), 907–918.

Franz, M., McLean, E., Tung, J., Altmann, J., & Alberts, S. C. (2015). Self-organizing dominance hierarchies in a wild primate population. *Proceedings of the Royal Society B: Biological Sciences, 282*(1814), 20151512.

Freshwater, K., Ainscough, C., & Toon, K. (2003). Confronting abusers: The opinions of clinicians and survivors. *Journal of Child Sexual Abuse, 11*(4), 35–52.

Gide, A. (2011). *Autumn leaves*. Philosophical Library. (Original work published 1950)

Gillece, J. B., & Russell, B. G. (2001). Maryland's programs for women offenders with mental illness and substance abuse disorders: Incarcerated and in the community. *Women, Girls & Criminal Justice, 2*(6), 84–89.

Goodman, J., & Packard, M. G. (2016). Memory systems and the addicted brain. *Frontiers in Psychiatry, 7*. www.frontiersin.org/articles/10.3389/fpsyt.2016.00024.

Gordon, J. S., Staples, J. K., He, D. Y., & Atti, J. A. A. (2016). Mind–body skills groups for posttraumatic stress disorder in Palestinian adults in Gaza. *Traumatology, 22,* 155–164.

Gray, M. J., Maguen, S., & Litz, B. T. (2007). Schema constructs and cognitive models of posttraumatic stress disorder. In L. P. Riso, P. L. du Toit, D. J. Stein, & J. E. Young (Eds.), *Cognitive schemas and core beliefs in psychological problems: A scientist-practitioner guide* (pp. 59–92). American Psychological Association.

Grey, N., Holmes, E., & Brewin, C. R. (2001). Peritraumatic emotional "hot spots" in memory. *Behavioural and Cognitive Psychotherapy, 29,* 367–372.

Griffin, E., Ledbetter, A., & Sparks, G. (2018). *A first look at communication theory* (10th ed.). McGraw-Hill.

Gu, S., Wang, F., Patel, N. P., Bourgeois, J. A., & Huang, J. H. (2019). A model for basic emotions using observations of behavior in drosophila. *Frontiers in Psychology, 10,* 781.

Hanney, L., & Kozlowska, K. (2002). Healing traumatized children: Creating illustrated storybooks in family therapy. *Family Process, 41,* 37–65.

Harned, M. S., & Linehan, M. M. (2008). Integrating dialectical behavior therapy and prolonged exposure to treat co-occurring borderline personality disorder and PTSD: Two case studies. *Cognitive and Behavioral Practice, 15*(3), 263–276.

Harris, M. (1998). *Trauma Recovery and Empowerment*. Free Press.

Harris, M., Fallot, R. D., & Berley, R. W. (2005). Special section on relapse prevention: Qualitative interviews on substance abuse relapse and prevention among female trauma survivors. *Psychiatric Services, 56*(10), 1292–1296.

Harsey, S. J., Zurbriggen, E. L., & Freyd, J. J. (2017). Perpetrator responses to victim confrontation: DARVO and victim self-blame. *Journal of Aggression, Maltreatment & Trauma, 26*(6), 644–663.

Hembree, E. A., & Foa, E. B. (2000). Posttraumatic stress disorder: Psychological factors and psychosocial interventions. *Journal of Clinical Psychiatry, 61,* 33–39.

Henig, R. M. (2004, April 4). The quest to forget. *New York Times*. www.nytimes.com/2004/04/04/magazine/the-quest-to-forget.html.

Herman, J. L. (1992). *Trauma and recovery*. Basic Books.

Herman, J. L. (2023). *Truth and repair: How trauma survivors envision justice*. Basic Books.

Hernández, P., Gangsei, D., & Engstrom, D. (2007). Vicarious resilience: A new concept in work with those who survive trauma. *Family Process, 46*(2), 229–241.

Hien, D. A., Cohen, L. R., Miele, G. M., Litt, L. C., & Capstick, C. (2004). Promising treatments for women with comorbid PTSD and substance use disorders. *American Journal of Psychiatry, 161*(8), 1426–1432.

Hoeppner, B. B., Hoeppner, S. S., Carlon, H. A., Perez, G. K., Helmuth, E., Kahler, C. W., & Kelly, J. F. (2019). Leveraging positive psychology to support smoking cessation in nondaily smokers using a smartphone app: Feasibility and acceptability study. *JMIR mHealth and uHealth, 7*(7), e13436.

Hoge, C. W., & Chard, K. M. (2018). A window into the evolution of trauma-focused psychotherapies for posttraumatic stress disorder. *Journal of American Medical Association, 319*(4), 343–345.

Honeycutt, J. M. (2003). *Imagined interactions: Daydreaming about communication*. Hampton Press.

Horowitz, R. (2002). Psychotherapy and schizophrenia: The mirror of countertransference. *Clinical Social Work Journal, 30*(3), 235–244.

Hotta, C., & Kawaguchi, J. (2009). Self-initiated use of thought substitution can lead to long term forgetting. *Psychologia: An International Journal of Psychological Sciences, 52,* 41–49.

Hundt, N. E., Ecker, A. H., Thompson, K., Helm, A., Smith, T. L., Stanley, M. A., & Cully, J. A. (2020).

"It didn't fit for me": A qualitative examination of dropout from prolonged exposure and cognitive processing therapy in veterans. *Psychological Services, 17,* 414–421.

Imel, Z. E., Laska, K., Jakupcak, M., & Simpson, T. L. (2013). Meta-analysis of dropout in treatments for posttraumatic stress disorder. *Journal of Consulting and Clinical Psychology, 81*(3), 394.

Imel, Z. E., Wampold, B. E., Miller, S. D., & Fleming, R. R. (2008). Distinctions without a difference: Direct comparisons of psychotherapies for alcohol use disorders. *Psychology of Addictive Behaviors, 22,* 533–543.

Imhof, J., Hirsch, R., & Terenzi, R. E. (1983). Countertransferential and attitudinal considerations in the treatment of drug abuse and addiction. *International Journal of Addiction, 18,* 491–510.

Israel, B., Wiprovnick, A. E., Belcher, A. M., Kleinman, M. B., Ramprashad, A., Spaderna, M., & Weintraub, E. (2022). Practical considerations for treating comorbid posttraumatic stress disorder in the addictions clinic: Approaches to clinical care, leadership, and alleviating shame. *Psychiatric Clinics of North America, 45*(3), 375–414.

Jackson, S. W. (1994). Catharsis and abreaction in the history of psychological healing. *History of Psychiatry, 17,* 471–491.

Jemmer, P. (2006). Abreaction-catharsis: Stirring dull roots with spring rain. *European Journal of Clinical Hypnosis, 7*(1), 26–36.

Jennings, A., & Ralph, R. O. (1997). *In their own words: Trauma survivors and professionals they trust tell what hurts, what helps, and what is needed for trauma services* [Maine Trauma Advisory Groups Report]. Maine Department of Mental Health, Mental Retardation and Substance Abuse Services, Office of Trauma Services.

Johnson, J. E., Pulsipher, D., Ferrin, S. L., Burlingame, G. M., Davies, D. R., & Gleave, R. (2006). Measuring group processes: A comparison of the GCQ and CCI. *Group Dynamics: Theory, Research, and Practice, 10,* 136–145.

Johnstone, L., & Boyle, M. (2018). *The Power Threat Meaning Framework: Towards the identification of patterns in emotional distress, unusual experiences and troubled or troubling behaviour, as an alternative to functional psychiatric diagnosis.* British Psychological Society.

Jung, C. G. (1966). *The practice of psychotherapy* (G. Adler & R. F. C. Hull, Trans.) (2nd ed.). Princeton University Press.

Kadden, R., Carroll, K., Donovan, D., Cooney, N., Monti, P., Abrams, D., . . . Hester, R. (1995). *Cognitive-behavioral coping skills therapy manual: A clinical research guide for therapists treating individuals with alcohol abuse and dependence* (Vol. 3). U.S. Department of Health and Human Services.

Kardiner, A. (1941). *The traumatic neuroses of war.* P.B. Hoeber.

Karpman, S. (1968). Fairy tales and script drama analysis. *Transactional Analysis Bulletin, 7*(26), 39–43.

Kasl, C. (1992). *Many roads, one journey.* HarperPerennial.

Keane, T. M. (1995). The role of exposure therapy in the psychological treatment of PTSD. *Clinical Quarterly (National Center for Posttraumatic Stress Disorder), 5,* 1, 3–6.

Keane, T. M., Fairbank, J. A., Caddell, J. M., & Zimering, R. T. (1989). Implosive (flooding) therapy reduces symptoms of PTSD in Vietnam combat veterans. *Behavior Therapy, 20*(2), 245–260.

Kelly, C. (2020, October 22). He posed as a doctor and a wilderness expert. Behind the facade was an accused child molester. *USA Today.* www.usatoday.com/in-depth/news/investigations/2020/10/22/how-accused-predator-gained-access-boy-scouts-young-marines/5634247002.

Kelly, J. F., Abry, A., Ferri, M., & Humphreys, K. (2020). Alcoholics Anonymous and 12-step facilitation treatments for alcohol use disorder: A distillation of a 2020 Cochrane Review for clinicians and policy makers. *Alcohol and Alcoholism, 55*(6), 641–651.

Knapp, C. (1996). *Drinking: A Love Story.* New York: Random House.

Krakow, B., Kellner, R., Neidhardt, J., Pathak, D., & Lambert, L. (1993). Imagery rehearsal treatment of chronic nightmares: With a thirty month follow-up. *Journal of Behavior Therapy and Experimental Psychiatry, 24*(4), 325–330.

Kubany, E. S., Hill, E. E., Owens, J. A., Iannce-Spencer, C., McCaig, M. A., Tremayne, K. J., & Williams, P. L. (2004). Cognitive trauma therapy for battered women with PTSD (CTT-BW). *Journal of Consulting & Clinical Psychology, 72*(1), 3–18.

Lambert, M. J. (2013). *Bergin and Garfield's handbook of psychotherapy and behavior change.* Wiley.

Lamott, A. (1994). *Bird by bird: Some instructions on writing and life*. Random House.
Leedom, L. J., Andersen, D., Glynn, M. A., & Barone, M. L. (2019). Counseling intimate partner abuse survivors: Effective and ineffective interventions. *Journal of Counseling & Development, 97,* 364–375.
Leeman, R. F., Hefner, K., Frohe, T., Murray, A., Rosenheck, R. A., Watts, B. V., & Sofuoglu, M. (2017). Exclusion of participants based on substance use status: Findings from randomized controlled trials of treatments for PTSD. *Behaviour Research and Therapy, 89,* 33–40.
Lenz, A. S., Henesy, R., & Callender, K. (2016). Effectiveness of Seeking Safety for co-occurring posttraumatic stress disorder and substance use. *Journal of Counseling & Development, 94*(1), 51–61.
Leslie, M. (Ed.). (2011). *The breaking the cycle compendium: Vol. 1. The roots of relationship* (rev. ed.). Mothercraft Press.
Levine, P. A. (2010). *In an unspoken voice: How the body releases trauma and restores goodness*. North Atlantic Books.
Lewis, A. (1980). *The quotable quotations book*. Ty Crowell.
Lewis, C., Roberts, N. P., Andrew, M., Starling, E., & Bisson, J. I. (2020). Psychological therapies for posttraumatic stress disorder in adults: Systematic review and meta-analysis. *European Journal of Psychotraumatology, 11*(1), 1729633.
Lewis, C., Roberts, N. P., Gibson, S., & Bisson, J. I. (2020). Dropout from psychological therapies for posttraumatic stress disorder (PTSD) in adults: Systematic review and meta-analysis. *European Journal of Psychotraumatology, 11*(1), Article No. 1709709.
Linley, P. A., & Joseph, S. (2002). Posttraumatic growth. *Counseling and Psychotherapy Journal, 13*(1), 14–17.
Litt, L., Cohen, L. R., & Hien, D. (2019). Seeking Safety: A present-focused integrated treatment for PTSD and substance use disorders. In A. A. Vujanovic & S. E. Back (Eds.), *Posttraumatic stress and substance use disorders* (pp. 183–207). Routledge.
Litz, B. T., Stein, N., Delaney, E., Lebowitz, L., Nash, W. P., Silva, C., & Maguen, S. (2009). Moral injury and moral repair in war veterans: A preliminary model and intervention strategy. *Clinical Psychology Review, 29*(8), 695–706.
Lowinson, J. H., Ruiz, P., Millman, R. B., & Langrod, J. G. (1997). *Substance abuse: A comprehensive textbook* (3rd ed.). Williams & Wilkins.
Luborsky, L., Singer, B., & Luborsky, L. (1976). Comparative studies of psychotherapies: Is it true that "everybody has won and all must have prizes"? *Proceedings of the Annual Meeting of the American Psychopathology Association, 64,* 3–22.
Maguen, S., Madden, E., Holder, N., Li, Y., Seal, K. H., Neylan, T. C., . . . Shiner, B. (2021). Effectiveness and comparative effectiveness of evidence-based psychotherapies for posttraumatic stress disorder in clinical practice. *Psychological Medicine, 53*(2), 1–10.
Maples-Keller, J. L., & Rauch, S. A. M. (2020). Habituation. In J. S. Abramowitz & S. M. Blakey (Eds.), *Clinical handbook of fear and anxiety: Maintenance processes and treatment mechanisms* (pp. 249–263). American Psychological Association.
Marich, J. (2012). *Trauma and the Twelve Steps: A complete guide for enhancing recovery*. Cornersburg Media.
Marks, J. (2015). *The hidden children: The secret survivors of the Holocaust*. Random House.
Marlatt, G. A., & Gordon, J. R. (1985). *Relapse prevention: Maintenance strategies in the treatment of addictive behaviors*. Guilford Press.
Marsh, T. N., Cote-Meek, S., Toulouse, P., Najavits, L. M., & Young, N. L. (2015). The application of two-eyed seeing decolonizing methodology in qualitative and quantitative research for the treatment of intergenerational trauma and substance use disorders. *International Journal of Qualitative Methods, 14*(5), 1–13.
Mate, G. (2022, June 11). *Trauma and addiction*. Paper presented at the Trauma Days Conference of the Polarity Center, Zurich, Switzerland.
Matthiessen, L. (2023). *First light: A journey out of darkness*. Arcade.
McCann, I. L., & Pearlman, L. A. (1990). *Psychological trauma and the adult survivor: Theory, therapy and transformation*. Brunner/Mazel.
McCullough, L. (2003). *Treating affect phobia: A manual for short-term dynamic psychotherapy*. Guilford Press.
McDermott, S. (2021, January 24). The homeless drug addict who became a professor. *BBC News*. www.bbc.com/news/stories-55559382.

McGovern, M. P., Lambert-Harris, C., Acquilano, S., Xie, H., Alterman, A. I., & Weiss, R. D. (2009). A cognitive behavioral therapy for co-occurring substance use and posttraumatic stress disorders. *Addictive Behaviors, 34*(10), 892–897.

McGovern, M. P., Lambert-Harris, C., Alterman, A. I., Xie, H., & Meier, A. (2011). A randomized controlled trial comparing integrated cognitive behavioral therapy versus individual addiction counseling for co-occurring substance use and posttraumatic stress disorders. *Journal of Dual Diagnosis, 7*(4), 207–227.

McKay, J. R. (2017). Making the hard work of recovery more attractive for those with substance use disorders. *Addiction, 112*(5), 751–757.

McLellan, A. T., Lewis, D. C., O'Brien, C. P., & Kleber, H. D. (2000). Drug dependence, a chronic medical illness: Implications for treatment, insurance, and outcomes evaluation. *Journal of American Medical Association, 284*(13), 1689–1695.

McLellan, A. T., Woody, G. E., Luborsky, L., & Goehl, L. (1988). Is the counselor an "active ingredient" in substance abuse rehabilitation?: An examination of treatment success among four counselors. *Journal of Nervous and Mental Disease, 176,* 423–430.

Megginson, L. C. (1963). Lessons from Europe for American business. *Southwestern Social Science Quarterly, 44*(1), 3–13.

Meisler, A. W. (1999). Group treatment of PTSD and comorbid alcohol abuse. In B. H. Young & D. D. Blake (Eds.), *Group treatments for post-traumatic stress disorder* (pp. 117–136). Brunner/Mazel.

Melzack, R. (1975). The McGill Pain Questionnaire: Major properties and scoring methods. *Pain, 1*(3), 277–299.

Meyer, E. C., Walser, R., Hermann, B., La Bash, H., DeBeer, B. B., Morissette, S. B., . . . Schnurr, P. P. (2018). Acceptance and commitment therapy for co-occurring posttraumatic stress disorder and alcohol use disorders in veterans: Pilot treatment outcomes. *Journal of Traumatic Stress, 31*(5), 781–789.

Micale, M. S. (1989). Hysteria and its historiography: A review of past and present writings (I). *History of Science, 27*(3), 223–261.

Miller, D., & Guidry, L. (2001). *Addictions and trauma recovery*. Norton.

Miller, W. R. (1999). *Integrating spirituality into treatment: Resources for practitioners*. American Psychological Association.

Miller, W. R. (2004). *Combined behavioral intervention manual: A clinical research guide for therapists treating people with alcohol abuse and dependence*. U.S. Department of Health and Human Services, National Institutes of Health.

Miller, W. R., Benefield, R. G., & Tonigan, J. S. (1993). Enhancing motivation for change in problem drinking: A controlled comparison of two therapist styles. *Journal of Consulting and Clinical Psychology, 61,* 455–461.

Miller, W. R., & C' de Baca, J. (2001). *Quantum change: When epiphanies and sudden insights transform ordinary lives*. Guilford Press.

Miller, W. R., & Rollnick, S. (1991). *Motivational interviewing: Preparing people to change addictive behavior*. Guilford Press.

Milosz, C. (1980, December 8). *The Nobel Prize in Literature 1980*. www.nobelprize.org/prizes/literature/1980/milosz/lecture.

Mohn, B. (1957, November 3). Talk with Isak Dinesen. *New York Times*. www.nytimes.com/1957/11/03/archives/talk-with-isak-dinesen.html.

Moreno, J. L. (1964). *Psychodrama*. Beacon House.

Morris, D. J. (2015, January 17). After PTSD, more trauma. *New York Times*. https://archive.nytimes.com/opinionator.blogs.nytimes.com/2015/01/17/after-ptsd-more-trauma.

Moser, J. S., Cahill, S. P., & Foa, E. B. (2010). Evidence for poorer outcome in patients with severe negative trauma-related cognitions receiving prolonged exposure plus cognitive restructuring: Implications for treatment matching in posttraumatic stress disorder. *Journal of Nervous and Mental Disease, 198*(1), 72–75.

Naipaul, V. S. (2019, December 30). The strangeness of grief. *The New Yorker*. www.newyorker.com/magazine/2020/01/06/the-strangeness-of-grief.

Najavits, L. M. (2002a). *A woman's addiction workbook*. New Harbinger.

Najavits, L. M. (2002b). Clinicians' views on treating posttraumatic stress disorder and substance use disorder. *Journal on Substance Abuse Treatment, 22,* 79–85.

Najavits, L. M. (2002c). *Seeking Safety: A treatment manual for PTSD and substance abuse.* Guilford Press.

Najavits, L. M. (2004). Assessment of trauma, PTSD, and substance use disorder: A practical guide. In J. P. Wilson & T. M. Keane (Eds.), *Assessment of psychological trauma and PTSD* (pp. 466–491). Guilford Press.

Najavits, L. M. (2007). *Creating Change Fidelity Scale.* Unpublished measure, Treatment Innovations, Newton Centre, MA.

Najavits, L. M. (2011). Treatments for PTSD and pathological gambling: What do patients want? *Journal of Gambling Studies, 27,* 229–241.

Najavits, L. M. (2014). Creating Change: A new past-focused model for PTSD and substance abuse. In P. Ouimette & J. P. Read (Eds.), *Trauma and substance abuse: Causes, consequences, and treatment of comorbid disorders* (pp. 281–303). American Psychological Association Press.

Najavits, L. M. (2015). The problem of dropout from "gold standard" PTSD therapies. *F1000Prime Reports, 7*(43).

Najavits, L. M. (2017). *Recovery from trauma, addiction, or both: Finding your best self.* Guilford Press.

Najavits, L. M. (2019). *Finding your best self: Recovery from addiction, trauma, or both* (rev. ed.). Guilford Press.

Najavits, L. M. (2022). Trauma and addiction: A clinician's guide to treatment. In U. Schnyder & M. Cloitre (Eds.), *Evidence based treatments for trauma-related psychological disorders: A practical guide for clinicians* (pp. 371–387). Springer.

Najavits, L. M., Clark, H. W., DiClemente, C. C., Potenza, M. N., Shaffer, H. J., Sorensen, J. L., . . . Zweben, J. E. (2020). PTSD/substance use disorder comorbidity: Treatment options and public health needs. *Current Treatment Options in Psychiatry, 7*(4), 544–558.

Najavits, L. M., Griffin, M. L., Luborsky, L., Frank, A., Weiss, R. D., Liese, B. S., . . . Simon Onken, L. (1995). Therapists' emotional reactions to substance abusers: A new questionnaire and initial findings. *Psychotherapy, 32,* 669–677.

Najavits, L. M., & Hien, D. A. (2013). Helping vulnerable populations: A comprehensive review of the treatment outcome literature on substance use disorder and PTSD. *Journal of Clinical Psychology: In Session, 69*(5), 433–479.

Najavits, L. M., Hyman, S. M., Ruglass, L. M., Hien, D. A., & Read, J. P. (2017). Substance use disorder and trauma. In S. Gold, J. Cook, & C. Dalenberg (Eds.), *Handbook of trauma psychology* (pp. 195–214). American Psychological Association.

Najavits, L. M., & Johnson, K. M. (2014). Pilot study of Creating Change, a new past-focused model for PTSD and substance abuse. *American Journal on Addictions, 23,* 415–422.

Najavits, L. M., Kivlahan, D., & Kosten, T. (2011). A national survey of clinicians' views of evidence-based therapies for PTSD and substance abuse. *Addiction Research and Theory, 19,* 138–147.

Najavits, L. M., Krinsley, K., Waring, M. E., Gallagher, M. W., & Skidmore, C. (2018). A randomized controlled trial for veterans with PTSD and substance use disorder: Creating Change versus Seeking Safety. *Substance Use & Misuse, 53*(11), 1788–1800.

Najavits, L. M., Runkel, R., Neuner, C., Frank, A., Thase, M., Crits-Christoph, P., & Blaine, J. (2003). Rates and symptoms of PTSD among cocaine-dependent patients. *Journal of Studies on Alcohol, 64,* 601–606.

Najavits, L. M., Schmitz, M., Gotthardt, S., & Weiss, R. D. (2005). Seeking Safety plus Exposure Therapy: An outcome study on dual diagnosis men. *Journal of Psychoactive Drugs, 37,* 425–435.

Najavits, L. M., & Strupp, H. H. (1994). Differences in the effectiveness of psychodynamic therapists: A process-outcome study. *Psychotherapy, 31,* 114–123.

Najavits, L. M., Sullivan, T. P., Schmitz, M., Weiss, R. D., & Lee, C. S. N. (2004). Treatment utilization of women with PTSD and substance dependence. *American Journal on Addictions, 13,* 215–224.

Najavits, L. M., & Weiss, R. D. (1994). Variations in therapist effectiveness in the treatment of patients with substance use disorders: An empirical review. *Addiction, 89,* 679–688.

Najavits, L. M., Weiss, R. D., & Shaw, S. R. (1997). The link between substance abuse and posttraumatic stress disorder in women: A research review. *American Journal on Addictions, 6,* 273–283.

Nass, G. C. M., van Rens, L. W., & Dijkstra, B. A. G. (2019). Clinicians' perceptions for indicating and contra-indicating integrated treatment for SUD and comorbid PTSD, a vignette study. *Substance Abuse Treatment, Prevention, and Policy, 14,* 7.

National Academy of Sciences. (2013). *Substance use disorders in the U.S. armed forces.* National Academies Press.

National Institute on Drug Abuse. (2018). *Principles of drug addiction treatment: A research-based guide* (3rd ed.). https://nida.nih.gov/sites/default/files/675-principles-of-drug-addiction-treatment-a-research-based-guide-third-edition.pdf.

National Institute on Drug Abuse. (2019, August 5). Genetics and epigenetics of addiction. *DrugFacts.* http://nida.nih.gov/publications/drugfacts/genetics-epigenetics-addiction.

Nichols, M. P., & Efran, J. S. (1985). Catharsis in psychotherapy: A new perspective. *Psychotherapy: Theory, Research, Practice, Training, 22*(1), 46.

Nichols, M. P., & Zax, M. (1977). *Catharsis in psychotherapy.* Gardner Press.

Norman, S. B., Trim, R., Haller, M., Davis, B. C., Myers, U. S., Colvonen, P. J., , , , Angkaw, A. C. (2019). Efficacy of integrated exposure therapy vs integrated coping skills therapy for comorbid posttraumatic stress disorder and alcohol use disorder: A randomized clinical trial. *JAMA Psychiatry, 76*(8), 791–799.

Nowinski, J., Baker, S., & Carroll, K. (1995). *Twelve Step facilitation therapy manual (Project MATCH): A clinical research guide for therapists treating individuals with alcohol abuse and dependence* (Vol. 1). National Institute on Alcohol Abuse and Alcoholism.

O'Brien, C. P., Childress, A. R., McLellan, T., & Ehrman, R. (1990). Integrating systematic cue exposure with standard treatment in recovering drug dependent patients. *Addictive Behaviors, 15,* 355–365.

Oliver, M. (1986). "Wild geese" [Poem]. *Atlantic Monthly Press,* p. 14.

Ouimette, P., & Read, J. P. (2014). *Handbook of trauma, PTSD and substance use disorder comorbidity.* American Psychological Association Press.

Palmer, S. E., & Schloss, K. B. (2010). An ecological valence theory of human color preference. *Proceedings of the National Academy of Sciences, 107*(19), 8877–8882.

Parson, E. R. (1984). The reparation of the self: Clinical and theoretical dimensions in the treatment of Vietnam combat veterans. *Journal of Contemporary Psychotherapy, 14*(1), 4–56.

Pearlman, L. A. (2007). *Time to say goodbye: How do we say goodbye in long-term relational trauma therapies?* Panel at the annual meeting of the International Society of Traumatic Stress Studies, Baltimore, MD.

Pearlman, L. A., & Saakvitne, K. W. (1995). *Trauma and the therapist: Countertransference and vicarious traumatization in psychotherapy with incest survivors.* Norton.

Pennebaker, J. W., & Evans, J. F. (2014). *Expressive writing: Words that heal.* Idyll Arbor.

Perez-Dandieu, B., & Tapia, G. (2014). Treating trauma in addiction with EMDR: A pilot study. *Journal of Psychoactive Drugs, 46*(4), 303–309.

Petry, N. M. (2000). A comprehensive guide to the application of contingency management procedures in clinical settings. *Drug and Alcohol Dependence, 58*(1), 9–25.

Pitman, R. K., Altman, B., Greenwald, E., Longpre, R. E., Macklin, M. L., Poiré, R. E., & Steketee, G. S. (1991). Psychiatric complications during flooding therapy for posttraumatic stress disorder. *Journal of Clinical Psychiatry, 52*(1), 17–20.

Popik, B. (2012, April 22). "The road to success is always under construction" [Business adage]. www.barrypopik.com/index.php/new_york_city/entry/the_road_to_success_is_always_under_construction.

Potter-Efron, R. (2006). Attachment, trauma and addiction. *Journal of Chemical Dependency Treatment, 8*(2), 71–87.

Prochaska, J. O., DiClemente, C. C., & Norcross, J. C. (1992). In search of how people change: Applications to addictive behaviors. *American Psychologist, 47,* 1102–1114.

Rad, R. R. (2010). *Rumi & self psychology.* Trafford.

Rando, T. A. (1993). *Treatment of complicated mourning.* Research Press.

Raphael, B. (2003). *The anatomy of bereavement: A handbook for the caring professions.* Routledge.

Rawson, R. A., & McCann, M. J. (2005). The matrix model of intensive outpatient treatment. *Behavioral Health Recovery Management, 3,* 1–37.

Resick, P. A., Monson, C. M., & Chard, K. M. (2008). *Cognitive processing therapy: Veteran/military version: Therapist manual.* Department of Veterans' Affairs. www.apa.org/ptsd-guideline/treatments/cognitive-processing-therapist.pdf.

Richards, S. E. (2003, May). Woman warrior. *Marie Claire*, p. 220.
Riemer, J., & Stampfer, N. (2015). *Ethical wills and how to prepare them: A guide to sharing your values from generation to generation*. Jewish Lights.
Rilke, R. M. (1986). *Letters to a Young Poet* (S. Mitchell, Trans.). Vintage. (Original work published 1929)
Roberts, N. P., Lotzin, A., & Schäfer, I. (2022). A systematic review and meta-analysis of psychological interventions for comorbid post-traumatic stress disorder and substance use disorder. *European Journal of Psychotraumatology, 13*(1), 2041831.
Rogers, C. (1995). *On becoming a person: A therapist's view of psychotherapy* (2nd ed.). HarperOne.
Rogers, F. (2013). *Life's journeys according to Mister Rogers: Things to remember along the way*. Hachette.
Rogers, N. (1993). *The creative connection: Expressive arts as healing*. Science and Behavioral Books.
Ross, C. A., & Gahan, P. (1988). Techniques in the treatment of multiple personality disorder. *American Journal of Psychotherapy, 42*(1), 40–52.
Røssberg, J., Eiring, Ø., & Friis, S. (2004). Work environment and job satisfaction: A psychometric evaluation of the Working Environment Scale-10. *Social Psychiatry and Psychiatric Epidemiology, 39*, 576–580.
Rothbaum, B. O., Hodges, L. F., Ready, D., Graap, K., & Alarcon, R. D. (2001). Virtual reality exposure therapy for Vietnam veterans with posttraumatic stress disorder. *Journal of Clinical Psychology, 62*(8), 617–622.
Rothschild, B. (2000). *The body remembers: The psychophysiology of trauma and trauma treatment*. Norton.
Ruglass, L. M., Lopez-Castro, T., Papini, S., Killeen, T., Back, S. E., & Hien, D. A. (2017). Concurrent treatment with prolonged exposure for co-occurring full or subthreshold posttraumatic stress disorder and substance use disorders: A randomized clinical trial. *Psychotherapy and Psychosomatics, 86*(3), 150–161.
Sannibale, C., Teesson, M., Creamer, M., Sitharthan, T., Bryant, R. A., Sutherland, K., . . . Peek-O'Leary, M. (2013). Randomized controlled trial of cognitive behaviour therapy for comorbid post-traumatic stress disorder and alcohol use disorders. *Addiction, 108*, 1397–1410.
Savage, A., & Russell, L. A. (2005). Tangled in a web of affiliation: Social support networks of dually diagnosed women who are trauma survivors. *Journal of Behavioral Health Services & Research, 32*(2), 199–214.
Schauer, M., Robjant, K., Elbert, T., & Neuner, F. (2020). Narrative exposure therapy. In J. D. Ford & C. A. Courtois (Eds.), *Treating complex traumatic stress disorders in adults: Scientific foundations and therapeutic models* (2nd ed., pp. 309–331). Guilford Press.
Schirmacher, W. (2003). *German 20th century philosophical writings*. A&C Black.
Schnurr, P. P., Friedman, M. J., Lavori, P. W., & Hsieh, F. Y. (2001). Design of Department of Veterans Affairs Cooperative Study No. 420: Group treatment of posttraumatic stress disorder. *Controlled Clinical Trials, 22*(1), 74–88.
Schwartz, R. C. (2013). Moving from acceptance toward transformation with internal family systems therapy (IFS). *Journal of Clinical Psychology, 69*(8), 805–816.
Seidel, R. W., Gusman, F. D., & Abueg, F. R. (1994). Theoretical and practical foundations of an inpatient post-traumatic stress disorder and alcoholism treatment program. *Psychotherapy, 31*, 67–78.
Shamai, M., & Levin-Megged, O. (2006). The myth of creating an integrative story: The therapeutic experience of Holocaust survivors. *Qualitative Health Research, 16*(5), 692–712.
Shapiro, F. (1995). *Eye movement desensitization and reprocessing: Basic principles, protocols, and procedures*. Guilford Press.
Shaw, L. M. (2023, April 10). *Love and forgiveness: Controversial healing tools for survivors and perpetrators of sexual abuse*. www.loveandforgiveness.com/chapter.php.
Shay, J. (1994). *Achilles in Vietnam: Combat trauma and the undoing of character*. Simon & Schuster.
Shem, S. (1978). *The house of God*. Richard Marek.
Sherman, A. D. F., Balthazar, M., Zhang, W., Febres-Cordero, S., Clark, K. D., Klepper, M., . . . Kelly, U. (2023). Seeking safety intervention for comorbid post-traumatic stress and substance use disorder: A meta-analysis. *Brain and Behavior, 13*(5), e2999.
Sherman, L. J., Lynch, S. E., Greeno, C. G., & Hoeffel, E. M. (2017). *Behavioral health workforce: Quality assurance practices in substance abuse treatment facilities* (The CBHSQ Report). U.S. Substance Abuse and Mental Health Services Administration.
Simmons, P. (2003). *Learning to fall: The blessings of an imperfect life*. Random House.
Simpson, T. L., Goldberg, S. B., Louden, D. K. N., Blakey, S. M., Hawn, S. E., Lott, A., . . . Kaysen, D.

(2021). Efficacy and acceptability of interventions for co-occurring PTSD and SUD: A meta-analysis. *Journal of Anxiety Disorders, 84,* 102490.

Simpson, T. L., Kaysen, D. L., Fleming, C. B., Rhew, I. C., Jaffe, A. E., Desai, S., . . . Resick, P. A. (2022). Cognitive processing therapy or relapse prevention for comorbid posttraumatic stress disorder and alcohol use disorder: A randomized clinical trial. *PLOS ONE, 17*(11), e0276111.

Solomon, S. D., Gerrity, E. T., & Muff, A. M. (1992). Efficacy of treatments for posttraumatic stress disorder. *Journal of the American Medical Association, 268,* 633–638.

Solomon, S. D., & Johnson, D. M. (2002). Psychosocial treatment of posttraumatic stress disorder: A practice-friendly review of outcome research. *Journal of Clinical Psychology, 58*(8), 947–959.

Somohano, V. C., & Bowen, S. (2022). Trauma-integrated mindfulness-based Relapse Prevention for women with comorbid post-traumatic stress disorder and substance use disorder: A cluster randomized controlled feasibility and acceptability trial. *Journal of Integrative and Complementary Medicine, 28*(9), 729–738.

Stampfl, T. G., & Levis, D. J. (1967). Essentials of implosive therapy: A learning-theory-based psychodynamic behavioral therapy. *Journal of Abnormal Psychology, 72*(6), 496.

Stapleton, J. A., Taylor, S., & Asmundson, G. J. (2006). Effects of three PTSD treatments on anger and guilt: Exposure therapy, eye movement desensitization and reprocessing, and relaxation training. *Journal of Traumatic Stress, 19*(1), 19–28.

Steele, K. H. (1989). A model for abreaction with MPD and other dissociative disorders. *Dissociation: Progress in the Dissociative Disorders, 2*(3), 151–159.

Steenkamp, M. M., Litz, B. T., & Marmar, C. R. (2020). First-line psychotherapies for military-related PTSD. *Journal of American Medical Association, 323*(7), 656–657.

Sterman, C. (2006). Traumatized addicted women: Treatment issues. *Journal of Chemical Dependency Treatment, 8*(2), 255–282.

Stone, D., & Heen, S. (2015). *Thanks for the feedback: The science and art of receiving feedback well.* Penguin.

Substance Abuse and Mental Health Services Administration. (2014). *Trauma-informed care in behavioral health services; Treatment Improvement Protocol (TIP) #57.* U.S. Government Printing Office. https://store.samhsa.gov/product/TIP-57-Trauma-Informed-Care-in-Behavioral-Health-Services/SMA14-4816.

Taylor, J. B. (2021). *Whole brain living: The anatomy of choice and the four characters that drive our life.* Hay House.

Taylor, S. (2006). *Clinician's guide to PTSD: A cognitive-behavioral approach.* Guilford Press.

Tedeschi, R. G. (2004). Posttraumatic growth: A new perspective on psychotraumatology. *Psychiatric Times, 4,* 58.

Thompson, K. (Director). (1990). *James Baldwin: The price of the ticket* [Video]. California Newsreel.

Tolman, C. W. (1996). *Problems of theoretical psychology* (Vol. 6). Captus Press.

Tolstoy, L. (1867). *War and peace.* Project Gutenberg (ebook). www.gutenberg.org/files/2600/2600-h/2600-h.htm#link2HCH0279.

Treaster, J. B., & Tabor, M. B. (1993, February 8). Little help for mentally ill addicts; two treatment bureaucracies compete to avoid them. *New York Times.* www.nytimes.com/1993/02/08/nyregion/little-help-for-mentally-ill-addicts-two-treatment-bureaucracies-compete-avoid.html.

Triffleman, E., Carroll, K., & Kellogg, S. (1999). Substance dependence posttraumatic stress disorder therapy. An integrated cognitive-behavioral approach. *Journal of Substance Abuse Treatment, 17*(1–2), 3–14.

Trotter, C. (1992). *Double bind.* Hazelden Press.

Twombly, S. (2021, January 8). Juggling my children, Their alcoholic sitter and my own sobriety. *New York Times.* www.nytimes.com/2021/01/08/well/family/alcoholic-babysitter-sobriety.html.

United States Special Operations Command. (2017, March 2). *PTSD affects brain circuitry.* www.socom.mil/POTFF/Pages/PTSD%20affects%20brain%20circuitry.aspx.

Vaish, A., Grossmann, T., & Woodward, A. (2008). Not all emotions are created equal: The negativity bias in social-emotional development. *Psychological Bulletin, 134*(3), 383–403.

van Dam, D., Ehring, T., Vedel, E., & Emmelkamp, P. M. (2013). Trauma-focused treatment for posttraumatic stress disorder combined with CBT for severe substance use disorder: A randomized controlled trial. *BMC Psychiatry, 13*(1), 172.

van de Ven, K., Ritter, A., & Roche, A. (2020). Alcohol and other drug (AOD) staffing and their workplace: Examining the relationship between clinician and organisational workforce characteristics and treatment outcomes in the AOD field. *Drugs: Education, Prevention and Policy, 27*(1), 1–14.

van der Hart, O., & Brown, P. (1992). Abreaction re-evaluated. *Dissociation, 5,* 127–140.

van der Hart, O., Brown, P., & van der Kolk, B. A. (1989). Pierre Janet's treatment of post-traumatic stress. *Journal of Traumatic Stress, 2,* 379–395.

van der Kolk, B. (2000). Posttraumatic stress disorder and the nature of trauma. *Dialogues in Clinical Neuroscience, 2*(1), 7–22.

van der Kolk, B. (2014). *The body keeps the score: Brain, mind and body in the healing of trauma.* Penguin Books.

van der Kolk, B., & van der Hart, O. (1990). Pierre Janet and the breakdown of adaptation in psychological trauma. *American Journal of Psychiatry, 146,* 1530–1540.

van der Kolk, B. A., McFarlane, A. C., & Weisaeth, L. (1996). *Traumatic stress: The effects of overwhelming experience on mind, body, and society.* Guilford Press.

van der Kolk, B. A., van der Hart, O., & Burbridge, J. (1995). The treatment of post traumatic stress disorder. In S. E. Hobfoll & M. W. de Vries (Eds.), *Extreme stress and communities: Impact and intervention* (pp. 421–443). Springer.

van Dijk, J. A., Schoutrop, M. J., & Spinhoven, P. (2003). Testimony therapy: Treatment method for traumatized victims of organized violence. *American Journal of Psychotherapy, 57*(3), 361–373.

Varker, T., Jones, K. A., Arjmand, H.-A., Hinton, M., Hiles, S. A., Freijah, I., . . . O'Donnell, M. (2021). Dropout from guideline-recommended psychological treatments for posttraumatic stress disorder: A systematic review and meta-analysis. *Journal of Affective Disorders Reports, 4,* 100093.

Velasquez, M. M., Maurer, G. G., Crouch, C., & DiClemente, C. C. (2001). *Group treatment for substance abuse: A stages-of-change therapy manual.* Hazelden.

Verduyn, P., & Lavrijsen, S. (2015). Which emotions last longest and why: The role of event importance and rumination. *Motivation and Emotion, 39*(1), 119–127.

Veronen, L. J., & Kilpatrick, D. G. (1983). Stress management for rape victims. In D. Meichenbaum & M. E. Jaremko (Eds.), *Stress reduction and prevention* (pp. 341–374). Plenum Press.

Vogelmann-Sine, S., Sine, L., Smyth, N. J., & Popky, A. J. (1998). *EMDR: Chemical dependency treatment manual.* Trauma Recovery HAP Store.

Vogel-Scibilia, S. E., McNulty, K. C., Baxter, B., Miller, S., Dine, M., & Frese, F. J. (2009). The recovery process utilizing Erikson's stages of human development. *Community Mental Health Journal, 45,* 405–414.

Volpicelli, J. R., Pettinati, H. M., McLellan, A. T., & O'Brien, C. P. (2001). *Combining medication and psychosocial treatments for addictions: The BRENDA approach.* Guilford Press.

Washington State Institute for Public Policy. (2018, April 28). *Benefit-cost results: Substance use disorders.* www.wsipp.wa.gov/BenefitCost/Program/307.

Washton, A. M., & Zweben, J. E. (2022). *Treating alcohol and drug problems in psychotherapy practice: Doing what works* (2nd ed.). Guilford Press.

Wattenberg, M. S., Gross, D. L., Niles, B. L., Unger, W. S., & Shea, M. T. (2021). *Present-centered group therapy for PTSD: Embracing today.* Routledge.

Watts, B. V., Shiner, B., Zubkoff, L., Carpenter-Song, E., Ronconi, J. M., & Coldwell, C. M. (2014). Implementation of evidence-based psychotherapies for posttraumatic stress disorder in VA specialty clinics. *Psychiatric Services, 65*(5), 648–653.

Weisaeth, L. (2002). The European history of psychotraumatology. *Journal of Traumatic Stress, 15*(6), 443–452.

Weiss, R., & Schneider, J. (2015). *Always turned on: Facing sex addiction in the digital age.* Gentle Path Press.

White, W. L. (1996). *Pathways: From the culture of addiction to the culture of recovery: A travel guide for addiction professionals.* Hazelden.

White, W. L. (1998). *Slaying the dragon: The history of addiction treatment and recovery in America.* Chestnut Health Systems/Lighthouse Institute.

White, W. L., & Kleber, H. D. (2008). Preventing harm in the name of help: A guide for addiction professionals. *Counselor, 9*(6), 10–17.

World Health Organization. (2019). *International classification of diseases* (11th ed.). https://icd.who.int.

Zisook, S., & Shear, K. (2009). Grief and bereavement: What psychiatrists need to know. *World Psychiatry, 8*(2), 67.

Zlotnick, C., Shea, T. M., Rosen, K., Simpson, E., Mulrenin, K., Begin, A., & Pearlstein, T. (1997). An affect-management group for women with posttraumatic stress disorder and histories of childhood sexual abuse. *Journal of Traumatic Stress, 10*(3), 425–436.

Zweig, C., & Abrams, J. (1991). *Meeting the shadow: The hidden power of the dark side of human nature*. Penguin.

Index

Addiction. *See also* Addiction and trauma
 12-step groups, 26, 43, 79
 addiction-informed care, 55, 78
 behavioral type, 2, 150, 321, 325, 329, 330, 332–334
 best treatment practices, 77–80, 152
 confrontational treatment, 35, 232
 contract to reduce, 78
 cross-training, 35, 79
 key concepts, 77
 key signs, 329–330
 link to trauma, 2–4
 medical clearance, 79
 motivation for treatment, 77, 78
 professional associations, 80
 reasons for, in relation to trauma, 3
 screening, 79
 stages of change, 110
 substance type, 79, 277, 330, 332–334
 symptom substitution, 79
 terminology, 79
 treatment, past-focused models, 26
 treatment, present-focused models, 22
 worsening, criteria for, 78
Addiction and trauma. *See also* Addiction; Trauma
 causal pathways, 3
 challenges, 32–34, 87–88
 defenses
  emotional, 167–171
  cognitive, 235–237
 factors, risk and protective, 158–159
 links between, 2–4, 154–155
 memory problems, 281–282
 narrative, 211
 physical problems, 264, 273–275
 power dynamics, 292–295
 progress, 34–35
 screening, 324
 silencing, 177–178
 societal impact on, 221–222, 227–229
Assessment
 addiction, 79, 324
 Agnew Relationship Measure—Client Version, 355
 Agnew Relationship Measure—Counselor Version, 352
 types, 40
 Creating Change Feedback Questionnaire, 43, 319
 Creating Change Fidelity Scale, 43
 End-of-Session Questionnaire, 70
 Excessive Behavior Scale, 332–334
 materials for sessions, 64–65
 posttraumatic stress disorder, 324
 progress and worsening, 47–48
 Safe Behavior Scale, 71–72
 screening, 127, 324
 Strengths and Challenges Questionnaire, 341–343
 trauma, 81, 324

B

Break the Silence topic, 173–182
 client pages, 187–193
 commitment ideas, 182
 counselor pages, 173–176
 Handout 1: Silencing in Trauma and Addiction, 177–178
 Handout 2: Feeling Heard, 179–180
 Handout 3: Sharing Outside of Treatment, 181
 quotation for, 177

C

Counselor role
  Agnew Relationship Scale—Client version, 355
  Agnew Relationship Scale—Counselor version, 352
  alliance, 87
  best treatment practices
    addiction, 77–80
    trauma, 80–81
  boundaries, 84
  emotional reactions, countertransfrence, 88–90
  empathy, 81–82
  interest in Creating Change, 91–92
  openness to feedback, 84
  positive processes, 81–92
  requirements, 8
  self-awareness, 88–90, 91–92
  self-care, 85
  self-disclosure, 85
  strengths, 91–92
  wounded healer concept, 82
Create Change topic, 109–119
  client pages, 113–119
  commitment ideas, 119
  counselor pages, 109–113
  Handout 1: Creating Change Skills, 113–116
  Handout 2: How Change Happens, 117–118
  quotation for, 113
Creating Change model. *See also* Implementation
  balancing positive and negative experiences, 9, 25
  development of, 16
  evidence, 16–18
  flexibility, 6, 10, 15, 29, 39
  key principles, 8–11
  list of topics, 6, 7
  narrative, approach to, 6
  other models, use with, 8, 58–59
  overall summary, 18–19, 99
  rationale, 11–14, 18–19
  safeguards, 10–11
  Seeking Safety, relation to, 4–6, 14–15
  Seeking Safety, use with, 2, 40, 57–58
  skills, 8–9, 113–116
  society, focus on, 9, 29
  title, meaning of, 15–16
  website, 75
Culture. *See also* the topic Influences: Family, Community, Culture; *See also* addiction-informed; trauma-informed
  "culture of silence," 173, 177
  Creating Change, adaptation for, 15, 46, 61
  emotional expression differences, 49, 166
  impact of, 9
  advantages and disadvantages, 159
  treatment setting, 55

D

Darkness and Light topic, 183–193
  client handouts, 187–193
  commitment ideas, 193
  counselor pages, 183–86
  Handout 1: Darkness and Light, 187–188
  Handout 2: Expression Exercises, 189–191
  Handout 3: Build Flexibility, 192
  quotation for, 187
Deepen Your Story topic, 300–311
  client pages, 304–311
  commitment ideas, 311
  counselor pages, 300–303
  Handout 1: Supporting Yourself, 304
  Handout 2: 30 Ways to Deepen Your Story, 305–307
  Handout 3: The Long View, 308–310
  quotation for, 304

E

Emergencies, 30, 47–48
  plan for, 105
Emotion. *See also* the topic Emotions and Healing
  approach to, 27–28, 48–51
Emotions and Healing topic, 194–205
  client pages, 198–205
  commitment ideas, 205
  counselor pages, 194–197
  Handout 1: Emotions and Healing Quiz, 198–200
  Handout 2: What Did You Learn about Feelings?, 201–202
  Handout 3: Shift Your Emotional Perspective, 203–204
Extra Topic: Recovery Strengths and Challenges, 336–347
  client pages, 341–347
  commitment ideas, 347
  counselor pages, 336–340
  Handout 1: Strengths and Challenges Questionnaire, 341–343
  Handout 2: Next Steps Plan, 344
  Handout 3: Mental Health Advance Directive, 345–346
  quotation for, 341

Index

Extra Topic: Understanding Trauma and Addiction, 321–335
  client pages, 326–335
  commitment ideas, 335
  counselor pages, 321–325
  Handout 1: What Is Trauma?, 326–328
  Handout 2: What Is Addiction?, 329–330
  Handout 3: Tip Sheet to Support the Client, 331
  Handout 4: Excessive Behavior Scale (Behavioral Addictions), 332–334
  quotation for, 326
Extra Topic: Your Relationships, 348–356
  client pages, 353–356
  commitment ideas, 356
  counselor pages, 348–352
  Handout 1: Strengthen Your Relationships, 353–354
  Handout 2: Agnew Relationship Measure–Client Version, 355
  quotation for, 353

G

Grounding
  option at end of session, 45, 67
Growth topic, 312–320
  client pages, 316–320
  counselor pages, 312–315
  Handout 1: From Pain to Growth, 316
  Handout 2: Progress, 317
  Handout 3: Past, Present, Future, 318
  Handout 4: Creating Change Feedback Questionnaire, 319
  idea for commitment, 320
  quotation for, 316

H

Handouts
  20 Questions—Tell Part of Your Addiction Story, 156
  30 Ways to Deepen Your Story, 305–307
  A Conversation in Real Life, 259–260
  About Creating Change, 99–104
  About Telling Your Story, 211
  Agnew Relationship Measure—Client Version, 355
  An Imaginary Conversation, 258
  Build Flexibility, 192
  Context That Helped or Harmed, 134–135
  Creating Change Feedback Questionnaire, 319
  Creating Change Skills, 113–116
  Creating Change Treatment Agreement, 106–107
  Darkness and Light, 187–188
  Deciding to Confront a Perpetrator, 261–262
  Emotional Defenses, 165–166
  Emotions and Healing Quiz, 198–200
  Excessive Behavior Scale (Behavioral Addictions), 332–334
  Explore a Photo or Other Reminder of Your Past, 246
  Expression Exercises, 189–191
  Feeling Heard, 179–180
  From Pain to Growth, 316
  Honor Your Survival, 133
  How Change Happens, 117–118
  How Do you Cope with Difficult Memories?, 283–284
  Identify Your Influences, 226–227
  Lifetime Advantages and Disadvantages, 158–159
  Memory Issues in Trauma and Addiction, 281–282
  Mental health advance directive, 345–346
  Messages About Your Body, 270
  Next Steps Plan, 344
  Open the Door to a New Perspective, 247–248
  Past, Present, Future, 318
  Power, Trauma, and Addiction, 292–295
  Practical Information about Your Treatment, 105
  Progress, 317
  Putting It into Words, 271–272
  Relationship Patterns, 143–146
  Relationship Wisdom, 147
  Remember a Time, 296–297
  Safe versus Unsafe People, 298
  Sharing Outside of Treatment, 181
  Shift Your Emotional Perspective, 203–204
  Silencing in Trauma and Addiction, 177–178
  Society–Helpful and Harmful, 227–229
  Strengthen Your Relationships, 353–354
  Strengths and Challenges Questionnaire, 341–343
  Supporting Yourself, 304
  Supportive Helplines, 127
  The Larger Context, 221–222
  The Long View, 308–310
  The Tangled Web of Addiction and Trauma, 154–155
  The Many Ways of *Knowing*, 238–239
  The Many Ways of *Not Knowing*, 235–237

Handouts (*cont.*)
    The Tree (Part I)—Your Past and Present, 223–224
    The Tree (Part II)—Your Future, 225
    Then versus Now, 157
    Timeline, 213–214
    Tip Sheet to Support the Client, 331
    Too Much or Too Little Memory—What You Can Do, 285–286
    Trauma, Addiction, and the Body, 273–275
    Trust versus Doubt, 124–126
    Ways of Surviving, 167–171
    What Did You Learn about Feelings?, 201–202
    What Do You Want People to Understand?, 256–257
    What Do You Want to Share?, 212
    What Is Addiction?, 329–330
    What Is Trauma?, 326–328
    What You Lived Through, 134–135
    Your Personal Truth, 245
    Your Relationship with Your Body, 268–269
Honor Your Survival topic, 129–138
    client pages, 133–138
    commitment ideas, 138
    counselor pages, 129–132
    Handout 1: Honor Your Survival, 133
    Handout 2: What You Lived Through, 134–135
    Handout 3: Context That Helped or Harmed, 136–137
    quotation for, 133

I

Implementation. *See also* specific treatment topics
    adaptation of the model, 39, 46, 61
    best treatment practices
        addiction, 77–80
        counselor processes, 81–92
        trauma, 80–81
    certificate of attendance, 74
    check-in, 59–61, 68
    check-out, 63–64, 68
    client complexity, 14, 55–57, 87–88
    client eligibility/readiness, 13–14, 40, 55–57, 341–343, *See also* the Extra Topic—Recovery Strengths and Challenges
    client empowerment, 80, 82–83, 86–87
    client engagement, 10, 12, 39, 41–42, 45–46, 62–63, 95
    commitment (homework), 60, 69
    emergencies, 127, 345–346

    emotions, working with, 27–28, 48–51; *See also* the topic Emotions and Healing
    group modality, 38, 52–54
    handouts, use of, 61
    how to begin, 2, 37–38, 41–44
    key questions, 38–40
    other models, use with, 58–59
    overview, 6–8
    progress and worsening, 30, 44, 78, 105
    quotation, 61
    Seeking Safety, use with, 2, 14–15, 40, 57–58
    session format, 40–41, 59–64, 66–67, 103
    setting, 54–55
    three-session try-out, 41, 73
    website for Creating Change, 75
Influences: Family, Community, Culture topic, 216–230
    client pages, 221–230
    commitment ideas, 230
    counselor pages, 216–20
    Handout 1: The Larger Context, 221–222
    Handout 2: The Tree (Part I)—Your Past and Present, 223–224
    Handout 3: The Tree (Part II)—Your Future, 225
    Handout 4: Identify Your Influences, 226–27
    Handout 5: Society—Helpful and Harmful, 227–229
    quotation for, 221
Integrated treatment
    challenges, 32–34
    definition, 35
    past-focused models, 26
    present-focused models, 22
    progress, 34–35
Introduction topic, 95–108
    client pages, 99–108
    commitment ideas, 108
    counselor pages, 95–98
    Handout 1: About Creating Change, 99–104
    Handout 2: Practical Information about Your Treatment, 105
    Handout 3: Creating Change Treatment Agreement, 106–107
    quotation for, 99

K

Knowing and Not Knowing topic, 231–240
    client pages, 235–240
    commitment ideas, 240
    counselor pages, 231–234

Handout 1: The Many Ways of *Not Knowing*, 235–237
Handout 2: The Many Ways of *Knowing*, 238–239
quotation for, 235

L

Language
    adapt for culture in Creating Change, 46
    addiction, use of terms 79
    avoidance versus self-protection, use of terms, 46, 233
    minimizing jargon, 11
    denial, use of term, 232, 233
    emotion terms, 194
    historical differences, 32
Listen to Your Body topic, 264–276
    client pages, 268–276
    commitment ideas, 276
    counselor pages, 264–267
    Handout 1: Your Relationship with Your Body, 268–269
    Handout 2: Messages about Your Body, 270
    Handout 3: Putting It into Words, 271–272
    Handout 4: Trauma, Addiction, and the Body, 273–275
    quotation for, 268

M

Memory. *See also* the topic Memory
    approach to, 28
Memory topic, 277–287
    client pages, 281–287
    commitment ideas, 287
    counselor pages, 277–280
    Handout 1: Memory Issues in Trauma and Addiction, 281–282
    Handout 2: How Do you Cope with Difficult Memories?, 283–284
    Handout 3: Too Much or Too Little Memory: What You Can Do, 285–286
    quotation for, 281

N

Narrative
    approach to, 6
    balancing positive and negative experiences, 9
    types of, 211

P

Past-focused models
    addiction, 26
    comparison to present-focused, 22–26
    trauma, current, 24
    description, 22–26
    trauma, historical, 23
    integrated, 26
    limitations, 4–6, 9, 11-14, 30, 31–32, 52
Posttraumatic stress disorder. *See also* trauma
    posttraumatic growth, 312
    rates in relation to substance use disorder, 3
    screening, 81, 324, 328
Power Dynamics topic, 288–299
    client pages, 292–299
    commitment ideas, 299
    counselor pages, 288–291
    Handout 1: Power, Trauma, and Addiction, 292–295
    Handout 2: Remember a Time, 296–297
    Handout 3: Safe versus Unsafe People, 298
    quotation for, 292

Q

Quotations for topics
    Albert Schweitzer, 353
    Alice Walker, 292
    André Gide, 187
    Anonymous, 154, 304, 341
    Carl Rogers, 165
    Clarissa Pinkola Estés, 113
    Clifford Beers, 221
    Czeslaw Milosz, 177
    Dante Alighieri, 198
    Frank Lloyd Wright, 245
    Frederick Douglass, 326
    George Eliot, 256
    Isak Dinesen, 211
    Jacob L. Moreno, 268
    Jalaluddin Rumi, 281
    James Baldwin, 124
    Mary Oliver, 99
    Philip E. Simmons, 316
    Pierre Janet, 133
    Rainer Maria Rilke, 235
    Virginia Satir, 143

R

Relationship Patterns topic, 139–148
    client pages, 143–148
    commitment ideas, 148

Relationship Patterns topic (*cont.*)
  counselor pages, 139–142
    Handout 1: Relationship Patterns, 143–146
    Handout 2: Relationship Wisdom, 147
  quotation for, 143
Relationships
  healthy versus unhealthy, 143–146, 298
Respect Your Defenses topic, 161–172
  client pages, 165–172
  commitment ideas, 172
  counselor pages, 161–164
    Handout 1: Emotional Defenses, 165–166
    Handout 2: Ways of Surviving, 167–171
  quotation for, 165

S

Seeking Safety model
  Creating Change, similarities and differences, 5, 14–15, 58, 100
  Creating Change, use with, 2, 40, 57–58
  pilot study with Creating Change, 18
  randomized controlled trial compared to Creating Change, 17
  session format identical to Creating Change, 40
Session format. *See also* Implementation
  check-in, 59–61, 66–67, 68
  check-out, 63–64, 66–67, 68
  commitment (homework), 63, 69
  commitment sheet, 69
  detailed guide to, 40–41
  elements, 103
  End-of-Session Questionnaire as option, 66–67, 70
  grounding option, 45, 67
  handouts, use of, 61, 62–63, 66–67
  purpose, 8
  quotation, 61, 66–67

T

Tell Your Story topic, 206–215
  client pages, 211–215
  commitment ideas, 215
  counselor pages, 206–210
    Handout 1: About Telling Your Story, 211
    Handout 2: What Do You Want to Share?, 212
    Handout 3: Timeline, 213–214
  quotation for, 211
Trauma
  best treatment practices, 80–81
  confronting a perpetrator, 80, 261–62
  context aspects, 136–137
  cross-training, 35, 81
  key concepts, 80
  link to addiction, 2–4
  moral injury, 83–84
  posttraumatic growth, 312
  problems from, 327–328
  professional associations, 81
  reenactments, 85
  screening, 81, 324
  trauma-informed care, 34, 81
  treatment, past-focused models, description and list of, 22–26
  treatment, present-focused models, description and list of, 21
  types of, 134–135, 326
Trauma and addiction. *See* Addiction and trauma
Treatment models
  comparison of, 2, 11, 13, 15, 58
  historical lessons, 27–32
  integrated for trauma and addiction
  past-focused, list of, 26
  present-focused, list of, 22
  past-focused, description and list of, 22–26
  present-focused, description and list of, 20–22
  self-help, 79
  stage-based, 4–6, 100
Treatment topics
  Break the Silence, 173–182
  Create Change, 109–119
  Darkness and Light, 183–193
  Deepen Your Story, 300–311
  Emotions and Healing, 194–205
  Extra Topic: Recovery Strengths and Challenges, 336–347
  Extra Topic: Understanding Trauma and Addiction, 321–335
  Extra Topic: Your Relationships, 348–356
  Growth, 312–320
  Honor Your Survival, 129–138
  Influences: Family, Community, Culture, 216–230
  Introduction, 95–108
  Knowing and Not Knowing, 231–240
  Listen to Your Body, 264–276
  Memory, 277–287
  Power Dynamics, 288–299
  Relationship Patterns, 139–148
  Respect Your Defenses, 161–172
  Tell Your Story, 206–215
  Trust versus Doubt, 120–128
  What You Want People to Understand, 250–263

Why Addiction?, 149–160
Your Personal Truth, 241–249
Trust versus Doubt topic
   client pages, 124–128
   commitment ideas, 128
   counselor pages, 120–123
   Handout 1: Trust versus Doubt, 124–126
   Handout 2: Supportive Helplines, 127
   quotation for, 124

W

What You Want People to Understand topic, 250–263
   client pages, 256–263
   commitment ideas, 263
   counselor pages, 249–255
   Handout 1: What Do You Want People to Understand?, 256–257
   Handout 2: An Imaginary Conversation, 258
   Handout 3: A Conversation in Real Life, 259–260
   Handout 4: Deciding to Confront a Perpetrator, 261–262
   quotation for, 256

Why Addiction? topic, 149–160
   client pages, 154–160
   commitment ideas, 160
   counselor pages, 149–153
   Handout 1: The Tangled Web of Addiction and Trauma, 154–155
   Handout 2: 20 Questions–Tell Part of Your Addiction Story, 156
   Handout 3: Then versus Now, 157
   Handout 4: Lifetime Advantages and Disadvantages, 158–159
   quotation for, 154

Y

Your Personal Truth topic, 241–249
   client pages, 245–249
   commitment ideas, 249
   counselor pages, 240–244
   Handout 1: Your Personal Truth, 245
   Handout 2: Explore a Photo or Other Reminder of Your Past, 246
   Handout 3: Open the Door to a New Perspective, 247–248
   quotation for, 245